Contributors

Audrey Knippa, MS, MPH, RN, CNE
Nursing Education Coordinator and
 Content Project Leader

Sheryl Sommer, PhD, MSN, RN
Director, Nursing Curriculum and
 Education Services

Brenda Ball, MEd, BSN, RN
Nursing Education Specialist

Lois Churchill, MN, RN
Nursing Education Specialist

Carrie B. Elkins, DHSc, MSN, PHCNS, BC
Nursing Education Specialist

Mary Jane Janowski, MA, BSN, RN
Nursing Resource Specialist

Karin Roberts, PhD, MSN, RN, CNE
Nursing Education Coordinator

Mendy G. Wright, DNP, MSN, RN
Nursing Education Specialist

Derek Prater, MS Journalism
Lead Product Developer and Editorial Project Leader

Erika A. Archer, BS Education, Foreign Language
Product Developer

Johanna Barnes, BA Journalism
Product Developer

Chris Crawford, BS Journalism
Product Developer

Hilary E. Groninger, BS Journalism
Product Developer

Megan E. Herre, BS Journalism
Product Developer

Amanda Lehman, BA English
Product Developer

Joanna Shindler, BA Journalism
Product Developer

Brant L. Stacy, BS Journalism, BA English
Product Developer

Consultants

Tracey Bousquet, BSN, RN

Christina D. Brazier, MSN, RN

Penny Fauber, PhD, RN

Terri Lemon, MSN, RN

Veronica Njie-Carr, PhD, APRN-BC

Gale P. Sewell, MSN, RN, CNE

Julie Skrabal, MSN, RN

INTELLECTUAL PROPERTY NOTICE

IMPORTANT NOTICE TO THE READER

USER'S GUIDE

Welcome to the Assessment Technologies Institute® Fundamentals for Nursing Review Module Edition 7.0. The mission of ATI's Content Mastery Series® review modules is to provide user-friendly compendiums of nursing knowledge that will:

- Help you locate important information quickly.

- Assist in your remediation efforts.

- Provide exercises for applying your nursing knowledge.

- Facilitate your entry into the nursing profession as a newly licensed RN.

Organization

This review module is organized into units covering the NCLEX® major client needs categories: Safe, Effective Care Environment, Health Promotion and Maintenance, Psychosocial Integrity, and Physiological Integrity. Chapters within these units conform to one of three organizing principles for presenting the content:

- Nursing concepts

- Growth and development

- Procedures

Nursing concepts chapters begin with an overview describing the central concept and its relevance to nursing. Subordinate themes are covered in outline form to demonstrate relationships and present the information in a clear, succinct manner.

Growth and development chapters cover expected growth and development, including physical and psychosocial development and age-appropriate activities, and health promotion, including immunizations, health screenings, nutrition, and injury prevention.

Procedures chapters include an overview describing the procedure(s) covered in the chapter. These chapters will provide you with nursing knowledge relevant to each procedure, including indications, interpretations of findings, client outcomes, nursing actions, and complications.

Application Exercises

Questions are provided at the end of each chapter so you can practice applying your knowledge. The Application Exercises include both NCLEX-style questions, such as multiple-choice and multiple-select items, and questions that ask you to apply your knowledge in other formats, such as short-answer and matching items. After the Application Exercises, an answer key is provided, along with rationales for the answers.

NCLEX® Connections

To prepare for the NCLEX-RN, it is important for you to understand how the content in this review module is connected to the NCLEX-RN test plan. You can find information on the detailed test plan at the National Council of State Boards of Nursing's Web site: https://www.ncsbn.org/. When reviewing content in this review module, regularly ask yourself, "How does this content fit into the test plan, and what types of questions related to this content should I expect?"

To help you in this process, we've included NCLEX Connections at the beginning of units and sections and with each question in the Application Exercises Answer Keys. The NCLEX Connections at the beginning of units and sections will point out areas of the detailed test plan that relate to the content within that unit or section. The NCLEX Connections attached to the Application Exercises Answer Keys will demonstrate how each exercise fits within the detailed content outline.

These NCLEX Connections will help you understand how the detailed content outline is organized, starting with major client needs categories and subcategories and followed by related content areas and tasks. The major client needs categories are:

- Safe and Effective Care Environment
  o Management of Care
  o Safety and Infection Control
- Health Promotion and Maintenance
- Psychosocial Integrity
- Physiological Integrity
  o Basic Care and Comfort
  o Pharmacological and Parenteral Therapies
  o Reduction of Risk Potential
  o Physiological Adaptation

An NCLEX Connection might, for example, alert you that content within a unit is related to:

- Basic Care and Comfort
  o Assistive Devices
    ▪ Assess client use of assistive devices.

Icons

Icons are used throughout the review module to draw your attention to particular areas. Keep an eye out for these icons:

This icon indicates an Overview, or introduction, to a particular subject matter. Descriptions and categories will typically be found in an Overview.

This icon is used for the Application Exercises and the Application Exercises Answer Keys.

This icon is used for NCLEX connections.

This icon is used for gerontological content. When you see this icon, take note of information that is specific to aging or the care of older adult clients.

This icon is used for content related to safety. When you see this icon, take note of safety concerns or steps that nurses can take to ensure client safety and a safe environment.

This icon is used for examples of how to apply math concepts, such as in dosage calculation.

This icon indicates that a media supplement, such as a graphic, an animation, or a video, is available. If you have an electronic copy of the review module, this icon will appear alongside clickable links to media supplements. If you have a hardcopy version of the review module, visit www.atitesting.com for details on how to access these features.

Feedback

ATI welcomes feedback regarding this review module. Please provide comments to: comments@atitesting.com.

Table of Contents

Section: Health Assessment

Unit 3 ✓ Psychosocial Integrity

Unit 4 ✓ Physiological Integrity

Section: ✓ Basic Care and Comfort

UNIT 1: SAFE, EFFECTIVE CARE ENVIRONMENT

Section: Management of Care

- Health Care Delivery Systems
- Members of the Interdisciplinary Team ✓
- Ethical Responsibilities
- Legal Responsibilities
- Information Technology
- Delegation and Supervision
- Nursing Process
- Critical Thinking and Clinical Judgment
- Admissions, Transfers, and Discharge

NCLEX® CONNECTIONS

When reviewing the chapters in this section, keep in mind the relevant sections of the NCLEX® outline, in particular:

CLIENT NEEDS: MANAGEMENT OF CARE

Relevant topics/tasks include:
- Collaboration with Interdisciplinary Team
  - ○ Identify the need for interdisciplinary conferences.
- Delegation
  - ○ Utilize the five rights of delegation.
- Ethical Practice
  - ○ Recognize ethical dilemmas and take appropriate action.
- Information Technology
  - ○ Use information technology to enhance the care provided to the client.
- Legal Rights and Responsibilities
  - ○ Identify legal issues affecting the client.

UNIT 1	SAFE, EFFECTIVE CARE ENVIRONMENT
Section	Management of Care
Chapter 1	Health Care Delivery Systems

Overview

- Health care delivery systems are comprised of interactions between health care providers and clients within the constraints of financing mechanisms and regulatory agencies.

- Health care systems are comprised of the individuals who participate, the settings in which health care takes place, the agencies that regulate health care, and mechanisms that provide financial support.

- Most nursing care is delivered within the context of health care systems. As these systems continue to become more business-driven and less service-oriented, the challenge to nursing today is to retain its caring values while practicing within a cost-containment structure.

Components of Health Care Systems

COMPONENTS OF HEALTH CARE SYSTEMS
People – Participants in the health care system

- Consumers (clients)
- Providers
  - Licensed providers such as:
    - Registered nurses
    - Licensed vocational/practical nurses
    - Advanced practice nurses
    - Medical doctors
    - Pharmacists
    - Dentists
    - Dietitians
    - Physical, respiratory, and occupational therapists
  - Unlicensed providers, such as assistive personnel

COMPONENTS OF HEALTH CARE SYSTEMS
Settings – Where health care is provided

- Hospitals
- Homes
- Skilled-nursing, assisted-living, and extended-care facilities
- Community/health departments
- Adult day care centers
- Schools
- Hospices
- Provider's offices
- Ambulatory care clinics
- Occupational health clinics

Regulatory agencies – Where regulations for practice are enforced

- U.S. Department of Health and Human Services
- U.S. Food and Drug Administration (FDA)
- State and local public health agencies
- State licensing boards – to ensure that health care providers and agencies comply with state regulations
- The Joint Commission (formerly JCAHO) – to set quality standards for accreditation of health care facilities
- Professional Standards Review Organizations (PSROs)
- Utilization review committees – to monitor for appropriate diagnosis and treatment of hospitalized clients

Health care financing mechanisms – How health care is funded

- Public federally funded programs
  - Medicare is for clients over 65 years of age or older and for those with permanent disabilities. Premiums can be applied to one of two mechanisms:
    - Insurance program – Reimburses providers based on diagnosis-related groups (DRGs).
    - Managed care organizations (MCOs) – Enrolled clients receive comprehensive care overseen by a primary care provider.
  - Medicaid is for clients with low incomes.
    - It is federally funded.
    - Individual states determine eligibility requirements.
- Private plans
  - Traditional insurance reimburses for services on a fee-for-service basis.
  - Managed care organizations (MCOs) – Comprehensive care is overseen by a primary care provider and focuses on prevention and health promotion.
  - Preferred provider organizations (PPOs) – The client chooses from a list of contracted providers. Using noncontracted providers increases the client's out-of-pocket costs.
  - Exclusive provider organizations (EPOs) – The client chooses from a list of providers within a contracted organization.
  - Long-term care insurance – This provides for long-term care expenses not covered by Medicare.

Levels of Health Care

- Preventive health care focuses on educating and equipping clients to reduce and control risk factors of disease. Examples include programs that promote immunization, stress management, and seat belt use.

- Primary health care emphasizes health promotion, and includes prenatal and well-baby care, nutrition counseling, and disease control. This level of care is based on a sustained partnership between the client and the provider. Examples include office or clinic visits and scheduled school or work-centered screenings (vision, hearing, obesity).

- Secondary health care includes the diagnosis and treatment of emergency, acute illness, or injury. Examples include care that is given in hospital settings (inpatient and emergency departments), diagnostic centers, or emergent care centers.

- Tertiary health care involves the provision of specialized highly technical care. Examples include oncology centers and burn centers.

- Restorative health care involves intermediate follow-up care for restoring health. Examples include home health care, rehabilitation centers, and skilled nursing facilities.

- Continuing health care is designed to address long-term or chronic health care needs. Examples include hospice, adult day care, and in-home respite care.

Relationship Between Health Care Systems and Levels of Care

- People – The level of care provided depends on the needs of the client. Licensed and unlicensed health care personnel work in every level of care.

- Setting – The settings for secondary and tertiary care are usually within a hospital or specific facility/agency. Other levels of care are delivered in a variety of settings.

- Regulatory agencies are involved with ensuring the quality and quantity of health care, and the protection of health care consumers.

- Health care finance influences the quality and type of care by setting parameters for cost containment and reimbursement.

The Future of Health Care

- The ultimate issue in designing and delivering health care is ensuring the health and welfare of the population.

- Professional nursing is important in the future of health care delivery.

CHAPTER 1: HEALTH CARE DELIVERY SYSTEMS

 Application Exercises

1. Match the type of service with the appropriate health care level.

_____	Hospice	A. Prevention
_____	Immunizations	B. Primary
_____	School-based screenings	C. Secondary
_____	Emergency services	D. Tertiary
_____	Regional cancer center	E. Restorative
_____	Home health care	F. Continuing

2. Which of the following are health care regulatory agencies? (Select all that apply.)

_____ American Nurses Association (ANA)

_____ The Joint Commission (formerly JCAHO)

_____ State Boards of Nursing

_____ National League for Nursing (NLN)

_____ Food and Drug Administration (FDA)

3. Which of the following health care financing mechanisms is federally funded? (Select all that apply.)

_____ Preferred provider organization (PPO)

_____ Medicare

_____ Long-term care insurance

_____ Exclusive provider organization (EPO)

_____ Medicaid

4. A hospital conducts a community blood pressure screening in its lobby. This is an example of what level of care?

A. Preventive

B. Primary

C. Secondary

D. Tertiary

5. A client in a managed care organization (MCO) requires hospitalization. The admission must first be approved by the

    A. emergency department physician.

    B. utilization review committee.

    C. provider.

    D. managed care administrator.

CHAPTER 1: HEALTH CARE DELIVERY SYSTEMS

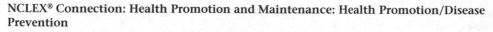 Application Exercises Answer Key

1. Match the type of service with the appropriate health care level.

F	Hospice	A. Prevention
A	Immunizations	B. Primary
B	School-based screenings	C. Secondary
C	Emergency services	D. Tertiary
D	Regional cancer center	E. Restorative
E	Home health care	F. Continuing

 NCLEX® Connection: Health Promotion and Maintenance: Health Promotion/Disease Prevention

2. Which of the following are health care regulatory agencies? (Select all that apply.)

       American Nurses Association (ANA)
  X   **The Joint Commission (formerly JCAHO)**
  X   **State Boards of Nursing**
       National League for Nursing (NLN)
  X   **Food and Drug Administration (FDA)**

The Joint Commission, State Boards of Nursing, and the FDA are all health care regulatory agencies. ANA and NLN are both professional nursing organizations. Even though ANA and NLN function to maintain high nursing practice standards, they do not regulate health care agencies.

NCLEX® Connection: Management of Care: Legal Rights and Responsibilities

3. Which of the following health care financing mechanisms is federally funded? (Select all that apply.)

       Preferred provider organization (PPO)
  X   **Medicare**
       Long-term care insurance
       Exclusive provider organization (EPO)
  X   **Medicaid**

Medicare and Medicaid are federally funded health care financing mechanisms. PPOs, long-term care insurance, and EPOs are privately funded.

NCLEX® Connection: Management of Care: Legal Rights and Responsibilities

4. A hospital conducts a community blood pressure screening in its lobby. This is an example of what level of care?

    A. Preventive

    B. Primary

    C. Secondary

    D. Tertiary

A screening is an attempt to detect an undiagnosed disease at its earliest stage, and it is an example of primary care. Preventive care includes immunizations or education for minimizing risk factors for illness. Secondary care includes hospital-based care that is performed on emergency department or hospitalized clients. Tertiary care includes specialized care usually located regionally, such as burn or cancer centers.

 NCLEX® Connection: Health Promotion and Maintenance: Health Promotion/Disease Prevention

5. A client in a managed care organization (MCO) requires hospitalization. The admission must first be approved by the

    A. emergency department physician.

    B. utilization review committee.

    C. provider.

    D. managed care administrator.

In an MCO, the provider oversees all of the client's care including hospitalizations. The emergency department physician may consult with the provider regarding a client, but the decision to admit the client and reimburse for the required services is left to the provider. Utilization review committees and the managed care administrator may review the appropriateness of the provider's treatment decisions, but they do not make admission decisions.

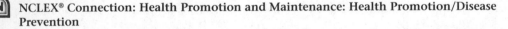

NCLEX® Connection: Health Promotion and Maintenance: Health Promotion/Disease Prevention

UNIT 1	SAFE, EFFECTIVE CARE ENVIRONMENT
Section	Management of Care
Chapter 2	Members of the Interdisciplinary Team

Overview

- Registered nurses and licensed practical/vocational nurses are integral members of the interdisciplinary health care team. Each discipline represented on an interdisciplinary team uses a set of skills that are within the scope of practice for the specific profession. In some instances, the scope of practice for one discipline overlaps with the scope of practice or set of skills for another profession. For example, the nurse and the respiratory care therapist both possess the knowledge and skill to perform chest physiotherapy (using postural drainage, percussion, and vibration to promote drainage of secretions from the lungs).

- The interdisciplinary health care team works collaboratively to provide holistic care to the client.

- The nurse is most often the manager of care and must understand the roles and responsibilities of other health care team members in order to collaborate in the care of the client and make appropriate referrals.

- The roles and responsibilities of nurses are based on knowledge and skill acquisition that is regulated by state nurse practice acts. Nursing care delivery models (primary care nursing) provide various formats for nurses to meet the needs of the client.

Interdisciplinary Personnel (Non-nursing)

- Clergy

  o Job description – Provide spiritual care to the client (pastors, rabbis, priests).

  o Example of when to refer – The client requests communion or the family asks for prayer prior to the client undergoing a procedure.

- Registered Dietitian

  o Job description – Assess, plan for, and educate the client regarding nutrition needs. Direct care of nutritional aides.

  o Example of when to refer – The client has a low albumin level and has experienced a recent unexplained weight loss.

- Laboratory Technician

  o Job description – Obtain specimens of the client's body fluids and perform the necessary diagnostic tests.

  o Example of when to refer – The provider orders a complete blood count (CBC) to be performed immediately.

- Occupational Therapist

  o Job description – Assess and plan for the client to regain activities of daily living skills, especially motor skills of the upper extremities. Direct care of occupational therapy assistants.

  o Example of when to refer – A client has difficulties using an eating utensil with her dominant hand following a stroke.

- Pharmacist

  o Job description – Provide and monitor medications for the client as prescribed by the provider. The pharmacist also supervises pharmacy technicians in states in which this practice is allowed.

  o Example of when to refer – A client is concerned about whether or not a new medication will interact with any of his other medications.

- Physical Therapist

  o Job description – Assess and plan for the client to increase musculoskeletal function, especially of the lower extremities, to maintain mobility. Direct care of physical therapy assistants.

  o Example of when to refer – Following a hip replacement, a client requires assistance learning to ambulate and regain strength.

- Provider

  o Job description – Assess, diagnose, and treat the client for disease and/or injury. Providers include medical doctors (MDs), doctors of osteopathy (DOs), advanced practice nurses (APNs), and physician assistants (PAs). State regulations vary in regard to the requirement for supervision of APNs and PAs by a physician (MDs and DOs).

  o Example of when to refer – A client experiences a change in vital signs. Temperature is 39° C (102.2° F). Client is achy, shaking, and reports "feeling cold."

- Radiologic Technologists

  o Job description – Position the client and perform x-rays and other imaging procedures for providers to review for diagnosis of disorders of various body parts.

  o Example of when to refer – A client reports severe pain in his hip after a fall, and the provider orders an x-ray of the client's hip.

- Respiratory Therapist

  o Job description – Evaluate respiratory status and provide prescribed respiratory treatments including oxygen therapy, chest physiotherapy, inhalation therapy, and artificial mechanical ventilation.

  o Example of when to refer – A client with respiratory disease is short of breath and requests a nebulizer treatment that has been ordered "as needed."

- Social Worker

  o Job description – Work with the client and the client's family by coordinating inpatient and community resources to meet psychosocial and environmental needs that are necessary for recovery and/or discharge.

  o Example of when to refer – A client who is dying of cancer wishes to go home but is no longer able to perform many activities of daily living. The spouse needs medical equipment in the home to care for the client.

- Speech Therapist

  o Job description – Evaluate and make recommendations regarding the functions of speech, language, and swallowing impacted by various client disorders or injuries. Teach the client techniques and exercises to improve function when possible.

  o Example of when to refer – A client is having difficulty swallowing a regular diet after trauma to the head and neck.

(M) View Media Supplement: Interdisciplinary Team (Video)

Nursing Personnel

- The nursing team is responsible for working together to advocate for and meet the needs of the client within the health care delivery system.

- The registered nurse is the lead team member, soliciting input from all nursing team members, setting priorities, sharing information with other disciplines, and coordinating the care of the client.

TITLE	EDUCATIONAL PREPARATION	ROLES/RESPONSIBILITIES
Registered Nurse (RN)	• Varies – Must meet requirements for licensure set by each state board of nursing • Requires completion of a diploma program, an associate degree, or baccalaureate degree in nursing prior to taking the licensure exam (licensed)	• Function legally under state nurse practice acts. • Perform assessments; establish nursing diagnoses, goals, and interventions; and conduct ongoing client evaluations. • Participate in developing interdisciplinary plans for client care. • Share appropriate information among team members; initiate referrals for client assistance, including health education; and identify community resources.
Licensed Practical Nurse (LPN)	• Varies – Must meet requirements set by each state board of nursing • Vocational or community college education required prior to taking the licensure exam (licensed)	• Work under the supervision of the RN. • Collaborate within the nursing process, coordinate the client plan of care, consult with other team members, and recognize the need for referrals to assist the client with actual or potential problems. • Possess technical knowledge and skills. • Participate in the delivery of nursing care, using the nursing process as a framework.
Unlicensed Assistive Personnel (UAP) including Certified Nurse Assistants (CNAs) and Certified Medical Assistants (CMAs), and non-nursing personnel such as dialysis technicians, monitor technicians, and phlebotomists	• Varies – Formal or informal training requirements as set by each state • Requirement by most states for training and examination to attain CNA status • Usually under the direct supervision of an RN or LPN	• Work under the direct supervision of an RN or LPN. • Specific tasks are usually outlined in a position description in the employing facility/agency. • Tasks may include feeding clients, preparing nutritional supplements, lifting, basic care (grooming, bathing, transferring, toileting, positioning), measuring and recording vital signs, and ambulating clients.

Expanded Nursing Roles

- Advanced Practice Nurse (APN) – Has a great deal of autonomy. APNs usually possess a minimum of a master's degree in nursing (or related field), advanced education in pharmacology and physical assessment, and certification in a specialized area of practice. Included in this role is the:

  - Clinical Nurse Specialist (CNS) – Typically specializes in a practice setting or a disease field.

  - Nurse Practitioner (NP) – Collaborates with one or more providers to provide nonemergency primary health care in a variety of settings.

  - Certified Registered Nurse Anesthetist (CRNA) – Administers anesthesia and provides care to the client during procedures. The RNA is under the supervision of an anesthesiologist.

  - Certified Nurse-Midwife (CNM) – Collaborates with one or more providers to provide care to maternal-newborn clients and their families.

- Nurse Educator – May teach at the associate degree, baccalaureate, master's, or doctoral level.

- Nurse Administrator – Provides leadership to nursing departments within a health care facility/agency.

- Nurse Researcher – Conducts research that will provide more nursing knowledge to improve the quality of client care.

Complementary or Alternative Medicine Therapists

- Interest in the use of complementary and alternative therapies continues to grow. These therapies are also referred to as complementary or alternative medicine (CAM). CAM therapies may be delivered by massage therapists, chiropractors, acupuncturists, reflexologists, and many other types of providers. CAM therapies may also be provided by nurses, physicians and other professionals who are associated with traditional allopathic medicine.

- Nurses should be receptive to learning about a client's alternative health beliefs and practices (home remedies, cultural practices, vitamin use, modification of prescriptions).

- The nurse who incorporates CAM therapy into her practice should be knowledgeable about the state laws in the state in which she practices to ensure that the therapies provided are within her scope of practice.

CHAPTER 2: MEMBERS OF THE INTERDISCIPLINARY TEAM

 Application Exercises

1. Match the following job titles to the activities each team member might perform.

D	Occupational therapist	A. Evaluates the client's nutritional status
G	Physical therapist	B. Dispenses medications as prescribed by the provider
E	Speech therapist	C. Draws blood specimens
F	Radiology technician	D. Provides the client a fork with an enlarged handle
C	Laboratory technician	E. Observes the client swallow gelatin
A	Registered dietitian	F. Removes the client's wristwatch prior to a magnetic resonance imaging (MRI) scan
B	Pharmacist	G. Teaches the client how to use a walker to ambulate

2. A nurse is caring for an older adult client who lives alone and is to be discharged in 3 days. He is assigned a prescribed diet but states that it is difficult to prepare adequate nutritious meals at home for just one person. To which of the following members of the health care team should he be referred?

A. Registered dietitian

B. Occupational therapist

C. Speech therapist

D. Social worker

CHAPTER 2: MEMBERS OF THE INTERDISCIPLINARY TEAM

 Application Exercises Answer Key

1. Match the following job titles to the activities each team member might perform.

__D__	Occupational therapist	A. Evaluates the client's nutritional status
__G__	Physical therapist	B. Dispenses medications as prescribed by the primary care provider
__E__	Speech therapist	C. Draws blood specimens
__F__	Radiology technician	D. Provides the client a fork with an enlarged handle
__C__	Laboratory technician	E. Observes the client swallow gelatin
__A__	Registered dietitian	F. Removes the client's wristwatch prior to a magnetic resonance imaging (MRI) scan
__B__	Pharmacist	G. Teaches the client how to use a walker to ambulate

NCLEX® Connection: Management of Care: Continuity of Care

2. A nurse is caring for an older adult client who lives alone and is to be discharged in 3 days. He is assigned a prescribed diet but states that it is difficult to prepare adequate nutritious meals at home for just one person. To which of the following members of the health care team should he be referred?

   A. Registered dietitian

   B. Occupational therapist

   C. Speech therapist

   D. Social worker

   A social worker can make arrangements for a meal delivery service to provide nutritious meals daily, or recommend a congregate meal site near the client's home. The registered dietitian usually performs the assessment of a client's nutritional status and provides teaching concerning appropriate diet. The occupational therapist can assist the client who is having problems manipulating eating/drinking utensils. The speech therapist can assist the client who is having swallowing problems.

   NCLEX® Connection: Management of Care: Continuity of Care

UNIT 1	SAFE, EFFECTIVE CARE ENVIRONMENT
Section	Management of Care
Chapter 3	Ethical Responsibilities

Overview

- Ethics has several definitions but the foundation of ethics is based on an expected behavior of a certain group in relation to what is considered right and wrong. It is the study of conduct and character.

- Morals are the values and beliefs held by people that guide their behaviors and decision-making.

- Ethical theory examines the different principles, ideas, systems, and philosophies used to make judgments about what is right and wrong and good and bad. Two common types of ethical theory are utilitarianism and deontology.

- Ethical principles are standards of what is right or wrong with regard to important social values and norms. Ethical principles pertaining to the treatment of clients include:

  o Autonomy – Ability of the client to make personal decisions, even when those decisions may not be in the client's own best interest.

  o Beneficence – Agreement that the care given is in the best interest of the client; taking positive actions to help others.

  o Fidelity – Agreement to keep one's promise to the client about care that was offered.

  o Justice – Fair treatment in matters related to physical and psychosocial care and use of resources.

  o Nonmaleficence – Avoidance of harm or pain as much as possible when giving treatments.

- Unusual or complex ethical issues may need to be dealt with by a hospital's ethics committee.

Ethical Decision Making in Nursing

- Ethical dilemmas are problems about which more than one choice can be made and the choice made is influenced by the values and beliefs of the decision makers. These are common in health care, and nurses must be prepared to apply ethical theory and decision making to ethical problems.

- A problem is an ethical dilemma if:

  ○ It cannot be solved solely by a review of scientific data.

  ○ It involves a conflict between two moral imperatives.

  ○ The answer will have a profound effect on the situation/client.

- Ethical decision making is a process that requires striking a balance between science and morality. There are several steps in ethical decision making:

  ○ Identify whether or not the issue is indeed an ethical dilemma.

  ○ State the ethical dilemma including all surrounding issues and individuals involved.

  ○ List and analyze all possible options for resolving the dilemma and review implications of each option.

  ○ Select the option that is in concert with the ethical principle applicable to this situation, the decision maker's values and beliefs, and the profession's values set forth for client care. Justify why that one option was selected in light of the previously mentioned variables.

  ○ Apply this decision to the dilemma and evaluate the outcomes.

- The *American Nurses Association Code of Ethics for Nurses* (2001) and The *International Council of Nurses' The ICN Code of Ethics for Nurses* (2006) are documents commonly accepted by professional nurses. The *Code of Ethics* for licensed practical/vocational nurses issued by the National Association for Practical Nurse Education and Service, Inc., also serves as a set of standards for nursing practice. Codes of ethics are available through the organizations' Web sites.

- The nurse's basic code of ethics and principles remains constant. These basic principles include:

  ○ Advocacy – Support of the cause of the client regarding health, safety, and personal rights

  ○ Responsibility – Willingness to respect obligations and follow through on promises

  ○ Accountability – Ability to answer for one's own actions

  ○ Confidentiality – Protection of privacy without diminishing access to quality care

- The Uniform Determination of Death Act (UDDA) is a document that can be used to assist with end-of-life and organ donor issues.

  ○ The UDDA provides two formal definitions of death that were developed by the National Conference of Commissioners on Uniform State Laws. Death is determined by one of two criteria:

    ▪ An irreversible cessation of circulatory and respiratory functions

    ▪ Irreversible cessation of all functions of the entire brain, including the brain stem

  ○ A determination of death must be made in accordance with accepted medical standards.

THE NURSE'S ROLE IN ETHICAL DECISION MAKING	
NURSE'S ROLE	EXAMPLES
An agent for the client facing an ethical decision	• Caring for an adolescent client who has to decide whether or not to undergo an abortion even though her parents believe it is wrong • Discussing options with a parent who has to decide whether or not to consent to a blood transfusion for a child when their religion prohibits such treatment
A decision maker in regard to nursing practice	• Assigning staff nurses a higher client load than recommended because administration has cut the number of nurses per shift • Witnessing a surgeon discuss only surgical options with a client without informing the client about more conservative measures available

CHAPTER 3: ETHICAL RESPONSIBILITIES

 Application Exercises

1. Match the ethical principle with the correct example.

_____	Justice	A. A client decides not to have open heart surgery despite significant blockages.
_____	Autonomy	B. A nurse offers pain medication to a client who is postoperative prior to ambulation.
_____	Beneficence	C. A nurse takes a client outdoors in a wheelchair after lunch as promised.
_____	Nonmaleficence	D. All clients waiting for a kidney transplant have to meet the same qualifications.
_____	Fidelity	E. A nurse questions a medication prescription as being too extreme in light of a client's advanced age and unstable condition.

2. Which of the following entities has a code of ethics that may be used to guide nursing practice? (Select all that apply.)

_____ The American Hospital Association

_____ The American Nurses Association

_____ The International Council of Nurses

_____ The National Association for Practical Nurse Education and Services, Inc.

_____ The Federation of Associations of Regulatory Boards

3. Which of the following is an ethical dilemma?

A. A nurse on a medical-surgical unit demonstrates signs of chemical impairment.

B. A nurse is overheard telling an older adult client that if he doesn't stay in bed, she will have to place him in a restraint.

C. A family has conflicting feelings about the initiation of nasogastric tube feedings for their father, who is terminally ill.

D. A client who is terminally ill is hesitant to name her spouse on her durable power of attorney form.

CHAPTER 3: ETHICAL RESPONSIBILITIES

Ⓐ Application Exercises Answer Key

1. Match the ethical principle with the correct example.

__D__	Justice	A. A client decides not to have open heart surgery despite significant blockages.
__A__	Autonomy	B. A nurse offers pain medication to a client who is postoperative prior to ambulation.
__B__	Beneficence	C. A nurse takes a client outdoors in a wheelchair after lunch as promised.
__E__	Nonmaleficence	D. All clients waiting for a kidney transplant have to meet the same qualifications.
__C__	Fidelity	E. A nurse questions a medication prescription as being too extreme in light of the client's advanced age and unstable condition.

Ⓝ **NCLEX® Connection: Management of Care: Advocacy**

2. Which of the following entities has a code of ethics that may be used to guide nursing practice? (Select all that apply.)

_____	The American Hospital Association
__X__	**The American Nurses Association**
__X__	**The International Council of Nurses**
__X__	**The National Association for Practical Nurse Education and Services, Inc.**
_____	The Federation of Associations of Regulatory Boards

The American Nurses Association, the International Council of Nurses, and the National Association for Practical Nurse Education and Services, Inc., are associations that advocate for high quality nursing care through published codes of ethics. The American Hospital Association is dedicated to serving hospitals and other types of facilities that provide health care and services. It does not have a code of ethics for nurses. The Federation of Associations of Regulatory Boards protects the public by promoting effective regulation across disciplines and jurisdictions inside the United States. It also does not have a code of ethics for nurses.

 NCLEX® Connection: Management of Care: Client Rights

3. Which of the following is an ethical dilemma?

    A. A nurse on a medical-surgical unit demonstrates signs of chemical impairment.

    B. A nurse is overheard telling an older adult client that if he doesn't stay in bed, she will have to place him in a restraint.

    C. A family has conflicting feelings about the initiation of nasogastric tube feedings for their father, who is terminally ill.

    D. A client who is terminally ill is hesitant to name her spouse on her durable power of attorney form.

Making the decision about initiating tube feedings is an example of an ethical dilemma. It cannot be solved solely by a review of scientific data. It is not easily solved. The answer will have a profound effect on the situation/client. A nurse who may be impaired is a legal issue. A nurse who threatens to restrain a client has committed assault, and it is a legal issue. The selection of a person to make health care decisions on a client's behalf is a legal decision.

(N) NCLEX® Connection: Management of Care: Ethical Practice

UNIT 1	SAFE, EFFECTIVE CARE ENVIRONMENT
Section	Management of Care
Chapter 4	Legal Responsibilities

Overview

- In order to be safe practitioners, nurses must understand the legal aspects of the nursing profession.

- Understanding the laws governing nursing practice allows nurses to protect clients' rights and to reduce the risk of nursing liability.

- Nurses are accountable for practicing nursing in accordance with the various sources of law affecting nursing practice. It is important that nurses know and comply with these laws. By practicing nursing within the confines of the law, nurses are able to:

    o Shield oneself from liability.

    o Advocate for clients' rights.

    o Provide care that is within the nurse's scope of practice.

    o Discern the responsibilities of nursing in relationship to the responsibilities of other members of the health care team.

    o Provide safe, competent care that is consistent with standards of care.

Sources of Law

- Federal Regulations

    o Federal regulations have a great impact on nursing practice. Some of the Federal laws impacting nursing practice include:

        ■ The Health Insurance Portability and Accountability Act (HIPAA)

        ■ The Americans with Disabilities Act (ADA)

        ■ The Mental Health Parity Act (MHPA)

        ■ The Patient Self-Determination Act (PSDA)

- Criminal and Civil Laws

  o Criminal law is a subsection of public law and relates to the relationship of an individual with the government. A nurse who falsifies a record to cover up a serious mistake may be found guilty of breaking a criminal law.

  o Civil laws protect the individual rights of people. One type of civil law that relates to the provision of nursing care is tort law.

UNINTENTIONAL TORTS	EXAMPLE
Negligence	A nurse fails to implement safety measures for a client who has been identified as at risk for falls.
Malpractice (Professional negligence)	A nurse administers a large dose of medication due to a calculation error. The client has a cardiac arrest and dies.
QUASI-INTENTIONAL TORTS	**EXAMPLE**
Breach of confidentiality	A nurse releases the medical diagnosis of a client to a member of the press.
Defamation of character	A nurse tells a coworker that she believes the client has been unfaithful to her spouse.
INTENTIONAL TORTS	**EXAMPLE**
Assault	The conduct of one person makes another person fearful and apprehensive (threatening to place a nasogastric tube in a client who is refusing to eat).
Battery	Intentional and wrongful physical contact with a person that involves an injury or offensive contact (restraining a client and administering an injection against her wishes).
False imprisonment	A person is confined or restrained against his will (using restraints on a competent client to prevent his leaving the health care facility).

- State Laws

  o The core of nursing practice is regulated by state law.

  o Each state has enacted statutes that define the parameters of nursing practice and gives the authority to regulate the practice of nursing to its state board of nursing.

  o In turn, the boards of nursing have the authority to adopt rules and regulations that further regulate nursing practice. Although the practice of nursing is similar among states, it is critical that nurses know the laws and rules governing nursing in the state in which they practice.

  o Boards of nursing have the authority to both issue and revoke a nursing license.

  o Boards also set standards for nursing programs and further delineate the scope of practice for registered nurses, licensed practical nurses, and advanced practice nurses.

- Licensure

  o In general, nurses must hold a current license in every state where they practice. The states (about half of them) that have adopted the nurse licensure compact are exceptions. This model allows licensed nurses who reside in a compact state to practice in other compact states under a multi-state license. Within the compact, nurses must practice in accordance with the statues and rules of the state in which they provide care.

Professional Negligence

- Professional negligence is the failure of a person with professional training to act in a reasonable and prudent manner. The terms "reasonable and prudent" are generally used to describe a person who has the average judgment, intelligence, foresight, and skill that would be expected of a person with similar training and experience.

- Negligence issues that prompt most malpractice suits include failure to:

  o Follow either professional or facility-established standards of care.

  o Use equipment in a responsible and knowledgeable manner.

  o Communicate effectively and thoroughly with the client.

  o Document care that was provided.

THE FIVE ELEMENTS NECESSARY TO PROVE NEGLIGENCE		
ELEMENT OF LIABILITY	EXPLANATION	EXAMPLE: CLIENT WHO IS A FALL RISK
1. Duty to provide care as defined by a standard	Care that should be given or what a reasonably prudent nurse would do	The nurse should complete a fall risk assessment for all clients upon admission, per facility protocol.
2. Breach of duty by failure to meet standard	Failure to give the standard of care that should have been given	The nurse does not perform a fall risk assessment during admission.
3. Foreseeability of harm	Knowledge that failing to give the proper standard of care may cause harm to the client	The nurse should know that failure to take fall risk precautions may endanger a client at risk for falls.
4. Breach of duty has potential to cause harm (combines elements 2 and 3)	Failure to meet the standard had potential to cause harm – relationship must be provable	If a fall risk assessment is not performed, the client's risk for falls is not determined and the proper precautions are not put in place.
5. Harm occurs	Actual harm to client occurs	The client falls out of bed and breaks his hip.

- Nurses can avoid being liable for negligence by:

  o Following standards of care.

  o Giving competent care.

  o Communicating with other health team members.

  o Developing a caring rapport with clients.

  o Fully documenting assessments, interventions, and evaluations.

CLIENT RIGHTS

Overview

- Nurses are accountable for protecting the rights of clients. Specific situations that provide nurses with the opportunity to protect clients' rights are informed consent, refusal or treatment, advance directives, confidentiality, and information security.

  o Clients' rights are the legal guarantees that clients have with regard to their health care.

  o Clients using the services of a health care institution retain their rights as individuals and citizens of the United States.

  o The American Hospital Association (AHA) identifies patients' rights in health care settings and is contained in "The Patient Care Partnership." For more information regarding this document, visit the organization's Web site (http://www.aha.org).

  o Further protection of rights are ensured for residents in nursing facilities that participate in Medicare programs from "Resident Rights" statutes that govern their operation.

Nursing Role in Client Rights

- Nurses must ensure that clients understand their rights, and nurses must also protect the rights of clients for whom they are providing care.

- Regardless of the age of the client, the client's nursing needs or the setting in which care is provided, the basic tenets are the same. The client has the right to:

  o Be informed about the aspects of care in order to be active in the decision-making process.

  o Accept, refuse, or request modification to the plan of care.

  o Receive care that is delivered by competent individuals who treat the client with respect.

INFORMED CONSENT

 Overview

- Informed consent is a legal process by which a client has given written permission for a procedure or treatment to be performed. Consent is considered to be informed when the client has been provided and understands:

    o The reason the treatment or procedure is needed

    o How the treatment or procedure will benefit the client

    o The risks involved if the client chooses to receive the treatment or procedure

    o Other options to treat the problem, including the option of not treating the problem

- The nurse's role in the informed consent process is to witness the client's signature on the informed consent form and to ensure that informed consent has been appropriately obtained.

View Media Supplement: Informed Consent (Video)

Informed Consent Guidelines

- Consent is required for all care that is given to the client in a health care facility. For most aspects of nursing care, "implied consent" is adequate. The client provides implied consent when the client adheres to the instructions provided by the nurse. For example, the nurse is preparing to administer a TB skin test and the client holds out his arm for the nurse.

- For an invasive procedure or surgery, the client is required to provide written consent.

- State laws prescribe who is able to give informed consent. Laws will vary regarding age limitations and emergencies. The nurse is responsible for knowing the laws in the state of practice.

- The form for informed consent must be signed by a competent adult. The person who signs the form must be capable of understanding the information provided by the health care professional who will be providing the service, such as a surgical procedure, and the person must be able to fully communicate with the health care professional. When the person giving the informed consent is unable to communicate due to a language barrier or due to a hearing impairment, a trained medical interpreter must be provided. Many health care facilities contract with professional interpreters who have additional skills in medical terminology to assist with providing information.

- Individuals who are authorized to grant consent for another person include:

    o Parent of a minor

    o Legal guardian

    o Court-specified representative

- An individual who has durable power of attorney authority for health care
- Emancipated minors (minors who are independent from their parents, such as a married minor) provide informed consent for themselves.

- The nurse must verify that consent is "informed" and may witness the client sign the consent form.

RESPONSIBILITIES FOR INFORMED CONSENT		
THE PROVIDER	THE CLIENT	THE NURSE
<ul><li>Obtains informed consent.</li><li>To do so, the provider must give the client:<ul><li>A complete description of the treatment/procedure</li><li>A description of the professionals who will be performing and participating in the treatment</li><li>A description of the potential harm, pain, and/or discomfort that might occur</li><li>Options for other treatments</li><li>The right to refuse treatment</li></ul></li></ul>	<ul><li>Gives informed consent.</li><li>To give informed consent, the client must:<ul><li>Give it voluntarily (no coercion involved).</li><li>Be competent and of legal age or be an emancipated minor. When the client is unable to provide consent, another authorized person must give consent.</li><li>Receive enough information to make a decision based on an understanding of what is expected.</li></ul></li></ul>	<ul><li>Witnesses informed consent.</li><li>This means the nurse must:<ul><li>Ensure that the provider gave the client the necessary information.</li><li>Ensure that the client understood the information and is competent to give informed consent.</li><li>Have the client sign the informed consent document.</li><li>Notify the provider if the client has more questions or appears not to understand any of the information provided. The provider is then responsible for giving clarification.</li><li>Document questions the client has and that the provider was notified. The nurse also documents any addition reinforcement of teaching. The nurse is responsible for recording the use of an interpreter in the client's medical record.</li></ul></li></ul>

Refusal of Treatment

- The Patient Self-Determination Act (PSDA) stipulates that on admission to a health care facility, all clients must be informed of their right to accept or refuse care. Competent adults have the right to refuse treatment, including the right to leave a health care facility without a discharge order from the provider.

- If the client refuses a treatment or procedure, the client is asked to sign a document indicating that he understands the risk involved with refusing the treatment or procedure and that he has chosen to refuse it.

- When a client decides to leave the facility without a discharge order, the nurse notifies the provider and discusses with the client the risks faced by leaving the facility prior to discharge.

- The nurse carefully documents the information that was provided to the client and that notification of the provider occurred.

- The client is asked to sign an "Against Medical Advice" form.

- If the client refuses to sign the form, this is also documented by the nurse.

Standards of Care (Practice)

- Nurses base practice on established standards of care or legal guidelines for care. These standards of care can be found in:
  - The nurse practice act of each state. Its legal guidelines for practice are established and enforced through a state board of nursing or other government agency.
    - Nurse practice acts vary from state to state, making it obligatory for the nurse to be informed about her state's nurse practice act as it defines the legal parameters of practice.
  - Published standards of nursing practice developed by professional organizations and specialty groups, including the American Nurses Association (ANA), the American Association of Critical Care Nurses (AACN), and the American Association of Occupational Health Nurses (AAOHN).

      ○   Health care facility policies and procedures maintained in the facility's policy and procedure manual.

          ■   Policies and procedures establish the standard of practice expected to be maintained by employees of that institution.

          ■   These manuals provide detailed information about how the nurse should respond to or provide care in specific situations and while performing client care procedures.

          ■   Nurses should be familiar with their facility's policies and procedures and provide client care in accordance with these policies. For example:

              □   Assess and document client findings postoperatively according to institutional policy.

              □   Change IV tubing and flush saline locks according to institutional policy.

- Standards of care define and direct the level of care that should be given by practicing nurses, and they are used in malpractice lawsuits to determine if that level was maintained.

- Nurses should refuse to practice beyond the legal scope of practice and/or outside of their areas of competence regardless of reason (staffing shortage, lack of appropriate personnel).

- Nurses should use the formal chain of command to verbalize concerns related to assignment in light of current legal scope of practice, job description, and area of competence.

Impaired Coworkers

- Impaired health care providers pose a significant risk to client safety.

- A nurse who suspects a coworker of using alcohol or abusing drugs while working has a duty to report the coworker to appropriate management personnel as specified by institutional policy.

- Institutional policies should provide guidelines for handling employees with a chemical abuse issue, and many provide peer assistance programs that facilitate the health care provider's entry into a treatment program.

- Each state has laws and regulations that govern the disposition of nurses who have been reported secondary to chemical abuse.

- Health care providers who are found guilty of misappropriation of controlled substances can also be charged with a criminal offense consistent with the infraction.

Advance Directives

- The purpose of advance directives is to communicate a client's wishes regarding end-of-life care should the client become unable to do so.

- The Patient Self-Determination Act (PSDA) requires that all clients admitted to a health care facility be asked if they have advance directives.

- o Clients without advance directives must be given written information that outlines their rights related to health care decisions and how to formulate advance directives.

- o A health care representative should be available to help with this process.

Types of Advance Directives

- Living Will

  - o A living will is a legal document that expresses the client's wishes regarding medical treatment in the event the client becomes incapacitated and is facing end-of-life issues.

  - o Most state laws include provisions that health care providers who follow the health care directives in a living will are protected from liability.

- Durable Power of Attorney for Health Care

  - o A durable power of attorney for health care is a document that designates a health care proxy, who is an individual authorized to make health care decisions for a client who is unable.

- Provider's Orders

  - o Unless a "do not resuscitate" (DNR) or "allow natural death" (AND) order is written, the nurse initiates cardiopulmonary resuscitation (CPR) when the client has no pulse or respirations. The written order for a DNR or AND must be placed in the client's medical record. The provider consults the client and the family prior to administering a DNR or AND.

Nursing Role in Advance Directives

- Nursing responsibilities regarding advance directives include:

  - o Provide written information regarding advance directives.

  - o Document the client's advance directives status.

  - o Ensure that the advance directives reflect the client's current decisions.

  - o Inform all members of the health care team of the client's advance directives.

Mandatory Reporting

- In certain situations, health care providers have a legal obligation to report their findings in accordance with state law.

- Abuse

  - o Nurses are mandated to report any suspicion of abuse (child or elder abuse, domestic violence) following facility policy.

- Communicable Diseases

  o Nurses are also mandated to report to the proper agency (local health department, state health department) when a client has been diagnosed with a communicable disease.

  o A complete list of reportable diseases and a description of the reporting system are available through the Centers for Disease Control and Prevention Web site (http://www.cdc.gov). Each state mandates which diseases must be reported in that state. There are more than 60 communicable diseases that must be reported to public health departments to allow officials to:

    ▪ Ensure appropriate medical treatment of diseases (tuberculosis).

    ▪ Monitor for common-source outbreaks (foodborne, hepatitis A).

    ▪ Plan and evaluate control and prevention plans (immunizations for preventable diseases).

    ▪ Identify outbreaks and epidemics.

    ▪ Determine public health priorities based on trends.

CHAPTER 4: LEGAL RESPONSIBILITIES

 Application Exercises

1. A nurse reviewing a client's chart discovers that the client's do-not-resuscitate (DNR) order has expired. The client's condition has not been stable today. Which of the following actions should the nurse take?

   A. Assume that the client still wishes to be a DNR client.

   B. Write a note on the front of the provider order sheet asking that the DNR be reordered.

   C. Notify the nurse manager that the DNR order has expired.

   D. Call the provider to get the order immediately reinstated.

2. Which of the following actions by a nurse can minimize her chances of being charged with negligence? (Select all that apply.)

   _____ Thoroughly explaining procedures prior to performing them

   _____ Approaching the client in a caring manner

   _____ Asking the client if she has any questions about her care

   _____ Providing care according to the plan of care

   _____ Documenting assessments in the client's medical record

   _____ Carrying out the provider's orders without question

3. A nurse witnesses an assistive personnel (AP) under her supervision reprimanding a client for not using the urinal properly. The AP threatens to put a diaper on the client if he does not use the urinal more carefully next time. Which of the following torts is the AP committing?

   A. Assault

   B. Battery

   C. False imprisonment

   D. Invasion of privacy

CHAPTER 4: LEGAL RESPONSIBILITIES

 Application Exercises Answer Key

1. A nurse reviewing a client's chart discovers that the client's do-not-resuscitate (DNR) order has expired. The client's condition has not been stable today. Which of the following actions should the nurse take?

   A. Assume that the client still wishes to be a DNR client.

   B. Write a note on the front of the provider order sheet asking that the DNR be reordered.

   C. Notify the nurse manager that the DNR order has expired.

   D. Call the provider to get the order immediately reinstated.

   DNR orders must be reinstated by the provider on an institutionally specified basis. Without a current DNR order, the nurse must institute CPR if the client goes into cardiopulmonary arrest. Since the client has been unstable today, the nurse should call the provider to get a current order reinstated. The nurse cannot assume that the client's wishes have not changed. Leaving a note on a medical record is unreliable, and there is no need to inform the charge nurse if the nurse contacts the provider immediately to confirm the client's or family's wishes and resolves the situation.

    NCLEX® Connection: Management of Care: Client Rights

2. Which of the following actions by a nurse can minimize her chances of being charged with negligence? (Select all that apply.)

__X__	**Thoroughly explaining procedures prior to performing them**
__X__	**Approaching the client in a caring manner**
__X__	**Asking the client if she has any questions about her care**
__X__	**Providing care according to the plan of care**
__X__	**Documenting assessments in the client's medical record**
_____	Carrying out the provider's orders without question

   All of these options except for the last option can help the client receive (and perceive that she is receiving) competent, caring, and thorough client care. If all of these criteria are met, the chances of negligence occurring are minimized. It is necessary to question a provider's order if the nurse deems it could have adverse effects on the client or if it is contraindicated secondary to another condition or treatment. If the nurse carries out an order that goes against what a reasonable and prudent nurse should know, he could be held liable for implementing the order.

   NCLEX® Connection: Management of Care: Legal Rights and Responsibilities

3. A nurse witnesses an assistive personnel (AP) under her supervision reprimanding a client for not using the urinal properly. The AP threatens to put a diaper on the client if he does not use the urinal more carefully next time. Which of the following torts is the AP committing?

A. Assault
B. Battery
C. False imprisonment
D. Invasion of privacy

By threatening the client, the AP is committing assault. Her threats could make the client become fearful and apprehensive. Since the AP has only verbally threatened the client, battery has not occurred. False imprisonment and invasion of privacy have not been committed.

Ⓝ **NCLEX® Connection: Management of Care: Legal Rights and Responsibilities**

UNIT 1	SAFE, EFFECTIVE CARE ENVIRONMENT
Section	Management of Care
Chapter 5	Information Technology

 Overview

- The client's chart or medical record is the legal record of care.

- The client's chart is a confidential, permanent, and legal document that is admissible in court. Nurses are legally and ethically responsible for ensuring that confidentiality is maintained. Access to the client's medical record should be restricted to only those health care providers who are involved directly in the client's care.

(M) View Media Supplement: Confidentiality (Video)

- The nursing care provided is recorded as documentation or charting and should reflect the nursing process.

- There is a rapidly growing trend for the client's records to be maintained electronically, which creates challenges in protecting the privacy and safety of the client's health information.

- Nursing documentation of the client's care must be recorded accurately.

- Information to chart includes:

  o   Assessments

  o   Medication administration

  o   Treatments given and the client's responses

  o   Client education

- Documentation is a standard for many accrediting agencies, including The Joint Commission (formerly JCAHO). The Joint Commission mandates the use of computerized databases to expedite the accreditation process. Health care facilities use the computerized data to manage budgets, quality improvement programs, research, and many other endeavors.

- Purposes for medical records include communication, legal documentation, financial billing, education, research, and auditing/monitoring.

- The purpose of reporting is to provide continuity of care when several nurses provide care to the client.

- Reporting should be conducted in a confidential manner.

Documentation

- Factual – Subjective and objective data can be documented.

  o Subjective data can be documented as direct quotes, within quotation marks, or summarized and identified as the client's statement.

  o Objective data should be descriptive and should include what the nurse sees, hears, feels, and smells. Document without derogatory words, judgments, or opinions. Document the client's behavior accurately. Instead of writing "client is agitated," write "client pacing back and forth in his room, yelling loudly."

- Accurate and Concise – Information that is documented must be precise. Facts should be documented (what the nurse sees, hears, feels, smells) without any interpretations of the situation. Only those abbreviations and symbols approved by The Joint Commission or by the facility are acceptable. If facility policy allows, use monitor strips when appropriate.

- Complete and Current – Information that is documented should be comprehensive and timely. Never pre-chart an assessment, intervention, or evaluation.

- Organized – Communicate information in a logical order.

Legal Guidelines

- Begin each entry with the date and time.

- Record entries legibly, in non-erasable black ink, and do not leave blank spaces in the nurses' notes.

- Do not use correction fluid or blacken out errors made while documenting in the client's record. Make corrections per facility protocol.

- Information inadvertently omitted may be added in the form of a "late entry." A late entry must include the time the charting was done and the specific time the charting reflects.

- All documentation must be signed with the signature and the title of the individual making the entry.

- Documentation should reflect assessments, interventions, and evaluations performed by the person signing the entry.

- Guidelines vary for electronic charting, and should include keeping the password private.

Documentation Formats

- Flow charts are used to record and show trends in vital signs, blood glucose levels, pain level, and other frequently performed assessments.

- Narrative documentation records information as a sequence of events.

- Charting by exception uses standardized forms that identify normal findings/values and allows selective documentation of abnormal findings.

- Problem-oriented medical records consist of a database, problem list, care plan, and progress notes. Various formats can be used to complete a progress note.

  - SOAPIE:
    - S – Subjective data
    - O – Objective data
    - A – Assessment (includes a nursing diagnosis based on the assessment)
    - P – Plan
    - I – Intervention
    - E – Evaluation

  - PIE:
    - P – Problem
    - I – Intervention
    - E – Evaluation

  - DAR (focus charting):
    - D – Data
    - A – Action
    - R – Response

- Computerized documentation has been developed to include a computer-based client care record.

  - Advantages include standardization, accuracy, confidentiality, and easy access for multiple users. In addition, acquisition and transfer of client information is expedited.

  - Challenges include learning the computerized system, knowing how to correct errors, and maintaining security.

  - Documentation rules and formats are the same as paper charting.

Reporting Formats

- Change-of-Shift Reports

  - This report is given at the conclusion of each shift by the nurse leaving to the nurse assuming responsibility for the client.

- o The report can be given face-to-face, audiotaped, or presented during walking rounds in the client's room.

- o An effective report should:

  - Include significant objective information about the client's health problems.

  - Be given in a logical order.

  - Be free of gossip and personal opinion.

  - Relate recent changes in medications, treatments, procedures, or the discharge plan.

- Telephone reports are useful when contacting the provider or other members of the interdisciplinary team.

  - o It is important to:

    - Have all the data prepared prior to contacting any member of the interdisciplinary team.

    - Use a professional demeanor.

    - Use exact, relevant, and accurate information.

    - Document the name of the person called, the time, content of the message, and the instructions or information received following the report.

- Telephone Orders (TO) or Verbal Orders (VO)

  - o This type of order should be avoided but may be necessary during emergencies and at unusual times.

Transcribing Medical Orders

- Use strategies to prevent errors when accepting a medical order that the provider gives verbally or by telephone.

  - o Have a second RN/LPN listen to a telephone order.

  - o Repeat back the order given, making sure to include the medication name (spell if necessary), dosage, time, and route.

  - o Document reading back the order and the presence of the second nurse on the telephone.

  - o Question any order that may seem contraindicated due to a previous order or to the client's condition.

- Transfer reports should include:

  - o Client's demographic information

  - o Client's medical diagnosis and providers

  - o An overview of the client's health status (physical and psychosocial), plan of care, and recent progress

- o   Any alterations that might become an urgent or emergent situation

- o   Directives for any assessments or client care essential within the next few hours

- o   Most recent vital signs

- o   Medications currently prescribed and last doses administered (including PRN)

- o   Allergies

- o   Diet and activity orders

- o   Presence of or need for special equipment or adaptive devices (oxygen, suction, wheelchair)

- o   Advance directives and resuscitation status

- o   Family involvement in care and health care proxy, if applicable

- Incident Reports (Unusual Occurrences)

  - o   Incident/variance reports are an important part of a facility's quality improvement plan.

  - o   An incident is the occurrence of an accident or an unusual event. Examples of incidents are medication errors, falls, and needle sticks.

  - o   The facts should be documented without judgment or opinion.

  - o   The incident report should not be referred to in the client's medical record.

  - o   Incident reports help improve health care quality by contributing to changes designed to make improvements.

Information Security

- Mandatory adherence with the Health Insurance Portability and Accountability Act of 1996 (HIPAA) was introduced in 2003 to help ensure that client information is kept confidential.

- A major component of HIPAA, the Privacy Rule, was introduced to promote the use of standard methods of maintaining the privacy of protected health information (PHI) among healthcare agencies.

- It is essential for the nurse to be aware of the rights of clients in regard to privacy and confidentiality. Facility policies and procedures are established in order to ensure adherence with HIPAA regulations.

- The Privacy Rule requires that the nurse protect all written and verbal communication about clients. Components of the privacy rule include:

  - o   Only health care team members directly responsible for the client's care should be allowed access to the client's record. Nurses may not share information with other clients or staff not involved in the care of the client.

  - o   Clients have a right to read and obtain a copy of their medical record, and facility policy should be followed when the client requests to read or have a copy of the record.

o   No part of the client chart can be copied except for authorized exchange of documents between health care institutions or health care providers.

o   Client medical records must be kept in a secure area to prevent inappropriate access to the information. Using public display boards to list client names and diagnoses is restricted.

o   Electronic records should be password protected and care must also be taken to prevent public viewing of the information.

- Health care workers should use only their own passwords to access information.

o   Client information may not be disclosed to unauthorized individuals/family members who request it or individuals who call on the phone.

- Many hospitals use a code system in which information is only disclosed to individuals who can provide the code.

- The nurse should ask any individual inquiring about a client's status for the code and disclose information on when the individual can give the code.

o   Communication about a client should only take place in a private setting where it cannot be overheard by unauthorized individuals. Change-of-shift reports can be done at the bedside as long as the client does not have a roommate and no visitors are present.

o   Health information systems (HIS) are used to manage administrative functions and clinical functions. The clinical portion of the system is often referred to as the clinical information system (CIA). The CIS may be used to coordinate essential aspects of client care.

o   In order to adhere to HIPAA regulations, each health care facility has specific policies and procedures designed to monitor staff adherence, technical protocols, computer privacy, and data safety.

o   Information security protocols include:

- Logging off from the computer before leaving the workstation to ensure that others cannot view protected health information on the monitor.

- Never sharing a user ID or password with anyone.

- Never leaving a client's chart or other printed or written PHI where others can access it.

- Shredding any printed or written client information used for reporting or client care after it is no longer needed.

CHAPTER 5: INFORMATION TECHNOLOGY

 Application Exercises

1. Which of the following actions places client information at risk for disclosure?

    A. Placing paper-based client charts behind the nurses' station

    B. Using a universal computer password for all staff on a unit

    C. Limiting information access to health care members directly involved in a client's care

    D. Reporting breaches in confidentiality

2. A nurse is preparing information for change-of-shift report. Which of the following should the nurse include in the report?

    A. The client's input and output for the shift

    B. The client's blood pressure from the previous day

    C. A bone scan that is scheduled for today

    D. The medication routine from the medication administration record

3. A nurse enters a client's room and finds him sitting in his chair. He states, "I fell in the shower but I got myself back up and into my chair." How should the nurse document this in the client's chart?

    A. The client fell in the shower.

    B. The client states he fell in the shower and was able to get himself back into his chair.

    C. This information should not be documented in the chart because the nurse did not witness the fall.

    D. The client fell in the shower but is now resting comfortably.

4. The skin barrier covering a client's intestinal fistula keeps falling off when she stands up to ambulate. The skin barrier has been applied twice during the current shift and remains intact only when the client is supine in bed. The nurse telephoned the physical therapist to tell her about the difficulties containing the drainage from the fistula, so the therapist did not work with the client today. The client sat in a chair during lunch with an absorbent pad over the fistula. A wound care nurse was called and states she will be coming in later today to see the client. The client states she is getting frustrated at not being able to work with her physical therapist. List the information the nurse should include in the change-of-shift report.

5. Which of the following legal guidelines should the nurse follow when documenting in the client's record? (Select all that apply.)

    _____   If an error is made, cover it with correction fluid and write in the correct information.

    _____   All entries should be dated and timed.

    _____   Document objective data, leaving out personal bias.

    _____   Use as many abbreviations as possible.

    _____   To save time, wait until the end of the shift to document any information.

CHAPTER 5: INFORMATION TECHNOLOGY

(A) Application Exercises Answer Key

1. Which of the following actions places client information at risk for disclosure?

    A. Placing paper-based client charts behind the nurses' station

    B. Using a universal computer password for all staff on a unit

    C. Limiting information access to health care members directly involved in a client's care

    D. Reporting breaches in confidentiality

    Access to information can be restricted by password. Therefore, it is necessary for all staff members to have their own passwords so that they will only have access to information regarding the clients to whom they are assigned. Placing paper-based charts behind the nurses' station will limit access. Limiting information access to health care members directly involved in a client's care protects client information. Reporting breaches in confidentiality will assist with identifying problems and finding solutions.

(N) **NCLEX® Connection: Management of Care: Confidentiality/Information Security**

2. A nurse is preparing information for change-of-shift report. Which of the following should the nurse include in the report?

    A. The client's input and output for the shift

    B. The client's blood pressure from the previous day

    C. A bone scan that is scheduled for today

    D. The medication routine from the medication administration record

    The bone scan is important because the nurse might have to modify the client's care to accommodate leaving the unit. Unless there is a significant change in the client's intake and output, blood pressure, or medication routine, the oncoming nurse can read that information in the chart.

(N) **NCLEX® Connection: Management of Care: Continuity of Care**

3. A nurse enters a client's room and finds him sitting in his chair. He states, "I fell in the shower but I got myself back up and into my chair." How should the nurse document this in the client's chart?

    A. The client fell in the shower.

    B. The client states he fell in the shower and was able to get himself back into his chair.

    C. This information should not be documented in the chart because the nurse did not witness the fall.

    D. The client fell in the shower but is now resting comfortably.

The nurse did not witness the fall, but it is important information to include in the chart. Because the nurse did not witness the fall, it cannot be documented as objective data. By writing what the client states, the information is considered subjective data. The nurse should also complete an incident report per facility/agency protocol.

 NCLEX® Connection: Safety and Infection Control: Reporting of Incident/Event/Irregular Occurrence/Variance

4. The skin barrier covering a client's intestinal fistula keeps falling off when she stands up to ambulate. The skin barrier has been applied twice during the current shift and remains intact only when the client is supine in bed. The nurse telephoned the physical therapist about the difficulties containing the drainage from the fistula, so the therapist did not work with the client today. The client sat in a chair during lunch with an absorbent pad over the fistula. A wound care nurse was called and states she will be coming in later today to see the client. The client states she is getting frustrated at not being able to work with her physical therapist. List the information the nurse should include in the change-of-shift report.

Client has an intestinal fistula.

Skin barrier stays intact when the client is supine, but the seal loosens when the client stands.

Physical therapist did not ambulate the client today.

Client sat in the chair during lunch.

Client states she is frustrated with not being able to work on improving mobility.

Wound care nurse was called and will see the client later today.

 NCLEX® Connection: Management of Care: Continuity of Care

5. Which of the following legal guidelines should the nurse follow when documenting in the client's record? (Select all that apply.)

_____ If an error is made, cover it with correction fluid and write in the correct information.

__X__ **All entries should be dated and timed.**

__X__ **Document objective data, leaving out personal bias.**

_____ Use as many abbreviations as possible.

_____ To save time, wait until the end of the shift to document any information.

All entries must be dated and timed. Documentation should be objective without personal bias. Correction fluid should never be used in a permanent record. The nurse should follow facility protocol for making corrections. Too many abbreviations may make the entry difficult to understand, and only institutionally accepted abbreviations should be used. Documentation should be kept current. Waiting until the end of the shift may result in omitted documentation.

NCLEX® Connection: Management of Care: Continuity of Care

UNIT 1	SAFE, EFFECTIVE CARE ENVIRONMENT
Section	Management of Care
Chapter 6	Delegation and Supervision

Overview

- Delegating is the process of transferring the authority and responsibility to another member of the health care team to complete a task, while retaining the accountability.

- Supervising is the process of directing, monitoring, and evaluating the performance of tasks by another member of the health care team. RNs are responsible for the supervision of client care tasks delegated to assistive personnel (AP) and licensed practical nurses (LPNs).

  ○ Licensed personnel are nurses who have completed a course of study and successfully passed either an LPN or RN examination, respectively.

  ○ Unlicensed personnel are individuals who are specially trained to function in an assistive role to licensed nurses in the provision of client care activities.

    ■ These individuals may be nursing personnel such as certified nursing assistants (CNAs) or certified medication assistants (CMAs), or they may be non-nursing personnel to whom nursing activities may be delegated, such as dialysis technicians, monitor technicians, or phlebotomists.

    ■ Some health care entities may differentiate between nurse and non-nurse assistive personnel or APs by using the acronym NAP for nursing assistive personnel.

Delegating and Supervising

- A licensed nurse is responsible for providing clear directions when a task is initially delegated and for periodic reassessment and evaluation of the outcome of the task.

  ○ RNs may delegate to other RNs, LPNs, and AP.

    ■ RNs must be knowledgeable about the applicable state nurse practice act and regulations regarding the use of LPNs and AP.

    ■ RNs must delegate tasks so that they can complete higher level tasks that only RNs can perform. This allows more efficient use of all members of the health care team.

  ○ LPNs may delegate to other LPNs and AP.

- Delegation Factors

  o Nurses can only delegate tasks appropriate for the skill and education level of the nurse who is receiving the assignment.

  o RNs cannot delegate the nursing process, client education, or tasks that require nursing judgment to LPNs or AP.

  o Task factors – Prior to delegating client care, the nurse should consider:

    ▪ Predictability of outcome

      □ Will the completion of the task have a predictable outcome?

      □ Is it a routine treatment?

      □ Is it a new treatment?

    ▪ Potential for harm

      □ Is there a chance that something negative may happen to the client (risk for bleeding, risk for aspiration)?

      □ Is the client unstable?

    ▪ Complexity of care

      □ Are complex tasks required as a part of the client's care?

      □ Is the delegatee legally able to perform the task and do they have the skills necessary?

    ▪ Need for problem solving and innovation

      □ Will a judgment need to be made while performing the task?

      □ Does it require nursing assessment skills?

    ▪ Level of interaction with the client

      □ Is there a need to provide psychosocial support or education during the performance of the task?

  o Delegatee factors – Considerations for selection of an appropriate delegatee include:

    ▪ Education, training, and experience

    ▪ Knowledge and skill to perform the task

    ▪ Level of critical thinking required to complete the task

    ▪ Ability to communicate with others as it pertains to the task

    ▪ Demonstrated competence

    ▪ Agency policies and procedures

    ▪ Licensing legislation (state nurse practice acts)

EXAMPLES OF TASKS THAT CAN BE DELEGATED TO LPNS AND AP (PROVIDED AGENCY POLICY AND STATE PRACTICE GUIDELINES PERMIT)	
TO LPNS	**TO AP**
• Monitoring client findings (as input to the RN's ongoing assessment of the client) • Reinforcing client teaching from a standard care plan • Performing tracheostomy care • Suctioning • Checking nasogastric tube patency • Administrating enteral feedings • Inserting a urinary catheter • Administrating medication (excluding intravenous medications in several states)	• Activities of daily living (ADLs) • Bathing • Grooming • Dressing • Toileting • Ambulating • Feeding (without swallowing precautions) • Positioning • Bed making • Specimen collection • Intake and output (I&O) • Vital signs (for stable clients)

- Delegation and Supervision Guidelines

  o Use the five rights of delegation to decide:

    - What tasks should be delegated (right task)

    - Under what circumstances (right circumstance)

    - To whom (right person)

    - What information should be communicated (right direction/communication)

    - How to supervise/evaluate (right supervision/evaluation)

(M) **View Media Supplement:** Delegation (Video)

  o Use professional judgment and critical thinking skills when delegating.

  o Right task

    - Identify what tasks are appropriate to delegate for each specific client.

      □ A right task is repetitive, requires little supervision, and is relatively noninvasive for a certain client.

    - Delegate activities to appropriate levels of team members (LPN, AP) based on professional standards of practice, legal and facility guidelines, and available resources.

RIGHT TASK	WRONG TASK
Delegate an AP to assist a client with pneumonia to use a bedpan.	Delegate an AP to administer a nebulizer treatment to a client with pneumonia.

- ○ Right circumstance
  - ■ Assess the health status and complexity of care required by the client.
  - ■ Match the complexity of care demands to the skill level of the health care team member.
  - ■ Consider the workload of the team member.

RIGHT CIRCUMSTANCE	WRONG CIRCUMSTANCE
Delegate an AP to assist in obtaining vital signs from a stable postoperative client.	Delegate an AP to assist in obtaining vital signs from a postoperative client who required naloxone (Narcan) for depressed respirations.

- ○ Right person
  - ■ Assess and verify the competency of the health care team member.
    - □ The task must be within the team member's scope of practice.
    - □ The team member must have the necessary competence/training.
  - ■ Continually review the performance of the team member and determine care competency.
  - ■ Assess team member performance based on standards and, when necessary, take steps to remediate any failure to meet standards.

RIGHT PERSON	WRONG PERSON
Delegate an LPN to administer enteral feedings to a client with a head injury.	Delegate an AP to administer enteral feedings to a client with a head injury.

- ○ Right direction/communication – Communicate either in writing or orally:
  - ■ Data to collect
  - ■ Method and timeline for reporting, including when to report concerns/assessment findings
  - ■ Specific task(s) to be performed; client-specific instructions
  - ■ Expected results, timelines, and expectations for follow-up communication

RIGHT DIRECTION/COMMUNICATION	WRONG DIRECTION/COMMUNICATION
Delegate an AP to assist the client in room 312 with a shower, to be completed by 0900.	Delegate an AP to assist the client in room 312 with morning hygiene.

- ○ Right supervision/evaluation – The delegating nurse must:
  - ■ Provide supervision, either directly or indirectly (assigning supervision to another licensed nurse).
  - ■ Provide clear directions and understandable expectations of the task(s) to be performed (timeframes, what to report).
  - ■ Monitor performance.

- Provide feedback.
- Intervene if necessary (unsafe clinical practice).
- Evaluate the client and determine if client outcomes were met.
- Evaluate client care tasks and identify needs for performance improvement activities and/or additional resources.

RIGHT SUPERVISION	WRONG SUPERVISION
Delegate an AP to assist in ambulating a client after completing the admission assessment.	Delegate an AP to assist in ambulating a client prior to performing an admission assessment.

- Supervision
  - Occurs after delegation
  - Oversees a staff's performance of delegated activities
  - Determines if:
    - Completion of tasks is on schedule
    - Performance was at a satisfactory level
    - Abnormal or unexpected findings were documented and reported
    - Assistance is needed to complete assigned tasks in a timely manner
    - Assignment should be re-evaluated and possibly changed

CHAPTER 6: DELEGATION AND SUPERVISION

 Application Exercises

1. A nurse on a medical-surgical unit has received change-of-shift report and has been assigned to care for four clients. Which of the following client's needs may be assigned to an assistive personnel (AP)?

    A. Feeding a client who was admitted 24 hr ago with aspiration pneumonia

    B. Reinforcing teaching for a client who is learning to walk using a quad cane

    C. Reapplying a condom catheter for a client who has urinary incontinence

    D. Applying a sterile dressing to a pressure ulcer

2. A nurse is delegating the ambulation of a client who had knee arthroplasty 5 days ago to an AP. Which of the following information should the nurse share with the AP? (Select all that apply.)

    _____ The client is in room 203 – Bed B.

    _____ The roommate is up independently.

    _____ The client ambulates with his slippers on over his antiembolic stockings.

    _____ The client uses a front-wheeled walker when ambulating.

    _____ The client had pain medication 30 min ago.

    _____ The client is allergic to codeine.

    _____ The client should ambulate at least 50 ft.

    _____ The client ate 50% of his breakfast this morning.

3. An RN is making assignments for client care to a licensed practical nurse (LPN) at the beginning of the shift. Which of the following assignments should the LPN question?

    A. Assisting a client who is 24 hr postoperative to use an incentive spirometer

    B. Collecting a clean-catch urine specimen from a client who was admitted on the previous shift

    C. Providing nasopharyngeal suctioning for a client with pneumonia

    D. Replacing the cartridge and tubing on a patient-controlled analgesia (PCA) pump

CHAPTER 6: DELEGATION AND SUPERVISION

 Application Exercises Answer Key

1. A nurse on a medical-surgical unit has received change-of-shift report and has been assigned to care for four clients. Which of the following client's needs may be assigned to an assistive personnel (AP)?

    A. Feeding a client who was admitted 24 hr ago with aspiration pneumonia

    B. Reinforcing teaching for a client who is learning to walk using a quad cane

    C. Reapplying a condom catheter for a client who has urinary incontinence

    D. Applying a sterile dressing to a pressure ulcer

The application of a condom catheter is a noninvasive, routine procedure that can be delegated to an AP. It would be inappropriate to delegate the feeding of a client who has aspiration pneumonia because the client is at risk for further aspiration. Reinforcing teaching should be done by either the RN or LPN. The application of a sterile dressing should also be completed by an RN or LPN.

Ⓝ NCLEX® Connection: Management of Care: Concepts of Management

2. A nurse is delegating the ambulation of a client who had knee arthroplasty 5 days ago to an AP. Which of the following information should the nurse share with the AP? (Select all that apply.)

__X__	**The client is in room 203 – Bed B.**
_____	The roommate is up independently.
__X__	**The client ambulates with his slippers on over his antiembolic stockings.**
__X__	**The client uses a front-wheeled walker when ambulating.**
__X__	**The client had pain medication 30 min ago.**
_____	The client is allergic to codeine.
__X__	**The client should ambulate at least 50 ft.**
_____	The client ate 50% of his breakfast this morning.

Correct direction/communication is necessary for safe delegation. The information checked is necessary for the AP to perform the task safely. The other information is not necessary to know for the task to be performed safely.

Ⓝ NCLEX® Connection: Management of Care: Concepts of Management

3. An RN is making assignments for client care to a licensed practical nurse (LPN) at the beginning of the shift. Which of the following assignments should the LPN question?

    A. Assisting a client who is 24 hr postoperative to use an incentive spirometer

    B. Collecting a clean-catch urine specimen from a client who was admitted on the previous shift

    C. Providing nasopharyngeal suctioning for a client with pneumonia

    D. Replacing the cartridge and tubing on a patient-controlled analgesia (PCA) pump

The RN is responsible for maintaining the PCA pump. Assisting a client to use an incentive spirometer, collecting a clean-catch urine specimen, and providing nasopharyngeal suctioning are within the scope of practice of the LPN.

Ⓝ NCLEX® Connection: Management of Care: Concepts of Management

UNIT 1	SAFE, EFFECTIVE CARE ENVIRONMENT
Section	Management of Care
Chapter 7	Nursing Process

Overview

- The Nursing Process:

  o Is a cyclical, critical thinking process that consists of five steps to follow in a purposeful, goal-directed, systematic way to achieve optimal client outcomes. The nursing process is a variation of scientific reasoning that allows the nurse to organize nursing care.

  o Is a client-centered, problem-solving, and decision-making framework that is foundational to nursing practice.

  o Provides a framework throughout which the nurse can apply knowledge, experience, judgment, and skills, as well as established standards of nursing practice to the formulation of a plan of nursing care. This plan is applicable to any client system, including individuals, families, groups, and communities.

  o Includes five sequential but overlapping steps – Assessment/data collection, analysis/ data collection, planning, implementation, and evaluation. Each step of the nursing process depends on the satisfactory completion of the preceding step(s). The accuracy and thoroughness of assessment/analysis/data collection and planning have a direct impact on implementation and evaluation. Use of the nursing process results in a comprehensive, individualized, client-centered plan of nursing care that can be delivered in a timely and reasonable manner.

  o Allows the nurse to integrate critical thinking creatively to make nursing judgments based on reason.

  o Promotes the professionalism of nursing while differentiating the practice of nursing from the practice of medicine and that of other health care professionals.

Assessment (RN)/Data Collection (PN)

- Assessment/Data collection involves the systematic collection of information about the client's present health status to identify the client's needs and to identify additional data to collect based on the nurse's findings. Client data can be collected during an initial assessment (baseline data), a focused assessment, and ongoing assessments.

- Methods of data collection include observation, interviews with the client and family, the medical history, a comprehensive or focused physical examination, diagnostic and laboratory reports, and collaboration.

To collect data effectively, a nurse must be able to ask the client appropriate questions, listen carefully to the client's responses, and have excellent head-to-toe physical assessment skills. The nurse must also be able to employ clinical judgment and critical thinking in accurately recognizing when to collect client assessment data. The nurse must also recognize the need to collect assessment data prior to interventions, including notification of the client's provider.

- Subjective data (symptoms) are usually obtained during a nursing history and include the client's own feelings, perceptions, and descriptions of health status. Subjective data are described, verified, and apparent only to the client.

- Objective data (signs) are usually obtained during a physical examination. The data are observable and measurable. Objective data are felt, seen, heard, or smelled by the nurse through observation or physical assessment of the client.

SOURCES OF DATA	SUBJECTIVE	OBJECTIVE
Primary sources of data	What the client tells the nurse: "My shoulder is really, really sore."	Data the nurse obtains through observation and examination: Client is observed grimacing when attempting to brush her hair with her left arm.
Secondary sources of data	What others tell the nurse based on what the client has told them: "She told me that her shoulder is sore every morning."	Data collected from other sources (family, friends, caregivers, health care professionals, literature review, medical records): Physical therapy note in chart indicates client has decreased range of motion of left shoulder.

- During this assessment/data collection, the nurse validates, interprets, and clusters data.

- Documentation of the assessment data must be thorough, concise, and accurate.

Analysis (RN)/Data Collection (PN)

- The nurse uses critical thinking skills (a diagnostic reasoning process) to identify the client's health status or problem(s), interpret or monitor the collected database, reach an appropriate nursing judgment about the client's health status and coping mechanisms, and provide direction for nursing care.

- Analysis/Data collection requires the nurse to look at the data and:

   o   Recognize patterns or trends.

   o   Compare the data with expected standards or reference ranges.

   o   Arrive at conclusions to guide nursing care.

- RNs make multiple analyses based on their interpretations of collected data. Each nurse decides, using reasoning and judgment, which data account for the client's health status or problems. At times, this requires further data collection and analysis. As the nurse again clusters the collected data, a specific finding might serve as an alert to a specific client problem that requires planning and intervention.

- As with the assessment/data collection step, complete and accurate documentation is essential. Documentation should focus on facts and should be highly descriptive.

Planning

- When planning client care (RN) or contributing to a client's plan of care (PN), the nurse must establish priorities and optimal outcomes of care that can be readily measured and evaluated. These established priorities and outcomes of client care then direct the nurse in selecting the nursing interventions to include in a client's plan of care to promote, maintain, or restore a client's health.

- The nurse engages in three types of planning. Initially, the nurse develops a comprehensive plan of care for clients based on comprehensive assessments that are completed, for example, on admission to a health care facility or to a home health organization.

- The nurse engages in ongoing planning throughout the provision of client care. While obtaining new information and evaluating the client's responses to care, the nurse modifies and individualizes the client's initial plan of care.

- Discharge planning is a process of anticipating and planning for a client's needs after discharge. To be effective, discharge planning must begin as soon as the client is admitted.

- Throughout the planning process, the nurse sets priorities, determines client outcomes, and selects specific nursing interventions.

- The nurse participates in priority setting when a preferential order of client problems is identified. This guides the delivery of nursing care. The nurse can use guidelines to set priorities, such as Maslow's hierarchy of basic needs.

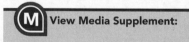 **View Media Supplement:** Maslow's Hierarchy (Image)

- The nurse works with the client to identify goals and client outcomes.

  - The goal will identify the optimal client status, whereas the client outcome will identify the observable criterion that will determine success or failure of the goal.

  - Often these terms are used interchangeably. With any format used, the goal/client outcome must be client-centered, singular, observable, measurable, time-limited, mutually agreed upon, and reasonable.

  - Concise, measurable goals allow the nurse and the client to evaluate progress toward the planned outcome and the effectiveness of nursing care.

- The nurse identifies nursing actions or nursing interventions that help achieve optimal client outcomes. Nursing interventions are any treatments or actions the nurse performs to enhance/achieve the client's outcomes.

  o Nursing interventions are based on scientific principles that provide the rationale for the action to be taken.

  o Interventions include:

    ▪ Nurse initiated/independent interventions – Autonomous actions based on scientific rationale that are expected to benefit the client. They are initiated by the nurse based on the client's identified problems and health care needs, and are within the nurse's scope of practice as identified by the ANA Standards of Practice, state nurse practice acts, and health care facility policies. The nurse performs or delegates the interventions. The nurse is accountable for these interventions, such as repositioning a client at least every 2 hr to prevent skin breakdown.

    ▪ Physician initiated/dependent interventions – Interventions the nurse initiates as a result of a provider's order (written, standing, or verbal) or the facility's protocol, such as blood administration procedures.

    ▪ Collaborative interventions – Interventions the nurse carries out in collaboration with other health care team professionals, such as assuring that the client receives and eats his evening snack.

- The nursing care plan (NCP) is the end product of the planning step. The NCP is organized for quick identification of the client's problems, outcomes, and interventions to be implemented.

Implementation

- In this step of the nursing process, the nurse provides client care based on assessment data gathered, analyses done, and the plan of care developed in the previous steps of the nursing process. In this step, the nurse must use problem-solving, clinical judgment, and critical thinking to select and implement appropriate therapeutic interventions based on nursing knowledge, priorities of care, and planned goals or outcomes to promote, maintain, or restore a client's health. The nurse also uses interpersonal skills (therapeutic communication) and technical skills (psychomotor performance) when implementing nursing interventions.

- Therapeutic interventions also include measures the nurse takes to minimize a client's risk and nursing responses to unplanned events, such as an observation of unsafe practice, a change in a client's status, or the emergence of a life-threatening situation.

- The nurse uses evidence-based rationale for the selection and implementation of all therapeutic interventions. Additionally, caring should be at the center of all therapeutic nursing interventions. The nurse demonstrates professional behavior in the delivery of all therapeutic nursing interventions.

- During implementation, the nurse may perform nursing actions, delegate tasks, supervise other health care staff, and document the care given and the client's responses.

Evaluation

- In this step of the nursing process, the nurse evaluates a client's response to nursing interventions and forms a clinical judgment about the extent to which goals and outcomes have been met.

- The nurse's evaluation of the progress made toward achievement of client outcomes is what determines whether or not to modify the client's plan of care.

- The nurse determines the effectiveness of the nursing care plan. The nurse collects data from the client based on the outcome criteria determined. The nurse compares what actually happened with the planned client outcome. This helps the nurse determine what further actions to take.

- Questions the nurse should consider include:

  o   "Were the planned client outcomes met?"

  o   "Were the nursing interventions appropriate/effective?"

  o   "Should I modify the outcomes and/or interventions?"

- Client outcomes that are stated in specific, measurable terms are easier to evaluate.

- Factors that can lead to lack of goal achievement include:

  o   An incomplete database

  o   Unrealistic client outcomes

  o   Nonspecific nursing interventions

  o   Inadequate time for the client to achieve the outcome

CHAPTER 7: NURSING PROCESS

(A) Application Exercises

1. Identify each of the following as subjective data (S) or as objective data (O).

	Respiratory rate of 22/min with respirations that are even and unlabored
	"I can only walk three blocks before my legs start to hurt."
	Pain rated at 3 on a scale of 0 to 10
	Skin pink, warm, and dry
	Urine output of 300 mL/8 hr
	"My wife doesn't come to visit very often."
	Dressing clean, dry, and intact

2. By the second postoperative day, a client has not achieved satisfactory pain relief. Based on this evaluation, what should the nurse do next based on the nursing process?

    A. Reassess the client to determine the reason satisfactory pain relief has not been achieved.

    B. Wait to see if the pain lessens over the next 24 hr.

    C. Change the plan to ensure that the client achieves adequate pain relief.

    D. Teach the client about the plan of care that is being implemented to manage his pain.

3. During evaluation, the nurse must gather information about the client to

    A. identify whether or not the client outcomes have been met.

    B. organize resources to proceed with implementing interventions.

    C. establish client-centered outcomes that are measurable and realistic.

    D. determine the priority of care and appropriate interventions.

4. For each of the following nursing interventions, identify whether the intervention is a nurse-initiated intervention (N) or a provider-initiated intervention (P).

	Give morphine sulfate 1 to 2 mg IV every 1 hr as needed for pain.
	Insert nasogastric tube.
	Apply moist heat to left arm.
	Listen actively to client's concerns.
	Perform daily bath after evening meal.
	Infuse 0.9% sodium chloride at 125 mL/hr.

CHAPTER 7: NURSING PROCESS

 Application Exercises Answer Key

1. Identify each of the following as subjective data (S) or as objective data (O).

O	Respiratory rate of 22/min with respirations that are even and unlabored
S	"I can only walk three blocks before my legs start to hurt."
S	Pain rated at 3 on a scale of 0 to 10
O	Skin pink, warm, and dry
O	Urine output of 300 mL/8 hr
S	"My wife doesn't come to visit very often."
O	Dressing clean, dry, and intact

 NCLEX® Connection: Health Promotion and Maintenance: Techniques of Physical Assessment

2. By the second postoperative day, a client has not achieved satisfactory pain relief. Based on this evaluation, what should the nurse do next based on the nursing process?

   A. Reassess the client to determine the reason satisfactory pain relief has not been achieved.

   B. Wait to see if the pain lessens over the next 24 hr.

   C. Change the plan to ensure that the client achieves adequate pain relief.

   D. Teach the client about the plan of care that is being implemented to manage his pain.

   The nurse should reassess the client to determine why the client has not achieved satisfactory pain relief. Various factors may be influencing the lack of pain relief. By the second postoperative day, the interventions implemented should have achieved the planned client outcome. Changing the plan may be necessary, but the nurse must first reassess the client to determine the reason for lack of outcome achievement. The current plan is not working, so teaching the client about this plan is providing false reassurance and does not address the client's current pain.

 NCLEX® Connection: Health Promotion and Maintenance: Techniques of Physical Assessment

3. During evaluation, the nurse must gather information about the client to

    A. identify whether or not the client outcomes have been met.

    B. organize resources to proceed with implementing interventions.

    C. establish client-centered outcomes that are measurable and realistic.

    D. determine the priority of care and appropriate interventions.

    Evaluation involves gathering information about the client to determine whether or not client outcomes have been met. Organizing resources takes place during the implementation step. Establishing client-centered outcomes and establishing priorities of care take place in the planning step.

 NCLEX® Connection: NCLEX Connection: Health Promotion and Maintenance: Techniques of Physical Assessment

4. For each of the following nursing interventions, identify whether the intervention is a nurse-initiated intervention (N) or a provider-initiated intervention (P).

P	Give morphine sulfate 1 to 2 mg IV every 1 hr as needed for pain.
P	Insert nasogastric tube.
P	Apply moist heat to left arm.
N	Listen actively to client's concerns.
N	Perform daily bath after evening meal.
P	Infuse 0.9% sodium chloride at 125 mL/hr.

 NCLEX® Connection: Management of Care: Continuity of Care

UNIT 1	SAFE, EFFECTIVE CARE ENVIRONMENT
Section	Management of Care
Chapter 8	Critical Thinking and Clinical Judgment

ⓐ Overview

- Nursing practice requires the application of knowledge from biological, social, and physical sciences; knowledge of pathophysiology; and knowledge of nursing procedures and skills. Consequently, nurses must use multiple thinking skills, including critical thinking skills such as interpretation, analysis, evaluation, inference, and explanation, to make clinical judgments about problems posed in nursing practice. A nursing knowledge base, developed through foundational thinking skills and including recall and comprehension, is a prerequisite to critical thinking in nursing.

- In nursing, critical thinking is an active, orderly, well though-out reasoning process that guides the nurse in various approaches to making a nursing judgment by applying knowledge and experience, problem-solving, and decision-making. A critical thinker prioritizes, explores various courses of action, keeps ethics in mind, and determines appropriate outcomes.

- To have a positive impact on a client's health status, the nurse must be able to think critically, correctly identify problems, and both identify and implement the best solutions (interventions). Critical thinking discourages the nurse from forming quick judgments that lead to single-focused solutions.

- Critical thinking requires lifelong learning and the acquisition of relevant experiences to reflect on continually for the purpose of improving one's ability to make appropriate nursing judgments.

- The components of critical thinking include knowledge, experience, critical thinking competencies, attitudes, and intellectual and professional standards.

- Critical thinking incorporates reflection, language, and intuition, and it evolves through three distinct levels as the nurse gains knowledge and experience while maturing into a competent nursing professional.

  - Reflection – Purposefully thinking back or recalling a situation to discover its meaning and gain insight into the event. The nurse should reflect on the following:

    - "Why did I say that or do this?"

    - "Did the original plan of care achieve optimal client outcomes?"

      - If so – "Which interventions were successful?"

      - If not – "Which interventions were unsuccessful?"

- Language – Precise, clear language demonstrating focused thinking and communicating unambiguous messages and expectations to both the client and other health care team members. The nurse should consider the following:

  - "Did I use language appropriate for the client?"

  - "Did I communicate the message clearly to the provider?"

- Intuition – An inner sensing that something is not currently supported with fact. Intuition should spark the nurse to search the data to confirm or disprove the "feeling." The nurse should ponder the following:

  - "Did the vital signs reflect any changes that would account for the client's present status?"

  - "When the client's status changed in this way last month, there was a specific reason for it. Is that what is happening here?"

Levels of Critical Thinking

- Basic Critical Thinking

  - The nurse trusts the experts and thinks concretely based on the "rules."

  - Basic critical thinking results from limited nursing knowledge and experience, as well as inadequate critical thinking experience.

    - Example – The client reports pain 1 hr after receiving a pain medication. Instead of reassessing the client's pain, the nurse tells the client he must wait 2 more hours before he can receive another dose.

- Complex Critical Thinking

  - The nurse begins to express autonomy by analyzing and examining data to determine the best alternative.

  - Complex critical thinking results from increased nursing knowledge, experience, intuition, and more flexible attitudes.

    - Example – The nurse realizes that the client is not ambulating as often as prescribed because of a fear of missing her daughter's phone call. The nurse assures the client that the staff will listen for and answer her phone when she is out of her room.

- Commitment

  - The nurse expects to have to make choices without help from others and fully assumes the responsibility for those choices.

  - Commitment results from an expert level of knowledge, experience, developed intuition, and reflective, flexible attitudes.

    - Example – The nurse increases the rate of an IV fluid infusion when the client's blood pressure indicates hypovolemic shock 24 hr after surgery.

Components of Critical Thinking

- Knowledge – Information specific to nursing and acquired through:

  - Basic nursing education

  - Continuing education courses

  - Advanced degrees and certifications

- Experience – Decision-making ability derived from opportunities to observe, sense, and interact with clients followed by active reflection. The nurse:

  - Demonstrates an understanding of clinical situations.

  - Recognizes and analyzes cues for relevance.

  - Incorporates experience into intuition.

- Competence – Cognitive processes a nurse uses to make nursing judgments, such as:

  - General critical thinking.

    - Scientific method

    - Problem-solving

    - Decision-making

    - Diagnostic reasoning and inference

    - Clinical decision-making – collaboration

(M) View Media Supplement: Priority Setting (Video)

  - Specific critical thinking in nursing.

    - The nursing process:

THE NURSING PROCESS	CRITICAL THINKING SKILLS
Assessment/Data Collection – Collect information about the client's present health status to identify the client's needs and to identify additional data to collect based on the nurse's findings.	• Observe. • Use correct techniques for collecting data. • Differentiate between relevant and irrelevant data and between important and unimportant data. • Organize, categorize, and validate data. • Interpret assessment data and draw a conclusion.
Analysis/Data Collection – Interpret or monitor the collected database, reach an appropriate nursing judgment about the client's health status and coping mechanisms, and provide direction for nursing care.	• Identify clusters and cues. • Detect inferences. • Recognize an actual or potential problem, or risk. • Defer from making judgments.

THE NURSING PROCESS	CRITICAL THINKING SKILLS
Planning – Establish priorities and optimal outcomes of care that can be readily measured and evaluated, then select the nursing interventions to include in a client's plan of care to promote, maintain, or restore a client's health.	• Identify goals and outcomes for client care. • Set priorities. • Determine appropriate strategies and/or interventions for inclusion on a client's plan of care or teaching plan. • Take knowledge and apply it to more than one situation. • Create outcome criteria. • Theorize. • Consider the consequences of implementation.
Implementation – Provide client care based on assessment data gathered, analyses done, and the plan of care developed in the previous steps of the nursing process.	• Use knowledge base. • Use appropriate skills and teaching strategies. • Test theories. • Delegate and supervise nursing care. • Communicate appropriately in response to a situation.
Evaluation – Examine a client's response to nursing interventions and form a clinical judgment about the extent to which goals and outcomes have been met.	• Determine accuracy of theories. • Evaluate outcomes based on specific criteria. • Determine understanding of teaching.

- Attitudes – Mindsets that affect how a nurse approaches a problem. Attitudes of critical thinkers include:

    o Confidence – Feels sure of abilities.

    o Independence – Analyzes ideas for logical reasoning.

    o Fairness – Is objective, nonjudgmental.

    o Responsibility – Practices according to standards of practice.

    o Risk taking – Takes calculated chances in finding better solutions to problems.

    o Discipline – Develops a systematic approach to thinking.

    o Perseverance – Continues to work at a problem until it is resolved.

    o Creativity – Uses imagination to find solutions to unique client problems.

    o Curiosity – Requires more information about clients and problems.

    o Integrity – Practices truthfully and ethically.

    o Humility – Acknowledges weaknesses.

- Standards – Model to which care is compared to determine acceptability, excellence, and appropriateness.

  o Intellectual standards ensure the thorough application of critical thinking.

  o Professional standards include:

    ▪ Nursing judgment based on ethical criteria.

    ▪ Evaluation that relies on evidence-based practice.

    ▪ Demonstration of professional responsibility.

CHAPTER 8: CRITICAL THINKING AND CLINICAL JUDGMENT

 Application Exercises

Scenario: A nurse is caring for a 35-year-old man who is 24 hr postoperative following an inguinal hernia repair. The client is tolerating clear liquids well, has active bowel sounds, and is expressing a desire for "real food." Preoperatively, he was cooperative and pleasant. Now, he is easily agitated. The nurse has explained the importance of coughing, deep breathing, and dangling, yet he remains nonadherent. The client has pain medication prescribed every 4 to 6 hr as needed. He has been accepting it every 6 to 7 hr. His vital signs prior to his last pain medication dose were heart rate 100/min, respiratory rate 16/min, temperature 37° C (98.6° F), and blood pressure 136/80 mm Hg. His surgical dressing is dry and intact.

1. The nurse tells the client that she will call the provider to see whether or not he can have the ice cream and tomato soup that he requested. The provider prescribes a full liquid diet. This is an example of which level of critical thinking? Provide rationale.

2. The nurse suspects that the client is experiencing pain. Analyze the above situation and provide data to support or refute that judgment.

3. Analyze the client's seeming nonadherence and provide alternative possibilities for his lack of adherence.

4. A client is experiencing hypertension, and the provider prescribes a newly approved antihypertensive medication. Prior to administering the medication, the nurse gathers information about the medication using an electronic database. The nurse is using which of the following components of critical thinking when reviewing the medication information?

   A. Knowledge
   B. Experience
   C. Intuition
   D. Competence

5. A nurse receives a prescription for an antibiotic for a 35-year-old man who has cellulitis. The nurse checks the client's chart, discovers that the client is allergic to the antibiotic, and phones the provider to obtain a prescription for a different antibiotic. What critical thinking attitude did the nurse exhibit?

   A. Fairness
   B. Responsibility
   C. Risk taking
   D. Creativity

6. Match the critical thinking attitude with the appropriate example.

_____ Confidence

_____ Discipline

_____ Perseverance

_____ Integrity

_____ Humility

A. A nurse mistakenly gives the wrong dose of medication to a client. The nurse calls the provider to notify her of the error.

B. A nurse tries three different pouches before finding one that will contain the draining wound.

C. A nurse uses a head-to-toe approach to conduct a physical assessment.

D. A nurse states that she has difficulties inserting IV catheters in clients who are dehydrated.

E. A nurse offers to put an IV catheter in a client who is dehydrated.

CHAPTER 8: CRITICAL THINKING AND CLINICAL JUDGMENT

 Application Exercises Answer Key

Scenario: A nurse is caring for a 35-year-old man who is 24 hr postoperative following an inguinal hernia repair. The client is tolerating clear liquids well, has active bowel sounds, and is expressing a desire for "real food." Preoperatively, he was cooperative and pleasant. Now, he is easily agitated. The nurse has explained the importance of coughing, deep breathing, and dangling, yet he remains nonadherent. The client has pain medication prescribed every 4 to 6 hr as needed. He has been accepting it every 6 to 7 hr. His vital signs prior to his last pain medication dose were heart rate 100/min, respiratory rate 16/min, temperature 37° C (98.6° F), and blood pressure 136/80 mm Hg. His surgical dressing is dry and intact.

1. The nurse tells the client that she will call the provider to see whether or not he can have the ice cream and tomato soup he requested. The provider prescribes a full liquid diet. This is an example of which level of critical thinking? Provide rationale.

   Basic critical thinking – Thinking is concrete and based on a set of rules (order for full liquids). Advanced experience and knowledge would allow the nurse to introduce full liquids based on active bowel sounds and the client's tolerance of clear liquids.

   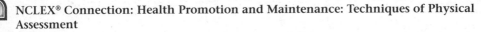 **NCLEX® Connection: Basic Care and Comfort: Nutrition and Oral Hydration**

2. The nurse suspects that the client is experiencing pain. Analyze the above situation and provide data to support or refute that judgment.

   Elevated blood pressure and pulse rate without elevated temperature, labored respirations, or signs of bleeding support that the client is in pain.

   Acceptance of pain medication only at or beyond the maximum time limit with atypical agitation also supports that the client is in pain.

   Refusal to comply with interventions that could increase his pain level (e.g., coughing, deep breathing) also supports that the client is in pain. Complex critical thinking would conclude that the client's pain management is unacceptable.

   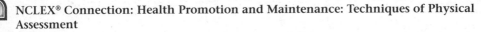 **NCLEX® Connection: Health Promotion and Maintenance: Techniques of Physical Assessment**

3. Analyze the client's seeming nonadherence and provide alternative possibilities for the lack of adherence.

The client is in pain and thus will not perform with potentially pain-inducing actions (coughing, deep breathing).

The client did not understand the nurse's explanation of the importance of coughing, deep breathing, and dangling. She should reflect on her presentation and readdress the educational issue.

The client is not able to retain instructions because of the pain he is experiencing; therefore, the pain must be managed appropriately and the education issue readdressed.

(N) **NCLEX® Connection: Basic Care and Comfort: Nonpharmacological Comfort Interventions**

4. A client is experiencing hypertension, and the provider prescribes a newly approved antihypertensive medication. Prior to administering the medication, the nurse gathers information about the medication using an electronic database. The nurse is using which of the following components of critical thinking when reviewing the medication information?

   A. Knowledge
   B. Experience
   C. Intuition
   D. Competence

By using the electronic database, the nurse takes initiative to increase her knowledge base, which is the first component of critical thinking. The nurse has had no prior experience with the medication, and intuition requires experience. Competence involves making judgments, but judgments cannot be made about the safe administration of a medication until knowledge is obtained.

(N) **NCLEX® Connection: Pharmacological and Parenteral Therapies: Medication Administration**

5. A nurse receives a prescription for an antibiotic for a 35-year-old man who has cellulitis. The nurse checks the client's chart, discovers that the client is allergic to the antibiotic, and phones the provider to obtain a prescription for a different antibiotic. What critical thinking attitude did the nurse exhibit?

   A. Fairness
   B. Responsibility
   C. Risk taking
   D. Creativity

The nurse is responsible for administering medications in a safe manner according to standards of practice. Fairness is using a nonjudgmental, objective approach in looking at clients and situations. Risk taking is a calculated approach to solving a problem that is not responding to traditional methods. Creativity is an approach that uses imagination to find solutions to unique client problems.

(N) **NCLEX® Connection: Pharmacological and Parenteral Therapies: Medication Administration**

6. Match the critical thinking attitude with the appropriate example.

__E__	Confidence	A. A nurse mistakenly gives the wrong dose of medication to a client. The nurse calls the provider to notify her of the error.
__C__	Discipline	B. A nurse tries three different pouches before finding one that will contain the draining wound.
__B__	Perseverance	C. A nurse uses a head-to-toe approach to conduct a physical assessment.
__A__	Integrity	D. A nurse states that she has difficulties inserting IV catheters in clients who are dehydrated.
__D__	Humility	E. A nurse offers to put an IV catheter in a client who is dehydrated.

(N) **NCLEX® Connection: Management of Care: Legal Rights and Responsibilities**

UNIT 1	SAFE, EFFECTIVE CARE ENVIRONMENT
Section	Management of Care
Chapter 9	Admissions, Transfers, and Discharge

Overview

- Responsibilities of nurses include ensuring continuity of care throughout the processes of admission, transfers, and discharge. Client information is organized and kept in a logical order for easy dissemination between nurses and other members of the health care team as clients are admitted, transferred, and discharged.

- The admission assessment provides baseline data to use in the development of the nursing care plan. Baseline data are compared with future assessments to monitor client status and response to treatment.

- Many clients experience anxiety and fear of the unknown at the time of admission to the hospital or health care facility. The feeling of independence and self-identity may be lost. Children may experience separation anxiety if parents are not present during the hospitalization. When nurses recognize clients' concerns and provides respectful, culturally sensitive care, the clients' experiences will be more positive.

- Discharge planning is an interdisciplinary process that is started by the nurse at admission. Nurses conduct discharge planning with both the client and client's family for optimal results.

- Nurses establish the ability of clients to participate in the admission assessment. Clients in distress or with mental status changes may need to have a family member provide necessary information.

- Nurses begin establishing the therapeutic relationship with clients and families during the admission process.

- Nurses promote professional communication between health care providers.

- Nurses use the nursing process as a guide to plan teaching and interventions for clients during discharge.

Admission Process

- Equipment

  - Prior to arrival of the client, take necessary equipment into the room. This should include appropriate documentation forms, equipment to obtain vital signs, pulse oximeter, and hospital attire for the client.

- Procedure

  o Introduce yourself to the client.

  o Explain the roles of other nursing staff.

  o If in a semiprivate room, introduce the client to his roommate.

  o Provide hospital attire and assist the client as necessary.

  o Position the client comfortably.

  o Apply the client's identification bracelet and allergy band, if needed.

  o Provide facility-specific brochures and informational material.

  o Provide information about advance directives.

  o Document the client's advance directives status in the medical record. (Place a copy in the medical record if it is available.)

  o Assess/collect the following data:

    ▪ Baseline data – Vital signs, height, weight, allergy status, home medications

    ▪ Biographical information on the client

    ▪ The client's reason for seeking health care

    ▪ Present illness and symptoms

    ▪ Health history of:

      □ Current illness

      □ Current medications (prescription and over-the-counter)

      □ Prior illnesses, chronic diseases

      □ Surgeries

      □ Previous hospitalizations

      □ Other relevant data

    ▪ Family history (hypertension, cancer, heart disease, diabetes mellitus)

    ▪ Psychosocial assessment

      □ Alcohol, tobacco, drug, and caffeine use

      □ History of mental illness

      □ History of abuse or homelessness

      □ Home situation/significant others

    ▪ Nutrition

      □ Current diet, any chewing or swallowing problems

      □ Recent weight gain/loss

- Spiritual health/quality-of-life concerns:
  - Religion
  - Advance directives/living will
- Review of systems
- Safety assessments:
  - History of falls
  - Sensory impairments (vision, hearing)
  - Use of assistive devices (walker, cane, crutches, or wheelchair)
- Discharge information
  - Family members in the home
  - Transportation for discharge
  - Any relevant phone numbers
  - Medical equipment needs at home

o Inventory any personal items brought by the client to the facility.

- Items to be inventoried usually include clothing, jewelry, money, credit cards, assistive devices (hearing aids, cane, dentures), medications, and religious articles.
- Document how items are disposed of to include leaving items at the bedside, storing items in the client's room closet, sending items home with family members, and locking up valuables in the facility's safe. The client should be discouraged from keeping valuables at the bedside.

o Orient the client and family to the room/facility. Share information with the client, including:

- Call light operation
- Electric bed operation
- Telephone services/television controls
- Overhead lighting operation
- Smoking policy
- Restroom locations
- Waiting areas
- Meal times
- Usual time for physician visits
- Dining/vending services
- Visiting policies

Transfer and Discharge Process

- Indications for Transfer and Discharge

    o The client's level of care has changed. For example, health status has improved so that intensive care is no longer needed.

    o Another setting is required to provide necessary care for the client. For example, the client is transferred from the medical unit to the surgical suite.

    o The facility does not offer the type of care the client now requires. For example, after the acute phase of a stroke, the client now requires care in a skilled facility.

    o The client no longer needs inpatient care and is ready to return home.

- Discharge Planning

    o This should begin when the client is admitted to the facility, unless the facility is to be the client's permanent residence (long-term care).

    o Assess whether or not the client will be able to return to his previous residence.

    o Determine whether or not the client will need and/or have someone to assist him at home.

    o Assess the residence to see if adaptations or specific equipment are required to accommodate the client prior to discharge.

    o Make a referral to the social worker to arrange for community services required by the client at discharge.

    o Communicate client health status and needs to community service providers.

    o The client's provider provides written documentation that the client may be discharged. Some clients leave the facility prior to being discharged. A client who is legally competent has the legal right to leave the facility at any time. The nurse notifies the client's provider, and if possible, has the client sign the proper forms and provides discharge teaching.

- Discharge Education

    o Discharge instructions are discussed with the client and written down for the client to have a copy at home.

    o Instructions should use clear, concise language that the client will understand.

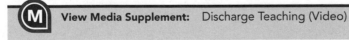

View Media Supplement: Discharge Teaching (Video)

    o Standards for discharge education include:

        ▪ Identifying safety concerns for the client at home.

        ▪ Reviewing signs and symptoms of potential complications and when to contact either emergency care or the provider.

        ▪ Providing the phone number of the provider.

- Providing names and phone numbers of community resources that will give care at the client's residence.

- Step-by-step instructions for performing continuing treatments, such as dressing changes.

- Dietary restrictions and guidelines, including those that pertain to medication administration.

- Amount and frequency of therapies the client is to perform to support continued independence at home.

- Directions on how to take medications and explanations for why each one is being prescribed.

- Equipment

  o Items to be transferred/discharged with the client include:

    - The client's personal belongings at the bedside (flowers, books, clothing, personal care items)

    - Valuables from the safe (if leaving the facility)

    - Medications (especially those belonging to the client or those that cannot be returned to the pharmacy for credit)

    - Assistive devices

    - Medical records or a transfer form

- Procedure

  o Responsibilities of the nurse include:

TRANSFERRING/DISCHARGING THE CLIENT	RECEIVING THE TRANSFERRED CLIENT
• On the day/time of transfer, confirm that the receiving facility/unit is expecting the client and that the room/bed is available. • Communicate the time the client will transfer to the receiving facility/unit. • Complete documentation (medical records, transfer form). • Give a verbal transfer report in person or via telephone. • Confirm the mode of transportation the client will be using to complete the transfer/discharge (cart, wheelchair, ambulance). • Make sure the client is dressed appropriately if going outside the facility. • Account for all of the client's valuables.	• Have any specialized equipment ready. • If appropriate, inform the client's roommate of the impending admission/transfer. • Inform other health care team members of the client's arrival and needs. • Meet with the client and family on arrival to complete the admission process and orient the client/family to the new facility/unit. • Assess how the client tolerates the transfer. • Review transfer documentation. • Implement appropriate nursing interventions in a timely manner.

- o Transfer documentation – Transfers within a facility usually require that the chart and other documentation accompany the client. Information should include:
  - Client medical diagnosis and care providers
  - Client demographic information
  - Overview of the client's health status, plan of care, and recent progress
  - Any alterations that may precipitate an immediate concern
  - Notification of any assessments or client care that will be needed within the next few hours
  - Most recent set of vital signs and medications including PRN given
  - Allergies
  - Diet and activity orders
  - Presence of or need for special equipment or adaptive devices (oxygen, suction, wheelchair)
  - Advance directives and emergency code status
  - Family involvement in care and health care proxy if applicable
- o Discharge documentation – Each client record should be closed with a discharge summary to include discharge instructions. Nursing documentation at discharge includes:
  - Type of discharge (ordered by the provider, against medical advice [AMA])
  - Actual date and time of discharge, who went with the client, and how the client was transported (wheelchair to a private car, stretcher to an ambulance)
  - Where the client was discharged to (home, long-term care facility)
  - A summary of the client's condition at discharge (steady gait, ambulating independently, in no apparent distress)
  - A description of any unresolved difficulties and procedures for follow-up
  - Disposition of valuables, client's medications brought from home, and/or prescriptions
  - A copy of the client's discharge instructions
- o Discharge instructions – The client's discharge instructions should include:
  - Step-by-step instructions for procedures to be done at home
  - Precautions to take when performing procedures or administering medications
  - Signs and symptoms of complications that should be reported
  - Names and numbers of health care providers and community services the client/ family can contact
  - Plans for follow-up care and therapies

CHAPTER 9: ADMISSIONS, TRANSFERS, AND DISCHARGE

(A) Application Exercises

1. Which of the following is a primary source for client data during the admission process?

    A. The client

    B. The family

    C. The emergency department staff

    D. The provider

2. A nurse is performing an admission assessment for an older adult client. After gathering the assessment data and performing the review of systems, which of the following actions is a priority for the nurse?

    A. Orient the client to his room.

    B. Conduct a client care conference.

    C. Review the client's medical orders.

    D. Develop a plan of care.

3. When transferring a client with a fractured radius from the emergency department to the orthopedic unit, which of the following information should the nurse include in the transfer report?

    A. The name of the client's partner

    B. Where the client was when the fracture occurred

    C. The time received and the amount of the last pain medication dose

    D. The client's occupation

4. Which of the following information should be included in a transfer report? (Select all that apply.)

    _____ The client is alert and oriented.

    _____ The client does not like spinach.

    _____ The client has an allergy to shellfish.

    _____ The client needs morphine every 4 hr.

    _____ The client has two cats at home.

5. Who is responsible for making sure all documentation is finished prior to transfer of a client to a new health care facility?

    A. Provider

    B. Certified nursing assistant

    C. Nurse transferring the client

    D. Social worker who set up the transfer

6. When does discharge planning begin in an acute care facility?

> A. Two days from discharge
>
> B. The day of discharge
>
> C. When the nurse gets the order for discharge
>
> D. When the client is admitted

7. What data should be included in a client's discharge summary? (Select all that apply.)

> _____ Interventions performed by the physical therapist 2 days ago
>
> _____ Where the client needs to go for follow-up care
>
> _____ Instructions given on medication and treatments
>
> _____ Summary of the client's condition at time of discharge
>
> _____ The phone number of the home health agency that will be making home visits

CHAPTER 9: ADMISSIONS, TRANSFERS, AND DISCHARGE

 Application Exercises Answer Key

1. Which of the following is a primary source for client data during the admission process?

A. The client

B. The family

C. The emergency department staff

D. The provider

The client is a primary source of data and is usually the best source of information. The family, the emergency department staff, and the provider will have valuable information to contribute, but only the client is a primary source for information.

 NCLEX® Connection: Health Promotion and Maintenance: Techniques of Physical Assessment

2. A nurse is performing an admission assessment for an older adult client. After gathering the assessment data and performing the review of systems, which of the following actions is a priority for the nurse?

A. Orient the client to his room.

B. Conduct a client care conference.

C. Review the client's medical orders.

D. Develop a plan of care.

The greatest risk to this client is injury from unfamiliar surroundings; therefore, the priority action is to orient the client to the room. Before the nurse leaves the room, the client should know how to use the call light and other equipment at the bedside. Conducting a client care conference, reviewing the client's medical orders, and developing a plan of care are all important, but are not the priority action for the nurse at this time.

 NCLEX® Connection: Management of Care: Continuity of Care

3. When transferring a client with a fractured radius from the emergency department to the orthopedic unit, which of the following information should the nurse include in the transfer report?

A. The name of the client's partner

B. Where the client was when the fracture occurred

C. The time received and the amount of the last pain medication dose

D. The client's occupation

It is important for the receiving nurse to know when and how much pain medication the client last received. The other information is not relevant to his immediate care at this time.

 NCLEX® Connection: Management of Care: Continuity of Care

4. Which of the following information should be included in a transfer report? (Select all that apply.)

    X   **The client is alert and oriented.**

    _____   The client does not like spinach.

    X   **The client has an allergy to shellfish.**

    X   **The client needs morphine every 4 hr.**

    _____   The client has two cats at home.

The client's level of consciousness, allergies, and need for pain medication are relevant to evaluating the client's health status and maintaining safety and comfort. Personal preferences, such as the client not liking spinach and keeping cats as pets, may sometimes be helpful, but neither is clinically significant for a transfer report.

 NCLEX® Connection: Management of Care: Continuity of Care

5. Who is responsible for making sure all documentation is finished prior to transfer of a client to a new health care facility?

    A. Provider

    B. Certified nursing assistant

    C. Nurse transferring the client

    D. Social worker who set up the transfer

The nurse who is transferring the client needs to complete the required documentation. The provider may write transfer orders for the client at the new facility. The certified nursing assistant can assist with the physical transfer of the client or belongings, but she cannot complete the transfer documentation. The social worker may assist in finding placement for the client, but the forms need to be completed by the nurse.

 NCLEX® Connection: Management of Care: Continuity of Care

6. When does discharge planning begin in an acute care facility?

    A. Two days from discharge

    B. The day of discharge

    C. When the nurse gets the order for discharge

    D. When the client is admitted

Discharge planning needs to begin when the client is admitted. Due to short hospital stays, this will allow for the maximum amount of time available to make all necessary arrangements and provide any necessary teaching.

 NCLEX® Connection: Management of Care: Continuity of Care

7. What data should be included in a client's discharge summary? (Select all that apply.)

	Interventions performed by the physical therapist 2 days ago
__X__	**Where the client needs to go for follow-up care**
__X__	**Instructions given on medication and treatments**
__X__	**Summary of the client's condition at time of discharge**
__X__	**The phone number of the home health agency that will be making home visits**

All of the above information, with the exception of interventions performed by the physical therapist 2 days ago, is pertinent information that should be included in the discharge summary. The physical therapist should have written a progress note on the day of care.

(N) NCLEX® Connection: Management of Care: Continuity of Care

UNIT 1: SAFE, EFFECTIVE CARE ENVIRONMENT

Section: Safety and Infection Control

- Medical and Surgical Asepsis
- Infection Control
- Client Safety
- Home Safety
- Ergonomic Principles
- Security and Disaster Plans

NCLEX® CONNECTIONS

When reviewing the chapters in this section, keep in mind the relevant sections of the NCLEX® outline, in particular:

CLIENT NEEDS: SAFETY AND INFECTION CONTROL

Relevant topics/tasks include:

- Accident/Injury Prevention
  - Identify deficits that may impede client safety.
- Ergonomic Principles
  - Assess the client's ability to balance, transfer, and use assistive devices prior to planning care.
- Reporting of Incident/Event/Irregular Occurrence/Variance
  - Acknowledge and document practice errors.
- Safe Use of Equipment
  - Facilitate appropriate and safe use of equipment.
- Standard Precautions/Transmission-Based Precautions/Surgical Asepsis
  - Apply principles of infection control.

UNIT 1	SAFE, EFFECTIVE CARE ENVIRONMENT
Section	Safety and Infection Control
Chapter 10	Medical and Surgical Asepsis

Overview

- Asepsis – The absence of illness-producing micro-organisms. Asepsis is maintained through the use of aseptic technique with hand hygiene as the primary behavior associated with asepsis/aseptic technique. There are two types of asepsis:

  - Medical asepsis – The use of precise practices to reduce the number, growth, and spread of micro-organisms from an object, person, or area. Previously referred to as "clean technique," medical asepsis is used for administering oral medication, managing nasogastric tubes, providing personal hygiene, and performing many other common nursing tasks.

  - Surgical asepsis – The use of precise practices to eliminate all micro-organisms from an object or area. Also known as "sterile technique," surgical asepsis is used for parenteral medication administration, insertion of urinary catheters, surgical procedures, sterile dressing changes, and many other common nursing procedures.

- Before beginning any task or procedure that requires aseptic technique, health care team members must check for latex allergies. If the client or any member of the team has a latex allergy, latex-free gloves, equipment, and supplies must be used.

Practices that Promote Medical Asepsis

- The No. 1 measure to reduce the growth and transmission of infectious agents is hand hygiene. The Centers for Disease Control and Prevention (CDC) states that "hand hygiene has been cited frequently as the single most important practice to reduce the transmission of infectious agents in health care settings. The term "hand hygiene" refers to both handwashing with an antimicrobial or plain soap and water as well as the use of alcohol-based products such as gels, foams, and rinses."

  - The three essential components of handwashing include:

    - Soap
    - Water
    - Friction

  - All health care personnel must perform hand hygiene, either with an alcohol-based product or with soap and water, before and after every client contact, after removing gloves, after contact with body fluids, and after using the restroom. When hands are visibly soiled, handwashing with soap and water is indicated.

     o   Perform hand hygiene using recommended antiseptic solutions when caring for clients who are immunocompromised or have infections with multidrug-resistant or extremely virulent microorganisms. These include chlorhexidine, povidone-iodine, or PCMX (parachlorometaxylenol).

     o   Hand hygiene is also recommended after contact with anything in the client's room and after touching any contaminated items, whether or not gloves are worn. Hand hygiene must be performed at once after gloves are removed and when otherwise indicated to avoid transfer of micro-organisms to other clients or environments. Performing hand hygiene may be necessary between tasks and procedures on the same client to prevent cross-contamination of different body sites.

     o   Handwashing must be done for at <u>least 15 seconds</u> to remove transient flora from the hands and <u>up to 2 min</u> when hands are more soiled. After washing, hands should be dried with a clean paper towel before turning off the faucet. If the sink does not have foot or knee pedals for turning off the water, using a clean, dry paper towel to turn off the faucet(s) is recommended.

     o   For hand hygiene with an alcohol-based product, dispense the manufacturer's recommended amount of product (usually 3 to 5 mL) in the palm of the hand. Rub vigorously, remembering to cover all surfaces of both hands and fingers. With an alcohol rub, continue to rub until both hands are completely dry.

- Additional examples of practices that reduce the growth and spread of micro-organisms are changing linens daily, cleaning floors and the client's bedside stand, and separating clean from contaminated materials.

- Use masks, gloves, gowns, and protective eyewear to help control the contact and spread of micro-organisms to both the health care staff and the client.

- Do not place items on the floor in the client's environment (even soiled laundry). The floor is considered "grossly" contaminated.

- Educate all clients on the importance of covering their mouths and noses when coughing or sneezing, using and disposing of tissues, and handwashing thoroughly to prevent spraying and spreading droplet infections.

- Do not shake linens, because doing so can spread micro-organisms in the air.

- Clean the least soiled areas first to prevent moving more contaminants into the cleaner areas.

- Use plastic bags for moist, soiled items, following facility protocol for bag selection, to prevent further contamination of items or of individuals handling the soiled items. Put all soiled items directly into the appropriate receptacle to avoid handling soiled items more than once.

- Pour any liquids used for client care directly into the drain, and avoid splattering that can spread droplets.

- All health care staff should:

  ○ Follow facility protocols for isolation and protection.

  ○ Wash their hair frequently and keep it short or pulled back to prevent contamination of the care area or the client.

  ○ Not wear artificial nails while providing care and should keep natural nails short and clean. The area around and under the nails can harbor micro-organisms.

  ○ Remove jewelry from hands and wrists to facilitate hand disinfection.

Practices that Maintain a Sterile Field

- Prolonged exposure to airborne micro-organisms can make sterile items nonsterile.

  ○ Avoid coughing, sneezing, and talking directly over a sterile field.

  ○ Air movement should be controlled by special ventilation.

- Only sterile items may be in a sterile field.

  ○ The outer wrappings and 1-inch edges of packaging that contains sterile items are not sterile. The inner surface of the sterile drape or kit, except for that 1-inch border around the edges, is the sterile field to which additional sterile items may be added. To position the field on the table surface, it is acceptable to grasp the 1-inch border before donning sterile gloves. Any object that comes into contact with the 1-inch border must be discarded.

  ○ Touch sterile materials only with sterile gloves.

  ○ Any object held below the waist or above the chest is considered contaminated.

  ○ Sterile materials may touch other sterile surfaces or materials; however, contact with nonsterile materials at any time renders a sterile area contaminated, no matter how short the contact.

- Microbes can move by gravity from a nonsterile item to a sterile item.

  ○ Do not reach across or above a sterile field.

  ○ Do not turn your back on a sterile field.

  ○ Hold items to be added to a sterile field at a minimum of 6 inches above the field.

- Any sterile, non-waterproof wrapper that comes in contact with moisture becomes nonsterile by a wicking action that allows microbes to travel rapidly from a nonsterile surface to the sterile surface.

  ○ Keep all surfaces dry.

  ○ Discard any sterile packages that become wet.

Nursing Interventions

- Equipment

  - Select a clean area in the client's environment (a bedside stand) to set up the sterile field.

  - Check that all sterile packages (additional dressings, sterile bowl, sterile gloves, and solution) are dry and have a future expiration date.

  - Make sure an appropriate waste receptacle is nearby.

- Procedure

  - Perform hand hygiene.

  - Open the plastic covering of the package per the manufacturer's directions, slipping the package onto the center of the workspace with the top flap of the wrapper opening away from the body.

  - Reach around the package to open the top flap of the package, grasp the outside flap between the thumb and the index finger, and unfold the top flap away from the body.

  - Next, open the side flaps, using the right hand for the right flap and the left hand for the left flap.

  - Grasp the last flap and turn it down toward the body.

  - Additional sterile packages

    - Open next to the sterile field by holding the bottom edge with one hand and pulling back on the top flap with the other hand. Place the packages that are to be used last furthest from the sterile field, and open these first.

    - Add them directly to the sterile field. Lift the package from the dry surface, holding it 15 cm (6 in) above the sterile field, pulling the two surfaces apart, and dropping it onto the sterile field.

  - Pour sterile solutions by:

    - Removing the bottle cap.

    - Placing the bottle cap face up on the surface.

    - Holding the bottle with the label in the palm of the hand so that the solution does not run down the label.

    - First pouring a small amount (1 to 2 mL) of the solution into an available receptacle.

    - Pouring the solution onto the dressing or site without touching the bottle to the site.

  - Once the sterile field is set up, don sterile gloves.

○ Sterile gloving includes opening the wrapper and handling only the outside of the wrapper. Don gloves by using the following steps.

- With the cuff side pointing toward the body, use the left hand and pick up the right-hand glove by grasping the folded bottom edge of the cuff and lifting it up and away from the wrapper.

- While picking up the edge of the cuff, pull the right glove onto the hand.

- With the sterile right-gloved hand, place the fingers of the right hand inside the cuff of the left glove, lifting it off the wrapper, and put the left hand into it.

- When both hands are gloved, adjust the fingers in the gloves if necessary.

- During that time, only the sterile gloved hand can touch the other sterile gloved hand.

- At the close of the sterile procedure, or if the gloves tear, remove the gloves. Take them off by grasping the outer part of one glove at the wrist, pulling the glove down over the fingers and into the hand that is still gloved. Then, place the ungloved hand inside the soiled glove and pull the glove off so that it is inside out and only the clean inside part is exposed. Discard into an appropriate receptacle.

CHAPTER 10: MEDICAL AND SURGICAL ASEPSIS

 Application Exercises

1. When entering a client's room to change a surgical dressing, a nurse notes that the client is coughing and sneezing. When preparing the sterile field, it is important that the nurse

   A. keep the sterile field on the far side of the client's room away from the bedside.

   B. instruct the client to refrain from coughing and sneezing during the dressing change.

   C. place a mask on the client to limit the spread of micro-organisms into the surgical wound.

   D. keep a box of tissues nearby for the client to use during the dressing change.

2. A nurse teaching a group of personal care assistants should emphasize that the most effective way to decrease the spread of infection is by

   A. wearing gloves with all clients.

   B. placing clients with infection in isolation.

   C. wearing gowns and masks at all times when in contact with a client's skin.

   D. performing hand hygiene.

3. While wearing sterile gloves, a nurse can touch any

   A. object on the sterile field.

   B. object on the bedside stand.

   C. part of the client's gown.

   D. sterile object below the waist.

4. Match each of the following practices to the best example.

   __D__ Medical asepsis practice   A. A nurse wears gloves each time he empties a bedpan.

   __A__ Standard precautions   B. A nurse drops a sterile dressing on the floor.

   __C__ Sterile field maintenance   C. A nurse keeps her sterile hands above her waist.

   __B__ Contamination   D. A nurse wipes off the client's bedside table.

5. Which of the following statements about surgical asepsis and a sterile field are correct? (Select all that apply.)

   _____ The nurse should turn her back on the sterile field if she needs to cough.

   _____ The 1-inch edge around a sterile field is also considered sterile.

   __✓__ A sterile item can touch another sterile item without contaminating it.

   __✓__ Sterile items must remain above the waist.

   __✓__ Surgical asepsis is also called "sterile technique."

6. Describe the proper procedure for pouring a sterile solution.

CHAPTER 10: MEDICAL AND SURGICAL ASEPSIS

 Application Exercises Answer Key

1. When entering a client's room to change a surgical dressing, a nurse notes that the client is coughing and sneezing. When preparing the sterile field, it is important that the nurse

    A. keep the sterile field on the far side of the client's room away from the bedside.

    B. instruct the client to refrain from coughing and sneezing during the dressing change.

    C. place a mask on the client to limit the spread of micro-organisms into the surgical wound.

    D. keep a box of tissues nearby for the client to use during the dressing change.

Placing a mask on the client prevents contamination of the surgical wound during the dressing change. It would be difficult for the nurse to maintain a sterile field on the far side of the room away from the bedside. The client may be unable to refrain from coughing and sneezing during the dressing change. Keeping tissues close by for the client to use still allows contamination of the surgical wound.

 NCLEX® Connection: Safety and Infection Control: Standard/Transmission-Based/Other Precautions

2. A nurse teaching a group of personal care assistants should emphasize that the most effective way to decrease the spread of infection is by

    A. wearing gloves with all clients.

    B. placing clients with infection in isolation.

    C. wearing gowns and masks at all times when in contact with a client's skin.

    D. performing hand hygiene.

Frequent hand hygiene is the best way to prevent the spread of infection. Wearing gloves is appropriate when in contact with any client's blood, body fluids, or nonintact skin, but hand hygiene is still important after removing the gloves. Placing clients with infections in isolation is important for certain types of infections, but it neglects the essential aspect of hand hygiene. Wearing gowns and masks is not necessary if the client's skin is intact.

 NCLEX® Connection: Safety and Infection Control: Standard/Transmission-Based/Other Precautions

3. While wearing sterile gloves, a nurse can touch any

> **A. object on the sterile field.**
>
> B. object on the bedside stand.
>
> C. part of the client's gown.
>
> D. sterile object below the waist.

> To maintain a sterile field, the nurse can only touch other sterile items when wearing sterile gloves without causing contamination. Touching an object on the bedside stand, touching the client's gown, and holding any sterile object below the waist makes the sterile field no longer sterile.

 NCLEX® Connection: Safety and Infection Control: Standard/Transmission-Based/Other Precautions

4. Match each of the following practices to the best example.

D	Medical asepsis practice	A. A nurse wears gloves each time he empties a bedpan.
A	Standard precautions	B. A nurse drops a sterile dressing on the floor.
C	Sterile field maintenance	C. A nurse keeps her sterile hands above her waist.
B	Contamination	D. A nurse wipes off the client's bedside table.

 NCLEX® Connection: Safety and Infection Control: Standard/Transmission-Based/Other Precautions

5. Which of the following statements about surgical asepsis and a sterile field are correct? (Select all that apply.)

> _____ The nurse should turn her back on the sterile field if she needs to cough.
>
> _____ The 1-inch edge around a sterile field is also considered sterile.
>
> __X__ **A sterile item can touch another sterile item without contaminating it.**
>
> __X__ **Sterile items must remain above the waist.**
>
> __X__ **Surgical asepsis is also called "sterile technique."**

> A sterile item can touch another sterile item without contaminating it. To maintain the sterility of an item, it must stay above the waist, and surgical asepsis is also called "sterile technique." If the nurse turns her back on the sterile field, the sterile field is considered contaminated. The nurse should step away but continue to face the sterile field. The 1-in edge around a sterile field is not considered sterile.

NCLEX® Connection: Safety and Infection Control: Standard/Transmission-Based/Other Precautions

6. Describe the proper procedure for pouring a sterile solution.

Remove the bottle cap and place the bottle cap face up on the surface.

Hold the bottle with the label in the palm of the hand so that the solution does not run down the label.

Pour a small amount of the solution into an available receptacle.

Pour the solution onto the dressing or site without touching the bottle to the site.

(N) NCLEX® Connection: Safety and Infection Control: Standard/Transmission-Based/Other Precautions

UNIT 1	SAFE, EFFECTIVE CARE ENVIRONMENT
Section	Safety and Infection Control
Chapter 11	Infection Control

Overview

- An infection occurs when the presence of a pathogen leads to a chain of events. All components of the chain must be present and intact for the infection to occur. The nurse uses infection control practices (medical asepsis, surgical asepsis, standard precautions) to break the chain and thus stop the spread of infection.

Risks of Infection

- The nurse should assess each client for the risks of infection specific to the client, the disease or injury, and the environment. The most common risks include:

    o Inadequate hand hygiene (client and caregivers)

    o Individuals who have compromised health or defenses against infection, which include:

        ▪ Those who are immunocompromised

        ▪ Those who have had surgery

        ▪ Those with indwelling devices

        ▪ A break in the skin (the body's best protection against infection)

        ▪ Those with poor oxygenation

        ▪ Those with impaired circulation

        ▪ Those who have chronic or acute disease

    o Use of poor medical or surgical asepsis by caregivers

    o Clients who have poor personal hygiene or poor nutrition, and those who are stressed

    o Clients who live in a very crowded environment

    o Older adult clients

    o Individuals who make poor lifestyle choices that put them at risk, which include:

        ▪ Clients who use IV drugs and share needles

        ▪ Clients who engage in unprotected sex

o   Clients who have recently been exposed to:

   ■   Poor sanitation

   ■   Mosquito-borne or parasitic diseases

   ■   Diseases endemic to the area visited, but not in the client's home country

Types of Infections

- Health-Care Associated Infections (HAIs)

  o   These are infections acquired while the client is receiving care in a health care setting. Formally called nosocomial infections, these can come from an exogenous source (from outside the client) or an endogenous source (inside the client when part of the client's flora becomes altered).

  o   The most common setting for HAIs is the intensive care unit.

  o   The best way to prevent HAIs is through frequent and effective hand hygiene.

  o   The most common site of HAIs is the urinary tract. The most common causative agents are *Escherichia coli*, *Staphylococcus aureus*, and enterococci.

  o   An iatrogenic infection is a type of HAI resulting from a diagnostic or therapeutic procedure.

  o   HAIs are not always preventable and are not always iatrogenic.

Signs and Symptoms of Infection

- The signs and symptoms, identifiable in the nursing assessment, of generalized or systemic infection include:

  o   Fever

  o   Increased pulse and respiratory rate (in response to the high fever)

  o   Malaise

  o   Anorexia, nausea, and/or vomiting

  o   Enlarged lymph nodes (repositories for "waste")

- Inflammation is the body's local response to injury or infection. The inflammatory response has three stages. Signs and symptoms during the first stage of the inflammatory response (local infection) include:

  o   Redness (from dilation of arterioles bringing blood to the area)

  o   Warmth of the area on palpation

  o   Edema

  o   Pain or tenderness

  o   Loss of use of the affected part

o   In the second stage, the micro-organisms have been are killed. Fluid containing dead tissue cells and WBCs accumulates and exudate appears at the site of infection. The exudate leaves the body by draining into the lymph system. The types of exudate are:

- Serous (clear)

- Sanguineous (contains red blood cells)

- Purulent (contains leukocytes and bacteria)

o   In the third stage, damaged tissue is replaced by scar tissue. Gradually, the new cells take on characteristics that are similar in structure and function to the old cells.

- In addition to the items found on physical assessment, laboratory results indicating infection include:

o   Leukocytosis (WBCs > 10,000/µL).

o   Increases in the specific types of WBCs on differential (left shift = an increase in neutrophils).

o   Elevated erythrocyte sedimentation rate (ESR).

o   Presence of micro-organisms on culture of the specific fluid/area.

- Components of the chain of infection include:

o   An infectious agent (bacteria, viruses, fungi, protozoa)

o   A reservoir where the infectious agent grows (wound drainage, food, oxygen tubing)

o   An exit portal of the infectious agent (skin, respiratory or gastrointestinal tracts)

o   A means of transmission (droplet, person-to-person contact, touching contaminated items)

o   An entry portal to a susceptible host (same as exit)

o   A host that must be susceptible to the infectious agent

Nursing Interventions

- General Guidelines

o   Use frequent and effective hand hygiene before and after care is given.

o   Educate the client about the required and recommended immunizations and where to obtain them. The target groups include children, older adults, those with chronic disease, and those who are immunocompromised and their families/contacts.

o   Educate the client and ask for a return demonstration of good oral hygiene. Good oral hygiene decreases the protein (which attracts micro-organisms) in the oral cavity, which thereby decreases the growth of micro-organisms that can migrate through breaks in the oral mucosa.

○ Encourage the client to consume an adequate amount of fluids. Adequate fluid intake prevents the stasis of urine by flushing the urinary tract and decreasing the growth of micro-organisms. Adequate hydration also keeps the skin from breaking down. Intact skin prevents micro-organisms from entering the body.

○ For immobile clients, ensure that pulmonary hygiene (turning, coughing, deep breathing, incentive spirometry) is done every 2 hr, or as prescribed. Good pulmonary hygiene decreases the growth of micro-organisms and the development of pneumonia by preventing stasis of pulmonary excretions, stimulating ciliary movement and clearance, and expanding the lungs.

○ Use of aseptic technique and proper personal protective equipment in the provision of care to all clients prevents unnecessary exposure to micro-organisms.

○ Teach and use respiratory hygiene/cough etiquette. It applies to anyone entering a health care setting: clients, visitors, and staff with signs or symptoms of illness, whether diagnosed or undiagnosed. This includes cough, congestion, rhinorrhea, or increased production of respiratory secretions. The components of respiratory hygiene/cough etiquette include:

  ▪ Covering the mouth and nose when coughing and sneezing.

  ▪ Using facial tissues to contain respiratory secretions, and disposing of them promptly into a hands-free receptacle.

  ▪ Wearing a surgical mask when coughing to minimize contamination of the surrounding environment.

  ▪ Turning the head when coughing and staying a minimum of 3 ft away from others, especially in common waiting areas.

  ▪ Performing hand hygiene after contact with respiratory secretions.

• Isolation Guidelines

  ○ Isolation guidelines are a group of actions that include hand hygiene and the use of barrier precautions, which are intended to reduce the transmission of infectious organisms.

  ○ The precautions apply to every client, regardless of the diagnosis, and must be implemented whenever contact with a potentially infectious material is anticipated.

  ○ Personal protective equipment is changed after contact with each client, and between procedures with the same client if in contact with large amounts of blood and body fluids.

 View Media Supplement: Precautions (Video)

o   Standard Precautions (Tier One)

- This tier of standard precautions applies to all body fluids (except sweat), nonintact skin, and mucous membranes.

- Hand hygiene using an alcohol-based waterless product is recommended after contact with the client, body fluids, and contaminated equipment/articles, and after removal of gloves.

- Alcohol-based waterless antiseptic is preferred unless the hands are visibly dirty, because the alcohol-based product is more effective in removing microorganisms.

- Clean gloves are worn when touching all body fluids, nonintact skin, mucous membranes, and contaminated equipment/articles.

- Gloves are removed and hand hygiene is completed between each client.

- Masks, eye protection, and/or face shields are required when care may cause splashing or spraying of body fluids.

- Gloves are worn when touching anything that has the potential to contaminate the hands of the nurse. This includes body secretions, excretions, blood and body fluids, non-intact, skin mucous membranes, and contaminated items.

- Hand hygiene is required after removal of the gown. A sturdy moisture-resistant bag should be used for soiled items, and the bag should be tied securely in a knot at the top.

- All equipment used for client care is to be properly cleaned; one-time use items are to be disposed of according to facility policy.

- Contaminated laundry should be bagged and handled to prevent leaking or contamination of clothing or skin.

- Safety devices on all equipment/supplies must be enabled after use; all sharps must be disposed of in a puncture-resistant container.

- A private room is not needed unless the client is unable to maintain appropriate hygienic practices.

o   Transmission Precautions (Tier Two)

- Airborne precautions are used to protect against droplet infections smaller than 5 mcg (measles, varicella, pulmonary or laryngeal tuberculosis). Airborne precautions require:

  □   A private room

  □   Masks/respiratory protection devices for caregivers and visitors

  ▸   An N95 or high-efficiency particulate air (HEPA) respirator is used if the client is known or suspected to have tuberculosis.

  □   Negative pressure airflow exchange in the room of at least six exchanges per hour

■ Droplet precautions protect against droplets larger than 5 mcg (streptococcal pharyngitis or pneumonia, scarlet fever, rubella, pertussis, mumps, mycoplasma pneumonia, meningococcal pneumonia/sepsis, pneumonic plague). Droplet precautions require:

□ A private room or a room with other clients with the same infectious disease

□ Masks for providers and visitors

■ Contact precautions protect visitors and caregivers against direct client/ environmental contact infections (respiratory syncytial virus, shigella, enteric diseases caused by micro-organisms, wound infections, herpes simplex, scabies, multidrug-resistant organisms). Contact precautions require:

□ A private room or a room with other clients with the same infection

□ Gloves and gowns worn by the caregivers and visitors

□ Disposal of infectious dressing material into a single, nonporous bag without touching the outside of the bag

- Transporting the Client

  o If movement of the client to another area of the facility is unavoidable, the nurse takes precautions to ensure that the environment is not contaminated. For example, a surgical mask is placed on the client with an airborne or droplet infection, and a draining wound is well covered.

- Guidelines for Cleaning Contaminated Equipment

  o Always wear gloves.

  o Rinse first in cold water. (Hot water coagulates proteins, making them adhere.)

  o Wash the article in hot water with soap.

  o Use a brush or abrasive to clean corners or hard-to-reach areas.

  o Rinse well in warm or hot water.

  o Dry the article – It is considered clean at this point.

  o Clean the equipment used in cleaning and the sink (still considered dirty unless a disinfectant is used).

  o Remove gloves and perform hand hygiene.

- Reporting Communicable Diseases

  o A complete list of reportable diseases and the reporting system are available through the Centers for Disease Control and Prevention's Web site (http://www.cdc.gov). There are more than 60 communicable diseases that must be reported to the public health departments to allow for officials to:

    ■ Ensure appropriate medical treatment of diseases (tuberculosis).

    ■ Monitor for common-source outbreaks (foodborne – hepatitis A).

    ■ Plan and evaluate control and prevention plans (immunizations for preventable diseases).

    ■ Identify outbreaks and epidemics.

    ■ Determine public health priorities based on trends.

CHAPTER 11: INFECTION CONTROL

 Application Exercises

1. Match the component of the chain of infection with the example of each component.

   B Infectious agent   A. Client

   C Reservoir   B. Bacteria, virus, fungi, protozoa

   D Means of transmission   C. Wound drainage, food, oxygen tubing

   E Exit and entry portal   D. Person-to-person contact

   A Host   E. Skin, respiratory, and gastrointestinal tracts

2. Which of the following are reasons health care professionals are required to report communicable/ infectious diseases? (Select all that apply.)

   ✓ Planning and evaluating control and prevention strategies

   ✓ Determining public health priorities

   ✓ Ensuring proper medical treatment

   ✗ Identifying endemic disease

   ✓ Monitoring for common-source outbreaks

3. A nurse is contributing to the plan of care for a client who is being admitted to the facility with a suspected diagnosis of pertussis. Which of the following should be included in the plan of care? (Select all that apply.)

   ✗ Place the client in a room that has negative air pressure of at least six exchanges per hour.

   ✓ Wear a mask when providing care within 3 ft of the client.

   ✓ Place a surgical mask on the client if transportation to another department is unavoidable.

   ✗ Use sterile gloves when handling soiled linen.

   ✓ Wear a gown when performing care that may result in contamination from secretions.

4. Place an (S) next to the signs and symptoms that indicate a systemic infection and an (L) in front of the signs and symptoms that indicate a local infection.

   S Fever

   L Edema

   L Pain or tenderness

   S Malaise

   L Warmth of the area on palpation

   S Increased pulse and respiratory rate

CHAPTER 11: INFECTION CONTROL

 Application Exercises Answer Key

1. Match the component of the chain of infection with the example of each component.

__B__	Infectious agent	A.	Client
__C__	Reservoir	B.	Bacteria, virus, fungi, protozoa
__D__	Means of transmission	C.	Wound drainage, food, oxygen tubing
__E__	Exit and entry portal	D.	Person-to-person contact
__A__	Host	E.	Skin, respiratory, and gastrointestinal tracts

 NCLEX® Connection: Safety and Infection Control: Standard/Transmission-Based/Other Precautions

2. Which of the following are reasons health care professionals are required to report communicable/infectious diseases? (Select all that apply.)

__X__ **Planning and evaluating control and prevention strategies**

__X__ **Determining public health priorities**

__X__ **Ensuring proper medical treatment**

_____ Identifying endemic disease

__X__ **Monitoring for common-source outbreaks**

Reporting of communicable/infectious diseases assists with planning and evaluating control and prevention strategies, determining public health policies, ensuring proper medical treatment is available, and monitoring for common-source outbreaks. Endemic disease is already prevalent within a population, so reporting is not necessary.

NCLEX® Connection: Safety and Infection Control: Standard/Transmission-Based/Other Precautions

3. A nurse is contributing to the plan of care for a client who is being admitted to the facility with a suspected diagnosis of pertussis. Which of the following should be included in the plan of care? (Select all that apply.)

          Place the client in a room that has negative air pressure of at least six exchanges per hour.

  X   **Wear a mask when providing care within 3 ft of the client.**

  X   **Place a surgical mask on the client if transportation to another department is unavoidable.**

          Use sterile gloves when handling soiled linen.

  X   **Wear a gown when performing care that may result in contamination from secretions.**

A client with known or suspected pertussis is placed on droplet precautions. A private room is required, but a room with negative air pressure is not required. A mask is worn when the nurse is within 3 ft of the client. A surgical mask is placed on the client during transport to another area of the facility. Gloves (clean) are worn when handling soiled linen, but sterile gloves are not necessary. A gown should be worn if the nurse's clothing or skin may be contaminated with body secretions or excretions.

NCLEX® Connection: Safety and Infection Control: Standard/Transmission-Based/Other Precautions

4. Place an (S) next to the signs and symptoms that indicate a systemic infection and an (L) in front of the signs and symptoms that indicate a local infection.

  S   Fever

  L   Edema

  L   Pain or tenderness

  S   Malaise

  L   Warmth of the area on palpation

  S   Increased pulse and respiratory rate

NCLEX® Connection: Reduction of Risk Potential: System Specific Assessment

UNIT 1	SAFE, EFFECTIVE CARE ENVIRONMENT
Section	Safety and Infection Control
Chapter 12	Client Safety

Ⓐ Overview

- Providing for safety and preventing injury are major nursing responsibilities. Many factors affect the client's ability to protect himself. Those factors include the client's:

  o Age, with the young and old at greater risk

  o Mobility cognitive

  o Sensory awareness

  o Emotional state

  o Lifestyle

  o Safety awareness

- All health care workers must be aware of:

  o How to assess for and recognize clients at risk for safety issues

  o Procedural safety guidelines

  o Protocols for responding to dangerous situations

  o Security plans

  o Identification and documentation of the incidents and responses per health care agency policy.

- It is the provider's responsibility to assess, report, and document client allergies and to provide client care that avoids exposure to allergens.

- Equipment should only be used by the nurse after a safety inspection and instruction.

Falls

(G) • Older adult clients may be at an increased risk for falls due to decreased strength, impaired mobility and balance, and endurance limitations combined with decreased sensory perception.

• Other clients at increased risk include those with decreased visual acuity, generalized weakness, urinary frequency, gait and balance problems (cerebral palsy, injury, multiple sclerosis) and cognitive dysfunction. Side effects of medications (orthostatic hypotension, drowsiness) can also increase the client's risk for falls.

• Clients are at greater risk for falls when more than one of the risk factors are present.

• Prevention of client falls is a major nursing priority. All clients admitted to health care institutions should be assessed for risk factors related to falls and, based on the assessment, preventative measures should be implemented.

(S) • Prevention of Falls

○ Complete a fall-risk assessment upon admission and at regular intervals on the client for individualization of the care plan to limit the risk of falls.

○ Document all identified risks and implement specific measures to reduce the risk for falls. The plan for each client is individualized based on the fall-risk assessment. For example, if the client has orthostatic hypotension, instruct the client to avoid getting up too quickly, to sit on the side of the bed for a few seconds prior to standing and to stand at the side of the bed for a few seconds prior to walking. General measures to prevent falls include the following:

■ Be sure the client knows how to use the call light, that it is in reach, and encourage its use.

■ Respond to call lights in a timely manner.

■ Orient the client to the setting (grab bars, call light) to ensure he knows how to use all assistive devices and can locate necessary items.

■ Place clients at risk for falls near the nursing station.

■ Ensure that bedside tables and over bed tables and frequently used items (telephone, water, tissues) are within the client's reach.

■ Maintain the bed in low position.

■ For clients who are sedated, unconscious, or otherwise compromised, the bed rails are kept up and the bed is kept in the low position.

■ Avoid the use of full side bedrails for clients who get out of bed or attempt to get out of bed without assistance.

■ Provide the client with nonskid footwear.

■ Keep the floor free from clutter with a clear path to the bathroom (no scatter rugs, cords, furniture).

■ Keep assistive devices nearby after validation of safe use by the client and family (glasses, walkers, transfer devices).

- Educate the client and family/caregivers on identified risks and the plan of care.

- Lock wheels on beds, wheelchairs, and carts to prevent the device from rolling during transfers or stops.

- Use chair or bed sensors for clients at risk for getting up unattended to alert staff of independent ambulation.

   o Report and document all incidents per the health care facility's policy. This provides valuable information that may be helpful in preventing similar incidents.

Seizures

- A seizure is a sudden surge of electrical activity in the brain. It may occur at anytime during a person's life and may be due to epilepsy, fever, or a variety of medical conditions. Partial seizures are due to electrical surges in one part of the brain, and generalized seizures involve the entire brain.

- Seizure precautions (measures to protect the client from injury should a seizure occur) are taken for clients who have a history of seizures that involve the entire body and/or result in unconsciousness.

   o Ensure rescue equipment is at the bedside to include oxygen, an oral airway, and suction equipment. A saline lock may be inserted for intravenous access if the client is at high risk for experiencing a generalized seizure.

   o Inspect the client's environment for items that may cause injury in the event of a seizure, and remove items that are not necessary for current treatment.

   o Assist the client at risk for a seizure with ambulation and transferring to reduce the risk of injury.

   o Advise all caregivers and family not to put anything in the client's mouth (except in status epilepticus, where an airway is needed) in the event of a seizure.

   o Advise all caregivers and family not to restrain the client in the event of a seizure, ensure the client's safety by lowering him to the floor or bed, protect his head, remove nearby furniture, provide privacy, put the client on his side with his head flexed slightly forward if possible, and loosen clothing to prevent injury.

   o In the event of a seizure, stay with the client and call for help.

   o Administer medications as ordered.

   o Note the duration of the seizure and the sequence and type of movement.

   o After a seizure, explain what happened to the client, and provide comfort, understanding, and a quiet environment for the client to recover.

   o Document the seizure in the client's record with any precipitating behaviors and a description of the event (movements, any injuries, length of seizure, aura, postictal state), and report it to the provider.

Seclusion and Restraints

- Nurses must know and follow federal/state/facility policies that govern the use of restraints.

- Use of seclusion rooms and/or restraints may be authorized for clients in some cases.

- In general, seclusion and/or restraints should be ordered for the shortest duration necessary and only if less restrictive measures are not sufficient. It is for the physical protection of the client or the protection of other clients or staff.

- A client may voluntarily request temporary seclusion in cases where the environment is disturbing or seems too stimulating.

- Restraints can be either physical or chemical, such as neuroleptic medication to calm the client.

- Seclusion and/or restraint must never be used for:

  o Convenience of the staff

  o Punishment for the client

  o Clients who are extremely physically or mentally unstable

  o Clients who cannot tolerate the decreased stimulation of a seclusion room

- Restraints should:

  o Never interfere with treatment

  o Restrict movement as little as is necessary to ensure safety

  o Fit properly

  o Be easily changed to decrease the chance of injury and to provide for the greatest level of dignity

- When all other less restrictive means have been tried to prevent a client from harming self or others, the following must occur in order for seclusion or restraint to be used:

  o The treatment must be prescribed by the provider in writing, based on a face-to-face assessment of the client.

    ▪ In an emergency situation in which there is immediate risk to the client or others, the nurse may place a client in restraints. The nurse must obtain an order from the primary care provided as soon as possible in accordance with agency policy (usually within 1 hr).

  o The prescription must include the reason for the restraint, the type of restraint, the location of the restraint, how long the restraint may be used, and the type of behaviors demonstrated by the client that warrant use of the restraint.

- o The provider must rewrite the prescription every 24 hr or the frequency of time specified by facility policy.

- o PRN prescriptions for restraints are not allowed.

- o Nursing responsibilities must be identified in the protocol, including how often the client should be:

  - Assessed – Including neurosensory checks of affected extremities (circulation, sensation, mobility). These checks are usually done at least every 2 hr.

  - Offered food and fluid.

  - Provided with means for hygiene and elimination.

  - Monitored for vital signs.

  - Offered range of motion of extremities.

- Frequency of client assessments in regard to food, fluids, comfort, and safety should be performed and documented every 15 to 30 min.

- Other responsibilities include:

  - o Always explain the need for the restraint to the client and family, emphasizing that the restraint is need to ensure the safety of the client and will be used only as long as it is necessary.

  - o Obtain signed consent from client or guardian, if required.

  - o Review the manufacturer's instructions for correct application.

  - o Remove or replace restraints frequently to ensure good circulation to the area and allow for full range of motion to the limb that has been restricted.

  - o Pad bony prominences.

  - o Use a quick-release knot to tie the restraint to the bed frame (loose knots that are easily removed) where it will not tighten when the bed is raised or lowered.

  - o Ensure that the restraint is loose enough for range of motion and with enough room to fit two fingers between the device and the client to prevent injury.

  - o Regularly assess the need for continued use of the restraints to allow for discontinuation of the restraint or limiting the restraint at the earliest possible time while ensuring the client's safety.

  - o Never leave the client unattended without the restraint.

  - o Complete documentation includes a description of the following:

    - Precipitating events and behavior of the client prior to seclusion or restraint

    - Alternative actions taken to avoid seclusion or restraint

    - The time restraints were applied and removed (if discontinued)

    - Type of restraint used and location

    - Client's behavior while restrained

- Type and frequency of care (range of motion, neuro, integumentary checks)

- Client's response when the restraint is removed

- Medication administration

○ An emergency situation must be present for the charge nurse restraints without first obtaining a provider's written order. If t initiated, the nurse must obtain the written order within a spec (usually within 1 hr).

Fire Safety

- Fires in health care facilities are usually due to problems related to electrical or anesthetic equipment. Unauthorized smoking may also be the case of a fire.

- All staff must be instructed in fire response procedures, which include knowing the:

  ○ Location of exits, fire extinguishers, and oxygen turn-offs valves

  ○ Evacuation plan for the unit and facility

- The fire response in the health care setting always follows this sequence (RACE):

  ○ Rescue – Protect and evacuate clients in close proximity to the fire.

  ○ Alarm – Report the fire by setting off the alarm.

  ○ Contain – Contain the fire by closing doors and windows as well as turning off any sources of oxygen. Clients who are on life support are ventilated with a bag-valve mask.

  ○ Extinguish – Extinguish the fire if possible using an appropriate fire extinguisher.

    - There are three classes of fire extinguisher:

      □ Class A is for paper, wood, upholstery, rags, or other types of trash fires.

      □ Class B is for flammable liquids and gas fires.

      □ Class C is for electrical fires.

    - To use a fire extinguisher:

      □ Pull the pin.

      □ Aim at the base of the fire.

      □ Squeeze the levers.

      □ Use a sweeping motion back and forth over the fire.

Application Exercises

1. A client is admitted to the emergency department after a head injury. He is combative and cursing. He has tried to hit and bite the staff. The nurse determines that restraints are necessary for the protection of the client and staff. Identify the appropriate nursing actions by documenting the actions as they would appear in the client's record.

2. A nurse enters a client's room and discovers flames in the trash can. Identify the sequence of actions in response to a fire in a client care area.

   _____ Report the fire (Alarm).
   _____ Protect and evacuate clients in immediate danger (Rescue).
   _____ Contain the fire (Contain).
   _____ Extinguish the fire (Extinguish).

3. Match the type of fire below with the appropriate class of fire extinguisher.

   _____ Gasoline   Class A
   _____ Cardboard   Class B
   _____ Electric wiring Class C

4. During his admission assessment, a client has a generalized tonic-clonic seizure. Which of the following nursing actions is appropriate?

   A. Go to the nurses' station to seek help.
   B. Place a padded tongue blade in the client's mouth.
   C. Turn the client onto his side.
   D. Keep the client awake after the seizure is over.

5. An older adult client was just admitted to the unit after falling at a nursing home. This client is oriented to person, place, and time and can follow directions. Which of the following actions by the nurse are appropriate to decrease the risk of a fall? (Select all that apply.)

   _____ Place a belt restraint on the client when he is sitting on the bedside commode.
   _____ Keep the bed in low position with full side rails up.
   _____ Ensure that the client's call light is within reach.
   _____ Provide the client with nonskid foot wear.
   _____ Complete a fall-risk assessment.

6. Identify the order of priority for completion of each of the following interventions for a newly admitted client who has a history of falls.

_____ Survey the client's belongings.

_____ Complete a fall-risk assessment.

_____ Complete a physical assessment.

_____ Make arrangements for a home safety survey.

_____ Educate the client and family on the fall risks.

CHAPTER 12: CLIENT SAFETY

 Application Exercises Answer Key

1. A client is admitted to the emergency department after a head injury. He is combative and cursing. He has tried to hit and bite the staff. The nurse determines that restraints are necessary for the protection of the client and staff. Identify the appropriate nursing actions by documenting the actions as they would appear in the client's record.

> **Upper extremity restraint (right and left wrist) applied at 1715 after the client repeatedly tried to hit and bite the staff. Client was not responsive to repeated requests to stop these behaviors. Client is alert but inappropriately responds to questions. Provider notified at 1725 of the need for restraints and reported he would be in to assess the client within the hour. Restraints applied per hospital protocol (loosely, with 2 fingerbreadths between the client and the device and to the frame of the bed). Client and family are aware of the need for the restraints relative to the client and staff safety. Client continues to try to strike out at the staff with both arms; therefore, unable to release the restraints. Initial circulatory and neurosensory checks show both upper extremities within normal limits and limited ROM relative to the restraints. Restraint care plan and flow chart initiated and added to client chart.**

 NCLEX® Connection: Safety and Infection Control: Use of Restraints/Safety Devices

2. A nurse enters a client's room and discovers flames in the trash can. Identify the sequence of actions in response to a fire in a client care area.

   __2__ Report the fire (Alarm).

   __1__ Protect and evacuate clients in immediate danger (Rescue).

   __3__ Contain the fire (Contain).

   __4__ Extinguish the fire (Extinguish).

 NCLEX® Connection: Safety and Infection Control: Accident/Injury Prevention

3. Match the type of fire below with the appropriate class of fire extinguisher.

   __B__ Gasoline   Class A

   __A__ Cardboard   Class B

   __C__ Electric wiring   Class C

 NCLEX® Connection: Safety and Infection Control: Safe Use of Equipment

4. During his admission assessment, a client has a generalized tonic-clonic seizure. Which of the following nursing actions is appropriate?

      A. Go to the nurses' station to seek help.

      B. Place a padded tongue blade in the client's mouth

      C. Turn the client onto his side.

      D. Keep the client awake after the seizure is over.

When a seizure occurs, the client is turned onto his side to allow for drainage of secretions and to keep the tongue from occluding the airway. The client should not be left alone. The nurse can use the call light to summon help. Nothing should be placed in the client's mouth. Attempting to place a tongue blade in the client's mouth could chip the client's teeth and could cause airway obstruction.

NCLEX® Connection: Physiological Adaptation: Alterations in Body Systems

5. An older adult client was just admitted to the unit after falling at a nursing home. This client is oriented to person, place, and time and can follow directions. Which of the following actions by the nurse are appropriate to decrease the risk of a fall? (Select all that apply.)

    _____ Place a belt restraint on the client when he is sitting on the bedside commode.

    _____ Keep the bed in low position with full side rails up.

    _X_ Ensure that the client's call light is within reach.

    _X_ Provide the client with nonskid foot wear.

    _X_ Complete a fall-risk assessment.

Ensuring that the call light is within reach enables the client to contact the nursing staff to ask for assistance and prevents the client from falling out of bed while reaching for the call light. Nonskid footwear may keep the client from slipping. A fall-risk assessment serves as the basis for an individualized plan of care. It is inappropriate to restrain this client and could be considered false imprisonment. Full side rails for this client may put the client at greater risk for a fall because he may attempt to climb over the bed rails to get out of bed.

NCLEX® Connection: Safety and Infection Control: Accident/Injury Prevention

6. Identify the order of priority for completion of each of the following interventions for a newly admitted client who has a history of falls.

__3__   Survey the client's belongings.

__1__   Complete a fall-risk assessment.

__2__   Complete a physical assessment.

__5__   Make arrangements for a home safety survey.

__4__   Educate the client and family on the fall risks.

1. The greatest risk to this client is injury from falling, therefore the first action is to determine his fall risk. The client's fall-risk assessment is used to find a safe room and guide how the client will be oriented to his room and the facility.

2. In addition to the report information from the emergency department, the physical assessment will help to identify further risks or injuries, as well as provide baseline physical data.

3. Surveying the client's belongings may provide further clues to fall risks (glasses, medications, hearing aids, canes, walkers).

4. It is important for family members and any visitors to be aware of the client's risk for falls. Providing instruction to the family will allow them to provide safety to the client.

5. The home safety survey is very important and should be completed prior to discharge. However, this survey does not take precedence over any of the other items that may impact safety during the hospital stay.

(N) NCLEX® Connection: Safety and Infection Control: Accident/Injury Prevention

UNIT 1	SAFE, EFFECTIVE CARE ENVIRONMENT
Section	Safety and Infection Control
Chapter 13	Home Safety

 Overview

- In addition to taking measures to prevent injury of clients in a health care setting, nurses play a pivotal role in promoting safety in the client's home and community. Nurses often collaborate with the client, family, and members of the interdisciplinary team (social workers, occupational therapists, and physical therapists) to promote the safety of the client.

- A number of factors contribute to the client's risk for injury. These factors include:

  o Age and developmental status

  o Mobility and balance

  o Knowledge about safety hazards

  o Sensory and cognitive awareness

  o Communication skills

  o Home and work environment

  o Community in which the client lives

- To initiate a plan of care, the nurse must identify risk factors using a risk assessment tool and complete a nursing history, a physical examination, and a home hazard appraisal.

Safety Risks Based on Age and Developmental Status

- The age and developmental status of the client creates specific safety risks. Some of the accident prevention measures for specific age groups are found below:

RISK	PREVENTION EDUCATION
	Infants and toddlers
Aspiration	• Keep all small objects out of reach. • Check toys for loose parts. • Do not feed the infant hard candy, peanuts, popcorn, or whole or sliced pieces of hot dog. • Do not place the infant in the supine position while feeding or prop the infant's bottle. • A pacifier (if used) should be constructed of one piece. • Provide parents with information about prevention of lead poisoning.
Suffocation	• Keep plastic bags out of reach. • Make sure crib mattress fits snugly and that crib slats are no more than 2⅜ inches apart. • Never leave an infant or toddler alone while in the bathtub. • Remove crib toys such as mobiles from over the bed as soon as the infant begins to push up. • Keep latex balloons away from infants and toddlers. • Fence swimming pools and use a locked gate. • Begin swimming lessons when the child's developmental status allows for protective responses such as closing her mouth under water. • Keep toilet lids down and bathroom doors closed.
Poisoning	• Keep house plants and cleaning agents out of reach. • Place poisons, paint, and gasoline in locked cabinet. • Keep medications in child-proof containers and locked up. • Dispose of medications which are not longer used or are out of date.
Falls	• Keep crib and playpen rails up. • Never leave the infant unattended on a changing table or other high surface. • Restrain when in high chair, swing, stroller, etc. • Place in a low bed when toddler starts to climb.
Motor vehicle/ Injury	• Use backward facing car seat until the infant/toddler is 1 year old and weighs at least 20 lb. • All car seats should be federally approved and be placed in the back seat.
Burns	• Test the temperature of formula and bath water. • Place pots on back burner and turn handle away from front of stove. • Supervise the use of faucets.

RISK	PREVENTION EDUCATION
Preschoolers and school-age children	
Drowning	• Be sure child has learned to swim and knows rules of water safety. • Place locked fences around home and neighborhood pools.
Motor vehicle/ Injury	• Use booster seats for children who are less than 4 feet 9 inches tall and weigh less than 40 lb. (Usually 4 to 8 years old). The child should be able to sit with his back against the car seat and his legs should dangle over the seat. • Use seat belts properly after booster seats are no longer necessary. • Use protective equipment when participating in sports or riding a bike or is a passenger on a bike. • Supervise and teach safe use of equipment. • Teach the child to play in safe areas. • Teach child safety rules of the road. • Teach child what to do if approached by stranger. • Begin sex education for school-age child.
Burns	• Reduce setting on water heater to no higher than 120° F. • Teach dangers of playing with matches, fireworks, fire arms. • Teach school-age child how to properly use microwave and other cooking instruments.
Poison	• Teach child about the hazards of alcohol, prescription, non-prescription, and illegal drugs. • Keep potentially dangerous substances out of reach.
Adolescents	
Motor vehicle/ Injury	• Ensure the teen has completed a driver education course. • Set rules on the number of people allowed to ride in cars, seat belt use, and to call for a ride home if a driver is impaired. • Reinforce teaching on proper use of protective equipment when participating in sports. • Be alert to signs of depression. • Teach about the hazards of firearms and safety precautions with firearms. • Teach to check water depth before diving.
Burns	• Teach to use sunblock and protective clothing. • Teach the dangers of sun bathing and tanning beds. • Educate on the hazards of smoking.

- Safety Risks and Prevention Measures for Young and Middle Age Adults

  o Motor vehicle crashes are the most common cause of death and injury to the adult. Occupational injuries contribute to the injury and death rate of the adult. High consumption of alcohol and suicide are also major concerns for adults.

- o Nurses can promote client safety for young and middle age adults by:
    - Reminding clients to drive defensively and to not drive after drinking alcohol.
    - Reinforcing teaching about the long term effects related to high alcohol consumption.
    - Being attuned to behaviors that suggest the presence of depression and/or thoughts of suicide and referring clients as appropriate.
    - Encouraging clients to become proactive about safety in the work place.
    - Ensuring that clients understand the hazards of excessive sun exposure and the need to protect the skin with the use of sun-blocking agents and protective clothing.

Safety Risks and Prevention Measures for Older Adults

- The rate at which age related changes occur varies greatly among older adults.
- Many older adults are able to maintain a lifestyle that promotes independence and the ability to protect themselves from safety hazards.
- Risk factors for falls in older adults include:
    - □ Physical, cognitive and sensory changes.
    - □ Changes in the musculoskeletal and neurological systems.
    - □ Impaired vision and/or hearing.
    - □ Frequent trips to the bathroom at night because of nocturia and incontinence.
- A decrease in tactile sensitivity may place the client at risk for burns and other types of tissue injury.
- When the client demonstrates factors that increases the risk for injury (regardless of age), a home hazard evaluation should be conducted by the nurse, a physical therapist, and/or occupational therapist. The client is made aware of the environmental factors that may pose a risk to safety and suggestion modifications to be made.
- Modifications that can be made to improve home safety include:
    - □ Removing items that could cause the client to trip, such as throw rugs and loose carpets
    - □ Placing electrical cords and extension cords that against a wall behind furniture
    - □ Making sure that steps and sidewalks are in good repair
    - □ Placing grab bars near the toilet and in the tub or shower and installing a stool riser
    - □ Using a non-skid mat in the tub or shower
    - □ Placing a shower chair in the shower
    - □ Ensuring that lighting is adequate both inside and outside of the home

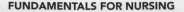

Fire Safety in the Home

- Home fires continue to be a major cause of death and injury for people of all ages.

- A home safety plan should include:

  o Keeping emergency numbers near the phone for prompt use in the event of an emergency of any type.

  o Ensuring that the number and placement of fire extinguishers and smoke alarms are adequate and that they are operable. Set a specific time to routinely change the batteries in the smoke alarms (for example: in the fall when the clocks are set back to standard time and spring when reset at Daylight Saving Time).

  o Having a family exit plan for fires that is reviewed and practiced regularly. Be sure to include closing windows and doors if able and to exit a smoke filled area by covering the mouth and nose with a damp cloth and getting down as close to the floor as possible.

  o Reviewing with clients of all ages that in the event that the client's clothing or skin is on fire, the mnemonic "stop, drop, and roll" should be used to extinguish the fire.

  o Reviewing oxygen safety measures. Because oxygen can cause materials to combust more easily and burn more rapidly, the client and family must be provided with information on use of the oxygen delivery equipment and the dangers of combustion. The following information should be included in the teaching plan:

    - Using and storing oxygen equipment according to the manufacturer's recommendations.

    - Placing a NO SMOKING sign in a conspicuous place near the front door of the home. A sign may also be placed on the door to the client's bedroom.

    - Informing the client and family of the danger of smoking in the presence of oxygen. Family members and visitors who smoke should do so outside the home.

    - Ensuring that electrical equipment is in good repair and well grounded.

    - Replacing bedding that can generate static electricity (wool, nylon, synthetics) with items made from cotton.

    - Keeping flammable materials away from the client when oxygen is in use such as heating oil and nail polish remover.

    - Following general measures for fire safety in the home, such as having a fire extinguisher readily available and an established exit route should a fire occur.

Additional Risks in the Home and Community

- Additional risks in the home and community include passive smoking, carbon monoxide poisoning, and food poisoning. Bioterrorism has also become a concern, making disaster plans a mandatory part of community safety.

- Nurses should teach clients about the dangers of these additional risks.

- Passive Smoking

o   Passive smoking is the unintentional inhalation of tobacco smoke.

o   Exposure to nicotine and other toxins places people at risk for numerous diseases including cancer, heart disease, and lung infections.

o   Low-birth weight infants, prematurity, stillbirths, and sudden infant death syndrome (SIDS) have been associated with maternal smoking.

o   Smoking in the presence of children is associated with the development of bronchitis, pneumonia, and middle ear infections.

o   For children with asthma, exposure to passive smoke can result in an increase in the frequency and the severity of asthma attacks.

o   The nurse should inform the client who smokes and his family about:

- The hazards of smoking

- Available resources to stop smoking (smoking cessation programs, medication support, self-help groups)

- The effect that visiting individuals who smoke or riding in the automobile of a smoker has on a non-smoker

- Carbon Monoxide

o   Carbon monoxide is a very dangerous gas because it binds with hemoglobin and ultimately reduces the oxygen supplied to the tissues in the body.

o   Carbon monoxide cannot be seen, smelled, or tasted.

o   Symptoms of carbon monoxide poisoning include nausea, vomiting, headache, weakness, and unconsciousness.

o   Death may occur with prolonged exposure.

o   Measures to prevent carbon monoxide poisoning include ensuring proper ventilation when using fuel-burning devices (lawn mowers, wood burning and gas fireplaces, charcoal grills).

o   Gas-burning furnaces, water heaters, and appliances should be inspected annually.

o   Flues and chimneys should be unobstructed.

o   Carbon monoxide detectors should be installed and inspected regularly.

- Food Poisoning

o   Food poisoning is a major cause of illness in the United States.

o   Most food poisoning is caused by some type of bacteria such as *Escherichia coli*, *Listeria monocytogenes*, and *Salmonella*.

o   Healthy individuals usually recover from the illness in a few days.

o   Very young, very old, pregnant women, and immunocompromised individuals are at risk for complications.

o   Clients who are especially at risk are instructed to follow a low-microbial diet.

- o Most food poisoning occurs because of unsanitary food practice.

- o Performing proper hand hygiene, ensuring that meat and fish are cooked to the correct temperature, handling raw and fresh food separately to avoid cross contamination, and refrigerating perishable items are measures that may prevent food poisoning.

- Bioterrorism

  - o Bioterrorism is the dissemination of harmful toxins, bacteria, viruses, and pathogens for the purpose of causing illness or death.

  - o Anthrax, variola, *Clostridium botulism*, and *Yersinia pestis* are examples of agents used by terrorists.

  - o Nurses as well as other health professionals must be prepared to respond to an attack by being proficient in early detection, recognizing the causative agent, identifying the affected community, and providing early treatment to affected persons.

CHAPTER 13: HOME SAFETY

 Application Exercises

1. A nurse is providing discharge instructions to a client who has a prescription for the use of oxygen in his home. Which of the following should the nurse teach the client about using oxygen safely in his home? (Select all that apply.)

_____ Family members who smoke must be at least 10 ft from the client when oxygen is in use.

_____ Nail polish should not be used near a client who is receiving oxygen.

_____ A "No Smoking" sign should be placed on the front door.

_____ Cotton bedding and clothing should be replaced with items made from wool.

_____ A fire extinguisher should be readily available in the home.

2. A nurse is providing home safety instructions to a group of older adult clients. Match the safety risk with the appropriate instruction.

_____ Passive smoking   A. Have water heaters inspected on an annual basis.

_____ Carbon monoxide poisoning   B. Cook all meat at an appropriate temperature.

_____ Food poisoning   C. Avoid enclosed areas with others who may be smoking.

CHAPTER 13: HOME SAFETY

 Application Exercises Answer Key

1. A nurse is providing discharge instructions to a client who has a prescription for the use of oxygen in his home. Which of the following should the nurse teach the client about using oxygen safely in his home? (Select all that apply.)

_____ Family members who smoke must be at least 10 ft from the client when oxygen is in use.

__X__ **Nail polish should not be used near a client who is receiving oxygen.**

__X__ **A "No Smoking" sign should be placed on the front door.**

_____ Cotton bedding and clothing should be replaced with items made from wool.

__X__ **A fire extinguisher should be readily available in the home.**

Nail polish and other flammable materials may cause a fire and should not be used. A "No Smoking" sign should be placed near the front door. A sign may also be placed on the client's bedroom door. A readily available fire extinguisher should be placed in all homes, including the home of a client who is receiving oxygen. Family members who smoke should do so outside. Woolen and synthetic materials create static electricity; cotton materials do not and should be used instead.

NCLEX® Connection: Safety and Infection Control: Home Safety

2. A nurse is providing home safety instructions to a group of older adult clients. Match the safety risk with the appropriate instruction.

__C__	Passive smoking	A. Have water heaters inspected on an annual basis.
__A__	Carbon monoxide poisoning	B. Cook all meat at an appropriate temperature.
__B__	Food poisoning	C. Avoid enclosed areas with others who may be smoking.

NCLEX® Connection: Safety and Infection Control: Home Safety

UNIT 1	SAFE, EFFECTIVE CARE ENVIRONMENT
Section	Safety and Infection Control
Chapter 14	Ergonomic Principles

Overview

- Ergonomics are the factors or qualities in an object's design and/or use that contribute to comfort, safety, efficiency, and ease of use.

- Using good body mechanics when positioning and moving clients promotes safety for the client as well as for health care providers.

- Before attempting to position or move a client, the nurse should perform a mobility assessment. Begin this assessment with the easiest movements (range of motion) and progress as long as the client tolerates it (balance, gait, and exercise).

Ergonomic Principles and Body Mechanics

- Body mechanics is the proper use of muscles to maintain balance, posture, and body alignment when performing a physical task. Nurses use body mechanics when providing care to clients by lifting, bending, and carrying out the activities of daily living.

- The risk of injury to the client and the nurse is reduced with the use of good body mechanics. Whenever possible, mechanical lift devices should be used to lift and transfer clients. Many health care agencies have "no manual lift" and "no solo lift" policies.

- Center of gravity

 View Media Supplement: Ergonomic Principles (Video)

- ○ The center of gravity is the center of a mass.

- ○ Weight is a quantity of matter acted on by the force of gravity.

- ○ To lift an object, the nurse must overcome the weight of the object and know the center of gravity of the object.

- ○ When the human body is in the upright position, the center of gravity is the pelvis.

- ○ When an individual moves, the center of gravity shifts.

- o The closer the line of gravity is to t[...]
  the individual is.
- o To lower the center of gravity, be[...]
- Lifting
  - o Use the major muscle groups t[...]
    muscles to increase support to [...]
  - o Distribute the weight betwee[...]
    strain on any one muscle gr[...]
  - o When lifting an object fron[...]
    thigh level, keeping the kn[...]
    the object as close as poss[...]
    increase stability and dec[...]
  - o Use assistive devices whe[...]
- When pushing or pulling a load:
  - o Widen the base of support.
  - o When opportunity allows, pull objects toward the center of gravity rathe[...]
    pushing away.
  - o If pushing, move the front foot forward, and if pulling, move the rear leg back to
    promote stability.
  - o Face the direction of movement when moving a client.
  - o Use own body as a counterweight when pushing or pulling to make the movement
    easier.
  - o Sliding, rolling, and pushing require less energy than lifting and offer less risk for
    injury.
  - o Avoid twisting the thoracic spine and bending the back while the hips and knees are
    straight.
- Guidelines to Prevent Injury
  - o Know your agency's policies regarding lifting.
  - o Plan ahead for activities that require lifting, transfer, or ambulation of a client, and ask
    others to be ready to assist at the planned time.
  - o Be aware that the safest way to lift a client may be with the use of assistive equipment.
  - o Rest between heavy activities to decrease muscle fatigue.
  - o Maintain good posture and exercise regularly to increase the strength of arm, leg,
    back, and abdominal muscles, so these activities will require less energy.
  - o Use smooth movements when lifting and moving clients to prevent injury through
    sudden or jerky muscle movements.

ERGONOMIC PRINCIPLES

When standing for [...]
rest. When sittin[...]
hips.

Avoid repeti[...]
to 20 min[...]

Mainta[...]
flexi[...]

Client Posit[...]

long periods of time, flex the hip and knee through use of a foot

for long periods of time, keep the knees slightly higher than the

tive movements of the hands, wrists, and shoulders. Take a break every 15

to flex and stretch joints and muscles.

n good posture (head and neck in straight line with pelvis) to avoid neck

n and hunched shoulders, which can cause impingement of nerves in the neck.

oid twisting the spine or bending at the waist (flexion) to minimize the risk for

injury.

oning

The nurse is responsible for positioning clients so that good body alignment is maintained. Many clients are able to reposition themselves when they are uncomfortable. It is especially important for the nurse to ensure proper positioning of clients who are unable to move themselves due to disability or injury.

- Transfers and Use of Assistive Devices

  o Assess the client's ability to help with transfers (balance, muscle strength, endurance).

  o Determine the need for additional personnel or assistive devices (transfer belt, hydraulic lift, sliding board).

  o Assess and monitor the client's proper use of mobility aids (canes, walkers, crutches).

  o Include assistance or mobility aids needed for safe transfers and ambulation in the plan of care.

Bed and Client Positions

POSITION	DESCRIPTION
Semi-Fowler's position	• The client lies supine with the head of the bed elevated approximately 30°, and his knees may be slightly elevated (about 15°). • This position is frequently used to prevent regurgitation of tube feedings and aspiration in clients with difficulty swallowing.
Fowler's position	• The client lies supine with the head of the bed elevated approximately 45°, and his knees may be slightly elevated (about 15°). • This position is frequently used during procedures such as nasogastric tube insertion and suctioning. It also allows for better chest expansion and ventilation, as well as better dependent drainage, after abdominal surgeries.

POSITION	DESCRIPTION
High-Fowler's position	• The client lies supine with the head of the bed elevated approximately 90°, and his knees may or may not be elevated. • This position promotes lung expansion by lowering the diaphragm and is used for clients experiencing severe dyspnea.
Supine or dorsal recumbent position	• The client lies on his back with his head and shoulders elevated on a pillow. The client's forearms may be placed on pillows or placed at the side. A foot support prevents footdrop and maintains proper alignment.
Prone position	• The client lies flat on his abdomen with his head to one side. • This position promotes drainage from the mouth for clients following throat or oral surgery, but inhibits chest expansion.
Lateral or side-lying position	• The client lies on his side with most of his weight on the dependent hip and shoulder. His arms should be flexed in front of the body. A pillow is placed under his head and neck, the upper arm, and under the leg and thigh to maintain body alignment. • This is a good sleeping position, but the client must be turned regularly to prevent development of pressure ulcers on the dependent areas. A 30° lateral position is recommended for clients at risk for pressure ulcers.
Sims' or semi-prone position	• The client is on his side halfway between lateral and prone positions. (Weight is on the anterior ileum, humerus, and clavicle.) The lower arm is behind the client while the upper arm is in front. Both legs are flexed, but the upper leg is flexed at a greater angle than the lower leg at the hip as well as at the knee. • This is a comfortable sleeping position for many clients, and it promotes oral drainage.
Orthopneic position	• The client sits in the bed or at the bedside. A pillow is placed on the over-bed table, which is placed across the client's lap. The client rests his arms on the over-bed table. • This position allows for chest expansion and is especially beneficial to clients with COPD.
Trendelenburg position	• The entire bed is tilted with the head of the bed lower than the foot of the bed. • This position is used during postural drainage, and it facilitates venous return.
Reverse Trendelenburg	• The entire bed is tilted with the foot of the bed lower than the head of the bed. This position promotes gastric emptying and prevents esophageal reflux.

CHAPTER 14: ERGONOMIC PRINCIPLES

 Application Exercises

1. A nurse is caring for a female client who has been placed in skeletal traction to treat a tibial fracture from a motor vehicle crash. Which of the following factors may place the client at risk for complications related to immobility?

    A. The client exercised regularly prior to her injury.

    B. The client has a head injury and is disoriented.

    C. The client has been taking a multivitamin daily.

    D. The client's 24-hr fluid intake is 2,000 mL.

2. A nurse is caring for a postoperative client who has an order for semi-Fowler's position. The nurse should recognize that

    A. the head of the bed should be raised 30°.

    B. the head of the bed should be raised 45°.

    C. the client should be placed in a side-lying position.

    D. a pillow should be placed between the client's knees.

3. Place the following steps of a mobility assessment in the correct sequence.

    _____ Exercise tolerance

    _____ Moving from supine to sitting on the side of the bed

    _____ Gait

    _____ Range of motion

4. Which of the following positions promotes drainage from the mouth for clients with throat or oral surgery but inhibits chest expansion?

    A. Fowler's position

    B. Semi-Fowler's position

    C. Prone position

    D. Reverse Trendelenburg

CHAPTER 14: ERGONOMIC PRINCIPLES

 Application Exercises Answer Key

1. A nurse is caring for a female client who has been placed in skeletal traction to treat a tibial fracture from a motor vehicle crash. Which of the following factors may place the client at risk for complications related to immobility?

> A. The client exercised regularly prior to her injury.
>
> **B. The client has a head injury and is disoriented.**
>
> C. The client has been taking a multivitamin daily.
>
> D. The client's 24-hr fluid intake is 2,000 mL.

> **Clients who have sensory impairment such as disorientation are at greater risk for complications due to immobility. The client's exercise program and intake of a multivitamin contribute to overall good health. A daily fluid intake of 2,000 mL is adequate.**

(N) **NCLEX® Connection: Basic Care and Comfort: Mobility/ Immobility**

2. A nurse is caring for a postoperative client who has an order for semi-Fowler's position. The nurse should recognize that

> **A. the head of the bed should be raised to 30°.**
>
> B. the head of the bed should be raised 45°.
>
> C. the client should be placed in a side-lying position.
>
> D. a pillow should be placed between the client's knees.

> **In the semi-Fowler's position, the client lies flat on his back. The head of the bed is raised 30°. He does not lie on his side and a pillow is not placed between his knees.**

(N) **NCLEX® Connection: Safety and Infection Control: Ergonomic Principles**

3. Place the following steps of a mobility assessment in the correct sequence.

> **4**   Exercise tolerance
>
> **2**   Moving from supine to sitting on the side of the bed
>
> **3**   Gait
>
> **1**   Range of motion

(N) **NCLEX® Connection: Basic Care and Comfort: Mobility/ Immobility**

4. Which of the following positions promotes drainage from the mouth for clients with throat or oral surgery but inhibits chest expansion?

    A. Fowler's position

    B. Semi-Fowler's position

    C. Prone position

    D. Reverse Trendelenburg

The prone position promotes drainage from the mouth for clients with throat or oral surgery, but it inhibits chest expansion. Fowler's and semi-Fowler's positions promote chest expansion. Reverse Trendelenburg promotes gastric emptying and prevents esophageal reflux.

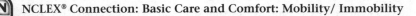 **NCLEX® Connection: Basic Care and Comfort: Mobility/ Immobility**

UNIT 1	SAFE, EFFECTIVE CARE ENVIRONMENT
Section	Safety and Infection Control
Chapter 15	**Security and Disaster Plans**

Overview

- A disaster is a mass casualty or intra-facility event that overwhelms or interrupts, at least temporarily, the normal flow of services of a hospital.

- Disasters that health care facilities face include internal and external emergencies.

  ○ Internal emergencies include loss of electric power or potable water and severe damage or casualties within the facility related to fire, weather (tornado, hurricane), an explosion, or a terrorist act. Internal emergency readiness includes safety and hazardous materials protocols and infection control policies and practices.

  ○ External emergencies include hurricanes, floods, volcano eruptions, earthquakes, pandemic flu, industrial accidents, chemical plant explosions, major transportation accidents, building collapse, and terrorist acts (including biological and chemical warfare). External emergency readiness includes a plan for participation in community-wide emergencies and disasters.

The Joint Commission and Emergency Preparedness

- The Joint Commission has established emergency preparedness management standards for various types of health care facilities. These standards mandate that an institutional emergency preparedness plan be developed by all health care institutions and that these plans include institution-specific procedures for:

  ○ Notifying and assigning personnel.

  ○ Notifying external authorities of emergencies.

  ○ Managing space and supplies and providing security.

  ○ Isolating and decontaminating radioactive or chemical agents (measures to contain contamination, decontamination at the scene of exposure).

  ○ Evacuating and setting up an alternative care site when the environment cannot support adequate client care and treatment. Critical processes when an alternative care site is necessary include:

    ■ Client information/care packaging (medications, admissions, medical records, and tracking).

    ■ Interfacility communication.

- Transportation of clients, staff, and equipment.
- Cross-privileging of medical staff.
  o Performing triage of incoming clients.
  o Managing clients during emergencies, including scheduling, modification or discontinuation of services, control of client information, and client discharge and transportation.
  o Interacting with family members and the news media.
  o Identifying backup resources (electricity, water, fire protection, fuel sources, medical gas and vacuum) for utilities and communication.
  o Orienting and educating personnel who will participate in implementation of the emergency preparedness plan.
  o Providing crisis support for health care workers (access to vaccines, infection control advice, mental health counseling).
  o Providing performance monitoring and evaluation related to emergency preparedness.
  o Conducting two emergency preparedness drills each year.
    - Drills should include an influx of clients beyond those being treated by the facility.
    - Drills should include either an internal or an external disaster (a situation beyond the normal capacity of the facility).

Nursing Role in Disaster Planning and Emergency Response Plans

- Emergency Response Plans

  o Each health care institution must have an emergency preparedness plan that has been developed by a planning committee. This committee reviews information regarding the potential for various types of natural and man-made emergencies depending on the characteristics of the community. Resources necessary to meet the potential emergency are also determined and a plan developed that takes into consideration all of the above factors.

  o Nurses, as well as a cross-section of other members of the health care team, should be involved in the development of a disaster plan for such emergencies. Criteria under which the disaster plan is activated should be clear. Roles for each employee should be outlined and administrative control determined. A designated area for the area command center should be established as well as a person to serve as the incident control manager.

- Triage

  o Principles of triage should be followed in health care institutions involved in a mass casualty event.

- These differ from the principles of triage that are typically followed during provision of day-to-day services in an emergency or urgent care setting. During mass casualty events, casualties are separated in relation to their potential for survival, and treatment is allocated accordingly.

- Categories of Triage During Mass Casualty Events

  - Emergent Category (Class I) – Highest priority is given to clients who have life-threatening injuries but also have a high possibility of survival once they are stabilized.

  - Urgent Category (Class II) – Second highest priority is given to clients who have major injuries that are not yet life threatening and can usually wait 45 to 60 min for treatment.

  - Nonurgent Category (Class III) – The next highest priority is given to clients who have minor injuries that are not life threatening and do not need immediate attention.

  - Expectant Category (Class IV) – The lowest priority is given to clients who are not expected to live and will be allowed to die naturally. Comfort measures may be provided, but restorative care will not.

- Discharge/Relocation of Clients

  - During an emergency such as a fire or a mass casualty event, decisions may need to be made regarding discharging clients or relocating them so their bed can be given to a client with higher priority needs.

  - Criteria should be followed when identifying clients who can be safely discharged.

    - Ambulatory clients requiring minimal care should be discharged or relocated first.

    - Clients requiring assistance should be next and arrangements should be made for continuation of their care.

    - Clients who are unstable and/or require nursing care should not be discharged or relocated unless they are in imminent danger.

- Fire

  - If a nurse discovers a fire that threatens the safety of a client, the nurse should use the RACE mnemonic to guide the order of actions.

  - If evacuation of the unit is necessary, horizontal evacuation is done first. Lateral evacuation is done if client safety cannot be maintained.

  - The RACE mnemonic is Rescue, Alarm, Contain, and Extinguish.

RACE MNEMONIC	
Rescue	• **Rescue** the client and other individuals from the area.
Alarm	• Sound the fire **alarm**, which will activate the EMS response system. • Systems that could increase fire spread are automatically shut down with activation of the alarm.

RACE MNEMONIC	
Contain	• Once the room or area has been cleared, the door leading to the area in which the fire is located as well as the fire doors should be kept closed in order to **contain** the fire. • Fire doors should be kept closed as much as possible when moving from area to area within the facility to avoid the spread of smoke and fire.
Extinguish	• Make an attempt to **extinguish** small fires using a single fire extinguisher, smothering them with a blanket, or dousing with water (except with an electrical or grease fire). • Complete evacuation of the area should occur if the nurse cannot put the fire out with these methods. • Attempts at extinguishing the fire should only be made when the employee has been properly trained in the safe use of a fire extinguisher and when only one extinguisher is needed.

- Severe Thunderstorm/Tornado

    o Draw shades and close drapes to protect against shattering glass.

    o Lower beds to the lowest position and move away from the windows.

    o Place blankets over all clients who are confined to beds.

    o Close all doors.

    o Move as many ambulatory clients as possible into the hallways (away from windows).

    o Do not use elevators.

    o Monitor for severe weather warnings using television, radio, or Internet.

- Biological Incidents

    o Take measures to protect self and others.

    o Recognize signs and symptoms of infection/poisoning and appropriate treatment.

INCIDENT	SIGNS AND SYMPTOMS	TREATMENT/PREVENTION
Inhalational anthrax	• Sore throat • Fever • Muscle aches • Severe dyspnea • Meningitis • Shock	• IV ciprofloxacin (Cipro)

INCIDENT	SIGNS AND SYMPTOMS	TREATMENT/PREVENTION
Botulism	• Difficulty swallowing • Progressive weakness • Nausea, vomiting, and abdominal cramps • Difficulty breathing	• Airway management • Antitoxin • Elimination of toxin
Smallpox	• High fever • Fatigue • Severe headache • Rash (starts centrally and spreads outward) that turns to pus-filled lesions • Vomiting • Delirium • Excessive bleeding	• Treatment: No cure • Supportive care: Hydration, pain medication, antipyretics • Prevention: Vaccine
Ebola	• Sore throat • Headache • High temperature • Nausea, vomiting, diarrhea • Internal and external bleeding • Shock	• Treatment: No cure • Supportive care: Minimize invasive procedures • Prevention: Vaccine

- Chemical Incidents

  o Take measures to protect self and to avoid contact.

  o Assess and intervene to maintain the client's airway, breathing, and circulation and administer first aid as needed.

  o Effectively remove the offending chemical by undressing the client, removing all identifiable particulate matter, and decontaminate the client by providing immediate and prolonged irrigations of contaminated areas.

  o Gather a specific history of the injury, if possible (name and concentration of the chemical, duration of exposure, previous client history).

  o In the event of chemical warfare, have knowledge of which facilities are open to exposed clients and which are only open to unexposed clients.

  o Follow the facility's emergency operations plans (for personal protection measures, the handling and disposal of wastes, use of space and equipment, reporting procedures).

- Hazardous Material Incidents

  o Take measures to protect self and to avoid contact.

  o Approach the scene cautiously.

  o Try to identify the material (emergency response guidebook, poison control centers). Have knowledge of where the material safety data sheets (MSDS) manual is located.

- o Try to contain the material as much as possible in one place prior to the arrival of the hazardous materials team.

- o If individuals are contaminated, decontaminate them as much as possible at the scene or as close as possible to the scene.

  - ■ With few exceptions, water is the universal antidote. For biological hazardous materials, wash skin with copious amounts of water and antibacterial soap.

  - ■ Wear gloves, gown, mask, and shoe covers to protect self from contamination.

  - ■ If clothing becomes contaminated, remove it carefully so that the hazardous material does not become airborne.

  - ■ Place all contaminated material into large plastic bags and seal them.

- Radiological Incidents

  - o Amount of exposure is related to time exposed, distance from source, and amount of shielding.

  - o The facility in which victims are cared for should activate interventions to prevent exposure of treatment areas (floors and furniture should be covered, air vents and ducts should be covered, radiation-contaminated waste should be disposed of according to procedural guidelines).

  - o Staff should wear water-resistant gowns, double glove, and fully cover their bodies with caps, shoe covers, masks, and goggles.

  - o Staff should wear radiation or dosimetry badges to monitor the amount of their radiation exposure.

  - o Clients should be initially be surveyed with a radiation meter to determine the amount of contamination.

  - o Decontamination should then occur prior to entering the hospital with soap and water and disposable towels. Water runoff will be contaminated and should be contained.

  - o After decontamination, clients should be resurveyed for residual contamination and washing continued until the client is clean of all contamination.

- Bomb Threat

  - o When a phone call is received:

    - ■ Lengthen the conversation as much as possible.

    - ■ Listen for distinctive background noises, such as music, voices, aircraft, or church bells.

    - ■ Be alert for distinguishing voice characteristics.

    - ■ Ask where the bomb will explode and at what time.

    - ■ Note if the caller indicates knowledge of the facility by his description of the location.

- o If what appears to be a bomb is found, do not touch it, clear the area, and obtain professional assistance. Try to isolate the object as much as possible by closing doors.

- o Notify authorities and key personnel (police, administrator, director of nursing or supervisor).

- o Cooperate with police and others – assist to conduct search as needed, provide copies of floor plans, have master keys available, and watch for and isolate suspicious objects such as packages and boxes.

- o Keep elevators available for authorities.

- o Remain calm and alert and try not to alarm clients.

SECURITY PLAN

Overview

- All health care facilities should have security plans in place that include preventive, protective, and response measures designed for identified security needs.

- Security issues faced by health care facilities include: admission of potentially dangerous individuals, vandalism, infant abduction, and information theft.

- The International Association for Healthcare Security & Safety (IAHSS) provides recommendations for the development of security plans.

Nursing Role in Security Plan

- Nurses should be aware that security measures include:

  - o An identification system that identifies employees, volunteers, physicians, students, and regularly scheduled contract services staff as authorized personnel of the health care facility.

  - o Electronic security systems in high-risk areas (the newborn nursery to prevent infant abductions, the emergency department to prevent unauthorized entrants). Examples include:

    - ▪ Security device attached to the umbilical cord of the newborn.

    - ▪ Key code access into and out of newborn nurseries.

    - ▪ Wristbands that electronically link the mother and her infant.

    - ▪ Alarms integrated with closed-circuit television cameras. Alarm activation may automatically integrate with the monitoring cameras, providing a view of the alarm location.

- Nurses should be aware that all health care institutions have color code designations for emergencies. These may vary between institutions, but some examples are:

  - o Code Red (fire).

  - o Code Pink (newborn abduction).

- o Code Orange (chemical spill).

- o Code Blue (mass casualty incident).

- o Code Gray (tornado).

- Nurses should be familiar with procedures and policies that outline proper measures to take when one of these emergencies is called.

- Nurses should be prepared to take immediate action when breaches in security occur. Time is of the essence in stopping an abduction or the stealing of confidential information.

CHAPTER 15: SECURITY AND DISASTER PLANS

 Application Exercises

1. A nurse who is employed by a large hospital in an urban community is serving on a committee that is updating its disaster plan. The nurse should recognize that in a mass casualty event, care of which of the following clients would receive the highest priority?

    A. A client who received crush injuries to the chest and abdomen and is expected to die

    B. A client who has a 4-in laceration to the head

    C. A client who has partial-thickness and full-thickness burns to his face, neck, and chest

    D. A client who has a fractured fibula and tibia

2. A nurse on a medical-surgical unit has been informed that a mass casualty event has occurred in the community and that it is necessary to discharge some of the clients to make beds available to the injury victims. Which of the following clients can be safely discharged? (Select all that apply.)

    _____ A client who is dehydrated and receiving IV fluid and electrolytes

    _____ A client who has a nasogastric tube in place to treat a small bowel obstruction

    _____ A client who is scheduled for a transurethral resection of the prostate (TURP)

    _____ A client who is 24-hr postoperative following a mastectomy

    _____ A client who is scheduled for an appendectomy

3. A nurse is caring for a client who has been admitted to the medical-surgical unit for the treatment of inhalational anthrax. The nurse should recognize that which of the following anti-infectives is an appropriate choice?

    A. Amoxicillin (Amoxil)

    B. Ciprofloxacin (Cipro)

    C. Sulfadiazine (Microsulfon)

    D. Ketoconazole (Nizoral)

4. A nurse who is working in a long-term care facility receives a bomb threat over the telephone. Which of the following actions should the nurse take? (Select all that apply.)

    _____ End the telephone call as soon as possible.

    _____ Listen for background noises.

    _____ Ask where the bomb is and when it will explode.

    _____ Notify the director of nursing.

    _____ Use the overhead paging system to warn residents and visitors of the threat.

5. Health care institutions have color-code designations for emergencies. Match the types of emergencies with the color code that is commonly used. Use each answer only once.

_____ Newborn abduction   A. Red

_____ Mass casualty incident   B. Pink

_____ Fire   C. Orange

_____ Chemical spill   D. Blue

_____ Tornado   E. Gray

CHAPTER 15: SECURITY AND DISASTER PLANS

 Application Exercises Answer Key

1. A nurse who is employed by a large hospital in an urban community is serving on a committee that is updating its disaster plan. The nurse should recognize that in a mass casualty event, care of which of the following clients would receive the highest priority?

   A. A client who received crush injuries to the chest and abdomen and is expected to die

   B. A client who has a 4-in laceration to the head

   C. A client who has partial-thickness and full-thickness burns to his face, neck, and chest

   D. A client who has a fractured fibula and tibia.

   The client who has the greatest chance of survival with prompt intervention should be given priority in a mass casualty event. If not treated immediately, a client who has burns to his face, neck, and chest is at risk for airway obstruction, but is still expected to live. Therefore, this client is the highest priority (Emergent Category – Class I). A client with major fractures would be the second priority (Urgent Category – Class II). A client with a minor injury that is not life-threatening, such as a laceration to the head, would have the third priority (Nonurgent Category – Class III). The lowest priority would be given to a client who is not expected to live. Comfort measures would be provided for this client (Expectant Category – Class IV).

    NCLEX® Connection: Safety and Infection Control: Emergency Response Plan

2. A nurse on a medical-surgical unit has been informed that a mass casualty event has occurred in the community and that it is necessary to discharge some of the clients to make beds available to the injury victims. Which of the following clients can be safely discharged? (Select all that apply.)

   _____ A client who is dehydrated and receiving IV fluid and electrolytes

   _____ A client who has a nasogastric tube in place to treat a small bowel obstruction

   __**X**__ **A client who is scheduled for a transurethral resection of the prostate (TURP)**

   __**X**__ **A client who is 24-hr postoperative following a mastectomy**

   _____ A client who is scheduled for an appendectomy

   A client who is scheduled for a TURP and a client who is 24-hr postoperative following a mastectomy could be safely discharged. A client who is dehydrated and receiving IV fluid and electrolytes is too unstable for discharge. A small bowel obstruction that is not treated could result in the death of the client. A client who has appendicitis needs immediate surgery to prevent rupture of the appendix and subsequent peritonitis.

    NCLEX® Connection: Safety and Infection Control: Emergency Response Plan

3. A nurse is caring for a client who has been admitted to the medical-surgical unit for the treatment of inhalational anthrax. The nurse recognizes that which of the following anti-infectives is the medication of choice?

    A. Amoxicillin (Amoxil)

    B. Ciprofloxacin (Cipro)

    C. Sulfadiazine (Microsulfon)

    D. Ketoconazole (Nizoral)

Ciprofloxacin is the drug of choice to treat inhaled anthrax. A tetracycline, such as doxycycline (Vibramycin), may also be used. The other medications are not used to treat inhaled anthrax. Amoxicillin is a type of penicillin and may be used to treat pneumonia and meningitis. Sulfadiazine is a sulfonamide used to treat urinary tract infections as well as other infectious conditions. Ketoconazole is used to treat fungal infections.

NCLEX® Connection: Safety and Infection Control: Handling Hazardous and Infectious Materials

4. A nurse who is working in a long-term care facility receives a bomb threat over the telephone. Which of the following actions should the nurse take? (Select all that apply.)

    _____ End the telephone call as soon as possible.

    X Listen for background noises.

    X Ask where the bomb is and when it will explode.

    X Notify the director of nursing.

    _____ Use the overhead paging system to warn residents and visitors of the threat.

In the event of a bomb threat, the caller should be kept on the line in order to trace the call and to collect as much information as possible. To help identify the location of the caller, the nurse should listen for background noises such as church bells, train whistles, or other noises. To promote safety, the caller is asked about the location of the bomb and the time it is set to explode. The director of nursing and/or the nursing home administrator are notified to be available to assist emergency personnel in location of the bomb and to prepare for evacuation of residents, if necessary. Announcing that a bomb threat has occurred using the paging system could cause mass panic and should be avoided.

NCLEX® Connection: Safety and Infection Control: Emergency Response Plan

5. Health care institutions have color-code designations for emergencies. Match the types of emergencies with the color code that is commonly used. Use each answer only once.

B	Newborn abduction	A. Red
D	Mass casualty incident	B. Pink
A	Fire	C. Orange
C	Chemical spill	D. Blue
E	Tornado	E. Gray

NCLEX® Connection: Safety and Infection Control: Emergency Response Plan

UNIT 2: HEALTH PROMOTION

Section: Nursing Throughout the Lifespan

- Health Promotion and Disease Prevention
- Client Education
- Infant (Birth to 1 Year)
- Toddler (1 to 3 Years)
- Preschooler (3 to 6 Years)
- School-Age Child (6 to 12 Years)
- Adolescent (12 to 20 Years)
- Young Adult (20 to 35 Years)
- Middle Adult (35 to 65 Years)
- Older Adult (65 Years and Older)

NCLEX® CONNECTIONS

When reviewing the chapters in this section, keep in mind the relevant sections of the NCLEX® outline, in particular:

CLIENT NEEDS: SAFETY AND INFECTION CONTROL	CLIENT NEEDS: HEALTH PROMOTION AND MAINTENANCE	CLIENT NEEDS: BASIC CARE AND COMFORT

Relevant topics/tasks include:
• Accident/Injury Prevention
  ○ Identify factors that influence accident/injury prevention.
• Home Safety
  ○ Educate the client on home safety issues.
	Relevant topics/tasks include:
	• Developmental Stages and Transitions
	  ○ Identify expected physical, cognitive, and psychosocial stages of development.
	• Health and Wellness
	  ○ Identify the client's health-oriented behaviors.
	• Health Promotion/Disease Prevention
	  ○ Educate the client on actions to promote/maintain health and prevent disease.
		Relevant topics/tasks include:
		• Mobility/Immobility
		  ○ Assess the client for mobility, gait, strength, and motor skills.

UNIT 2	HEALTH PROMOTION
Section	Nursing Throughout the Lifespan
Chapter 16	Health Promotion and Disease Prevention

Overview

- Nurses play an important role in promoting health and wellness, as well as disease prevention. A client's beliefs about health affect his health behaviors. Nurses can contribute greatly to the health of clients and population groups using health promotion and disease prevention strategies. In addition to traditional nursing measures, nurses include complementary therapies such as guided imagery, massage, relaxation, and music in the provision of care.

- Levels of prevention address health-related activities and are classified as primary, secondary, and tertiary. Levels of prevention are not the same as levels of care.

- Health promotion and disease prevention activities occur throughout the health care delivery system.

Risk Factor Assessment

- Genetics – A predisposition for various illnesses can be attributed to heredity (family history of heart disease, cancers, certain mental illnesses).

- Gender – Some specific diseases are more common in one gender than in the other. For example, there is a higher incidence of autoimmune disorders in females. Males have a higher suicide rate.

- Physiologic factors – Various physiologic states place the client at an increased risk for health problems (body mass index [BMI] greater than 25, pregnancy).

- Environmental factors – The presence of toxic substances and chemicals can affect health where clients live and work. Water quality, pesticide exposure, and air pollution should be commonly assessed.

- Lifestyle-risk behaviors – Lifestyle refers to the choices an individual makes about his manner of living. Individuals have control over their lifestyle, and making positive choices can reduce risk factors. Risk behaviors to screen for include stress, substance abuse, diet deficiencies, lack of exercise, and sun exposure.

- Age – Early disease detection and intervention is facilitated by following screening guidelines developed in a joint effort of the American Diabetes Association, the American Heart Association, and the American Cancer Society. Ages may vary based on individual practices (A female client who has become sexually active before the age of 20 should start screenings at the age when sexual activity begins).

- Frequency of exams and screening for clients who are asymptomatic and do not have risk factors:

TEST	FEMALE	MALE
Routine physical	Starting at age 20, every 1 to 3 years; beginning at 40 annually	Starting at age 20, every 5 years; beginning at 40 annually
Dental assessments	Every 6 months	Every 6 months
Blood pressure	Starting at age 20, each routine health care visit, minimum of every 2 years	Starting at age 20, each routine health care visit, minimum of every 2 years
Body mass index (BMI)	Starting at age 20, each routine health care visit	Starting at age 20, each routine health care visit
Blood cholesterol	Starting at age 20, a minimum of every 5 years	Starting at age 20, a minimum of every 5 years
Blood glucose	Starting at age 45, a minimum of every 3 years	Starting at age 45, a minimum of every 3 years
Colorectal screening	Fecal occult blood test annually starting at age 50 And Flexible sigmoidoscopy every 5 years Or colonoscopy every 10 years Or Double contrast barium enema every 5 years	Fecal occult blood test annually starting at age 50 And Flexible sigmoidoscopy every 5 years Or colonoscopy every 10 years Or Double contrast barium enema every 5 years
Colonoscopy	Starting at age 50, every 1 to 10 years, depending on test used by provider	Starting at age 50, every 1 to 10 years, depending on test used by provider

TEST	FEMALE	MALE
Pap test	• Starting at age 21 (or earlier if sexually active), annually, or every 2 years • After age 30, every 1 to 3 years, depending on test used by provider, and at provider's discretion	
Clinical breast exam	• Starting at age 20, 3 years • Starting at age 40 – yearly	
Mammogram	Starting at age 40 – yearly	
Clinical testicular exam		Starting at age 20, every year
Prostate-specific antigen test and digital rectal exam		Starting at age 50, as indicated by the provider

Prevention

- The terms primary prevention, secondary prevention, and tertiary prevention can be used to describe the focus of activities and the level of prevention.

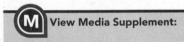 **View Media Supplement:** Health Screening (Video)

LEVEL OF PREVENTION	EXAMPLES OF PREVENTION ACTIVITIES
Primary prevention addresses the needs of healthy clients to promote health and prevent disease with specific protections.	• Immunization programs • Child car seat education • Nutrition and fitness activities • Health education in schools
Secondary prevention focuses on early identification of individuals or communities experiencing illness, providing treatment, and conducting activities that are geared to prevent a worsening health status.	• Communicable disease screening and case finding • Early detection and treatment of diabetes • Exercise programs for older adult clients who are frail
Tertiary prevention aims to prevent the long-term consequences of a chronic illness or disability and to support optimal functioning.	• Prevention of pressure ulcers as a complication of spinal cord injury • Promoting independence for the client who has traumatic brain injury

Nursing Interventions

- Nurses assist clients with many health promotion and disease prevention activities by providing education and guidance. The client's risk factors are examined to identify the aspects that can be modified to attain a healthier lifestyle. The nurse collaborates with the client to adopt mutually agreed upon goals, and identify support systems to attain goals (client will give up unhealthy behaviors and/or adopt healthy behaviors).

  - The nurse identifies and makes appropriate referrals to educational/community/ support resources, based upon assessment information.

  - In order for a client to be successful in achieving a more positive lifestyle, he must recognize the benefits of his actions (recognizing that not smoking reduces the risk of lung cancer) and be able to overcome barriers (he can afford his medication for hypertension).

- Use behavior-change strategies.

  - Identify the client's readiness to receive and act upon health information.

  - Identify interventions acceptable to the client.

  - Help motivate the client to change by setting realistic timelines.

  - Reinforce steps the client makes toward change.

  - Encourage the client to maintain the change.

- Promote healthy lifestyle behaviors by instructing clients to:

  - Minimize or reduce stress.

  - Get adequate sleep and rest.

  - Eat a nutritious diet to achieve and maintain a healthy weight.

  - Avoid saturated fats

  - Participate in regular physical activity most days of the week.

  - While outdoors, wear protective clothing, use sunscreen, and avoid sun exposure between 10 a.m. and 4 p.m.

  - Wear safety gear (bike helmets, knee and elbow pads) when participating in physical activity.

  - Avoid substances such as tobacco products, alcohol, and illegal drugs.

  - Practice safer sex.

  - Seek medical care when necessary, and visit the provider for routine screenings.

CHAPTER 16: HEALTH PROMOTION AND DISEASE PREVENTION

 Application Exercises

1. Match the appropriate level of health care prevention with the preventive activity. Each level can be used more than once.

1. Primary prevention	_____ Blood pressure screening at a senior center
	_____ Driver's education
2. Secondary prevention	_____ Monitored exercise therapy at a cardiac rehabilitation center
	_____ Community cholesterol screening
3. Tertiary prevention	_____ Teaching self-catheterization to a client with a spinal cord injury
	_____ Newborn immunizations

2. A 19-year-old female client has come to the college health clinic for a Pap test. It is her first visit. Which of the following interventions should the nurse perform first to determine the client's need for health promotion and disease prevention?

   A. Measure the client's vital signs.

   B. Encourage the client to be screened for HIV.

   C. Determine the client's risk factors.

   D. Instruct the client to use condoms for birth control.

3. A 21-year-old male client presents to the health clinic for a sore throat. The client tells the nurse that he has not seen a doctor since high school. Which of the following health screenings should the nurse anticipate will be performed for this client?

   A. Testicular cancer

   B. Blood glucose

   C. Fecal occult blood

   D. Prostate-specific antigen

CHAPTER 16: HEALTH PROMOTION AND DISEASE PREVENTION

 Application Exercises Answer Key

1. Match the appropriate level of health care prevention with the preventive activity. Each level can be used more than once.

1. Primary prevention   __2__   Blood pressure screening at a senior center

                               __1__   Driver's education

2. Secondary   __3__   Monitored exercise therapy at a cardiac rehabilitation center
   prevention

                               __2__   Community cholesterol screening

3. Tertiary prevention   __3__   Teaching self-catheterization to a client with a spinal cord injury

                               __1__   Newborn immunizations

 NCLEX® Connection: Health Promotion and Maintenance: Health Promotion/Disease Prevention

2. A 19-year-old female client has come to the college health clinic for a Pap test. It is her first visit. Which of the following interventions should the nurse perform first to determine the client's need for health promotion and disease prevention?

    A. Measure the client's vital signs.

    B. Encourage the client to be screened for HIV.

    C. Determine the client's risk factors.

    D. Instruct the client to use condoms for birth control.

    Using the nursing process, the first action the nurse should take is to assess the client. Assessment of risk factors must occur before health promotion or disease prevention interventions are developed. The nurse should conduct an interview with the client before performing any physical exam. This allows the nurse time to establish rapport with the client prior to any invasive procedures. Stressing the need for HIV screening and instructing the client in the use of birth control may be necessary if the assessment reveals any related risk factors.

 NCLEX® Connection: Health Promotion and Maintenance: Health Promotion/Disease Prevention

3. A 21-year-old male client presents to the health clinic for a sore throat. The client tells the nurse that he has not seen a doctor since high school. Which of the following health screenings should the nurse anticipate will be performed for this client?

    A. Testicular cancer

    B. Blood glucose

    C. Fecal occult blood

    D. Prostate-specific antigen

    The nurse can expect that the client will be screened for testicular cancer. The nurse can also anticipate that the client's blood pressure will be checked, along with his BMI and blood cholesterol. Blood glucose testing begins at 45, and testing for fecal occult blood and prostate-specific antigen usually begins at age 50.

    (N) NCLEX® Connection: Health Promotion and Maintenance: Health Screening

UNIT 2	HEALTH PROMOTION
Section	Nursing Throughout the Lifespan
Chapter 17	**Client Education**

 Overview

- Nurses provide education to individual clients, families, and communities. Factors influencing client education needs include health status, educational level, socioeconomic status, cultural influences, and developmental stage. The nurse may provide information regarding health promotion, illness prevention, and health restoration.

> **(M) View Media Supplement:** Client Education (Video)

- Teaching is an interactive process that is driven by specific client goals.

- Learning is an intentional gain of new information and represents a change in behavior.

- Motivation influences how much and how quickly a person learns.

- Information technology can be used to enhance access to and delivery of knowledge.

- Purposes of client teaching include:

  ○ Providing clients with information and skills to maintain and promote health, and to prevent illness (immunizations, lifestyle changes, prenatal care).

  ○ Providing clients with information about how to restore health (teaching a client how to administer insulin).

  ○ Providing clients with information about how to adapt to permanent illness or injury (ostomy care, learning swallowing techniques, speech therapy).

- Domains of learning:

  ○ Cognitive learning means obtaining new information, being able to apply the information, and being able to evaluate the information. For example, cognitive learning takes place when a client is taught the signs and symptoms of hypoglycemia, and then can verbalize when to notify the provider.

  ○ Affective learning involves feelings, beliefs, and ideals. For example, affective learning takes place when a client listens to the nurse explain life changes necessary to manage diabetes and then discusses feelings regarding the diagnosis.

- o Psychomotor learning is learning how to complete a physical activity or motor skill. For example, psychomotor learning takes place when a client practices preparing insulin injections.

Assessment/Data Collection

- Assess/monitor the client's learning needs.

- Assess the learning environment.

- Assess/monitor the client's learning style (auditory, visual, kinesthetic).

- Identify areas of concern.

- Assess/monitor available resources (financial, social, community).

- Identify the client's developmental stage.

- Determine the client's physical and cognitive ability.

- Identify special needs (visual impairment, decreased manual dexterity).

- Determine the client's motivation and readiness to learn.

Planning

- Identify mutually agreed upon client outcomes.

- Prioritize the learning objectives with the client's needs in mind.

- Use methods that emphasize the client's learning style.

- Select age-appropriate teaching methods/material.

- Provide electronic educational resources as appropriate (CDs, DVDs, computer/PDA software programs).

- Demonstrate use of the Internet in regard to accessing information and support services and how to recognize reliable sources.

- Organize learning activities to move from simple to more complex tasks, and known to unknown concepts.

- Incorporate active participation in the learning process.

- Schedule teaching sessions to coincide with the client's daily activities.

Implementation

- Create an environment conducive to learning (minimize distractions and interruptions, provide for privacy).

- Use therapeutic communication to develop a trusting relationship that allows the client to express areas of concern (active listening, empathy).

- Review previous knowledge and experiences.

- Explain the therapeutic regimen or procedure.

- Present steps building to more complex tasks.

- Demonstrate psychomotor skills.

- Allow time for return demonstrations.

- Provide positive reinforcement.

Evaluation

- Ask the client to explain the information in his own words.

- Observe the client demonstrating the learned activity (best for evaluation of psychomotor learning).

- Use written tools to measure the accuracy of information.

- Request the client's self-evaluation of progress.

- Observe verbal and nonverbal communication.

- Determine the client's ability to use the information over time, but re-evaluate the learning during follow-up telephone calls or during follow-up contacts, such as home health visits or appointments with the provider.

- Revise the care plan as needed.

Factors Affecting Learning

FACTORS THAT ENHANCE LEARNING	BARRIERS TO LEARNING
• Perceived benefit • Cognitive and physical ability • Health and cultural beliefs • Active participation • Age/educational level-appropriate methods	• Fear, anxiety, depression • Physical discomfort, pain, fatigue • Environmental distractions • Health and cultural beliefs • Sensory and perceptual deficits • Psychomotor deficits

CHAPTER 17: CLIENT EDUCATION

 Application Exercises

1. When a nurse is teaching a client how to draw up and mix insulin injections, which of the following best demonstrates that psychomotor learning has taken place?

    A. The client is able to discuss the appropriate technique.

    B. The client is able to demonstrate the appropriate technique.

    C. The client states that he understands.

    D. The client is able to write the steps on a piece of paper.

2. A nurse in a provider's office is collecting data from the mother of a 1-year-old child. The client states that her child is old enough for toilet training. Following an educational session by the nurse, the client now states that her earlier ideas have changed. She is now willing to postpone toilet training until the child is older. Learning has occurred in which of the following domains of learning?

    A. Cognitive

    B. Affective

    C. Psychomotor

    D. Kinesthetic

3. A nurse is providing preoperative teaching for a client who is scheduled for a mastectomy the next day. Which of the following client statements indicates that the client is ready to learn?

    A. "I don't want my spouse to see my incision."

    B. "Will you be able to give me pain medicine after the surgery?"

    C. "Can you tell me about how long the surgery will take?"

    D. "My roommate listens to everything I say."

CHAPTER 17: CLIENT EDUCATION

 Application Exercises Answer Key

1. When a nurse is teaching a client how to draw up and mix insulin injections, which of the following best demonstrates that psychomotor learning has taken place?

>   A. The client is able to discuss the appropriate technique.
>
>   **B. The client is able to demonstrate the appropriate technique.**
>
>   C. The client states that he understands.
>
>   D. The client is able to write the steps on a piece of paper.
>
>   **Demonstrating the appropriate technique indicates that psychomotor learning has taking place. Discussing the appropriate technique, stating understanding, and writing down steps will demonstrate learning, but only actual demonstration by the client will allow the nurse to evaluate psychomotor learning.**

(N) **NCLEX® Connection: Health Promotion and Maintenance, Principles of Teaching/Learning**

2. A nurse in a provider's office is collecting data from the mother of a 1-year-old child. The client states that her child is old enough for toilet training. Following an educational session by the nurse, the client now states that her earlier ideas have changed. She is now willing to postpone toilet training until the child is older. Learning has occurred in which of the following domains of learning?

>   A. Cognitive
>
>   **B. Affective**
>
>   C. Psychomotor
>
>   D. Kinesthetic
>
>   **Affective learning has taken place, as evidenced by the client's changed ideas regarding toilet training. Cognitive learning would be demonstrated if the client could state the behaviors that her child will demonstrate when ready to toilet train. Psychomotor learning would be demonstrated if the client performed the proper techniques for introducing her child to toilet training. Kinesthetic learning is a learning style, not a domain of learning.**

(N) **NCLEX® Connection: Promotion and Maintenance, Principles of Teaching/Learning**

3. A nurse is providing preoperative teaching for a client who is scheduled for a mastectomy the next day. Which of the following client statements indicates that the client is ready to learn?

    A. "I don't want my spouse to see my incision."

    B. "Will you be able to give me pain medicine after the surgery?"

    C. "Can you tell me about how long the surgery will take?"

    D. "My roommate listens to everything I say."

Asking a concrete question about the surgery indicates that the client is ready to discuss the surgery. The client's new diagnosis of cancer may cause anxiety, fear, or depression, all of which can interfere with the learning process. The client's concern about her spouse seeing the incision may indicate anxiety or depression. The client's request for pain medicine may indicate fear and anxiety. The lack of privacy due to the presence of a roommate may be a barrier to learning.

NCLEX® Connection: Health Promotion and Maintenance, Principles of Teaching/Learning

UNIT 2	HEALTH PROMOTION
Section	Nursing Throughout the Lifespan
Chapter 18	Infant (Birth to 1 Year)

Expected Growth and Development

- Physical Development

  ○ The infant's posterior fontanel closes by 2 to 3 months of age.

  ○ The infant's anterior fontanel closes by 12 to 18 months of age.

  ○ The infant's size is tracked by weight, height, and head circumference.

    ■ Weight: The infant gains about 150 to 210 g (about 5 to 7 oz) per month in the first 6 months. Birth weight should double by 4 to 6 months and the infant triples birth weight by the end of the first year.

    ■ Height: The infant grows about 2.5 cm (1 in) per month in the first 6 months, and then about 1.25 cm (0.5 in) per month until the end of the first year.

    ■ Head circumference: The circumference of the infant's head increases about 1.25 cm (0.5 in) per month in the first 6 months and then about 0.5 cm (0.2 in) between 6 to 12 months.

  ○ Dentition – 6 to 8 teeth erupt in the infant's mouth by the end of the first year.

    ■ Teething pain can be eased using cold teething rings, over-the-counter teething gels, or acetaminophen (Tylenol) and/or ibuprofen (Advil). Ibuprofen should only be given to children over the age of 6 months.

    ■ Clean the infant's teeth using a cool, wet washcloth.

    ■ Bottles should not be given to infants when they are falling asleep. This will help to avoid prolonged exposure to milk or juice that can cause dental caries (bottle mouth syndrome).

  ○ Fine and Gross Motor Development

AGE	GROSS MOTOR SKILLS	FINE MOTOR SKILLS
1 month	Demonstrates head lag	Has a present grasp reflex
2 months	Lifts head off mattress	Holds hands in an open position
3 months	Raises head and shoulders off mattress	No longer has a grasp reflex Keeps hands loosely open
4 months	Rolls from back to side	Places objects in mouth
5 months	Rolls from front to back	Uses palmar grasp dominantly

AGE	GROSS MOTOR SKILLS	FINE MOTOR SKILLS
6 months	Rolls from back to front	Holds bottle
7 months	Bears full weight on feet	Moves objects from hand to hand
8 months	Sits unsupported	Begins using pincer grasp
9 months	Pulls to a standing position	Has a crude pincer grasp
10 months	Changes from prone to sitting position	Grasps rattle by its handle
11 months	Walks while holding on to something	Can place objects into a container
12 months	Sits down from a standing position without assistance	Tries to build a two-block tower without success

- Cognitive Development
  - Piaget – Sensorimotor stage (birth to 24 months)
    - There are three things that occur during this time: separation, object permanence, and mental representation.
      - Separation is when infants learn to separate themselves from other objects in the environment.
      - Object permanence occurs at about 9 months of age. Object permanence is the process by which an infant knows that the object still exists when it is hidden from view.
      - Mental representation is the recognition of symbols.
  - Language Development
    - Responds to noises
    - Vocalizes with "ooos" and "aahs"
    - Laughs and squeals
    - Turns head to the sound of a rattle
    - Pronounces single-syllable words
    - Begins speaking two and then three-word phrases
- Psychosocial Development
  - An infant's stage of psychosocial development, according to Erikson, is trust vs. mistrust.
    - Infants trust that their feeding, comfort, stimulation, and caring needs will be met.
    - Social development is initially influenced by the infant's reflexive behavior and includes attachment, separation recognition/anxiety, and stranger fear.

- Attachment is seen when the infant begins to bond with his parents. This development occurs within the first month, but actually begins before the birth of the child. The process is enhanced when the infant and parents are in good health, have positive feeding experiences, and receive adequate rest.

- Separation recognition occurs during the first year as the infant learns his physical boundaries from that of other people. Learning how to respond to people in his environment is the next phase of development. Positive interactions with parents, siblings, and other caregivers help to establish trust.

- Separation anxiety develops between 4 and 8 months of age. Infants will protest loudly when separated from parents, which can cause considerable anxiety for the parents.

- Stranger fear becomes evident between ages 6 to 8 months, when children are less likely to accept strangers.

- Self-Concept Development

  - By the end of the first year, infants will be able to distinguish themselves as being separate from their parents.

- Body-Image Changes

  - The infant discovers that his mouth is a pleasure producer.

  - Hands and feet are seen as objects of play.

  - The infant discovers that smiling causes others to react.

- Age-Appropriate Activities

  - Infants have short attention spans and do not interact with other children during play (solitary play). Appropriate toys and activities that stimulate the senses and encourage development include:

    - Rattles.

    - Mobiles.

    - Teething toys.

    - Nesting toys.

    - Playing pat-a-cake.

    - Playing with balls.

    - Reading books.

Health Promotion

- Immunizations

  - 2010 Centers for Disease Control and Prevention (CDC) immunization recommendations (see www.cdc.gov for updates) for healthy infants less than 12 months include:

    - Birth – hepatitis B (Hep B)

- 2 months – Diphtheria and tetanus toxoids and pertussis (DTaP), rotavirus vaccine (RV), inactivated poliovirus (IPV), *Haemophilus influenzae* type B (Hib), pneumococcal vaccine (PCV), and Hep B

- 4 months – DTaP, RV, IPV, Hib, PVC

- 6 months – DTaP, IPV (6 to 18 months), PVC, Hep B (6 to 12 months). RotaTeq, an alternative formulation for RV, requires 3 doses that must be completed by 32 weeks.

- 6 to 12 months – Seasonal influenza vaccination yearly. The trivalent inactivated influenza vaccine (TIV) is available as an intramuscular injection.

- Nutrition

  ○ Feeding alternatives for an infant:

    - Breastfeeding provides a complete diet for the infant during the first 6 months of life and is recommended by health care providers.

    - Iron-fortified formula is an acceptable alternative to breast milk. Cow's milk is not recommended.

  ○ Solids can be introduced between 4 and 6 months of age.

    - Indicators for readiness include voluntary control of the head and trunk, hunger less than 4 hr after vigorous nursing or intake of 8 oz of formula, and interest of the infant.

    - Iron-fortified rice cereal should be offered first.

    - New foods should be introduced one at a time over a 5- to 7-day period to observe for signs of allergy or intolerance, which may include fussiness, rash, vomiting, diarrhea, or constipation. Vegetables or fruits are first started between 6 and 8 months of age, and after both have been introduced, meats may be added.

    - Milk, eggs, wheat, citrus fruits, peanuts, peanut butter, and honey should be delayed until the first year of life.

    - Table foods that are cooked, chopped, and unseasoned are appropriate by 9 months of age.

    - Appropriate finger foods include ripe bananas, toast strips, graham crackers, cheese cubes, noodles, and peeled chunks of apples, pears, and peaches.

    - Breast milk/formula should be decreased as intake of solid foods increases.

    - Parents should be encouraged to use iron-enriched foods after the infant is 6 months of age.

  ○ Weaning can be accomplished when the infant is able to drink from a cup (sometime after 6 months).

    - Replace one of the infant's feedings with breast milk or formula in a cup.

    - The infant's bedtime feeding is the last one to be replaced.

- Injury Prevention
  - Aspiration of Foreign Objects
    - Avoid small objects, such as grapes, coins, and candy, that can become lodged in the throat.
    - Provide age-appropriate toys.
    - Check clothing for safety hazards (loose buttons)
  - Bodily harm
    - Keep sharp objects out of the infant's reach.
    - Keep the infant away from heavy objects that can be pulled down onto her.
    - Do not leave infants alone with animals.
    - Monitor for shaken baby syndrome.
  - Burns
    - Check the temperature of bath water.
    - Turn down the thermostat on the hot water heater.
    - Have working smoke detectors in the home.
    - Turn handles of pots and pans to the back of the stove.
    - Apply sunscreen when outdoors during daylight hours.
    - Cover electrical outlets.
  - Drowning
    - Do not leave the infant unattended in the bathtub.
  - Falls
    - Keep the crib mattress in the lowest position with the rails all the way up.
    - Use restraints in infant seats.
    - Place the infant seat on the ground or floor if used outside of the car, and do not leave it unattended or on elevated surfaces.
    - Use safety gates across stairs.
  - Poisoning
    - Avoid exposing the infant to lead paint.
    - Keep toxins and plants out of the infant's reach.
    - Keep safety locks on cabinets that contain cleaners and other household chemicals.
    - Keep a poison control number near the phone.
    - Keep medications in childproof containers away from the infant's reach.
    - Have a working carbon monoxide detector in the home.

    o   Motor-vehicle Injuries

- Use an approved rear-facing car seat in the back seat, preferably in the middle, (away from air bags and side impact) to transport the infant. Infants should be in rear-facing car seats for the first year of life and until they weigh 9.1 kg (20 lb). It is recommended to have the infant ride rear facing until he has reached the weight limit allowed for the car seat (as long as the top of the infant's head is below the top of the seat back). In addition, a five-point harness or T-shield should be part of the convertible restraint.

    o   Suffocation

- Avoid plastic bags.
- Keep balloons away from infants.
- Be sure the crib mattress fits tightly.
- Ensure crib slats are no farther apart than 6 cm (2.4 in).
- Remove crib mobiles or crib gyms by 4 to 5 months of age.
- Do not use pillows in the crib.
- Place the infant on the back for sleep.
- Keep toys that have small parts out of reach.
- Remove drawstrings from jackets and other clothing.

CHAPTER 18: INFANT (BIRTH TO 1 YEAR)

(A) Application Exercises

Scenario: A 6-month-old infant is brought to the provider for a well-infant check. The infant weighed 3.2 kg (7 lb) at birth. Currently, he weighs 7.7 kg (17 lb).

1. Is the infant's weight appropriate for this age?

2. The nurse is providing teaching to the infant's mother about gross motor development. Which of the following gross motor skills are expected findings in the next 3 months? (Select all that apply.)

_____ Rolls from back to front

_____ Bears weight on legs

_____ Walks holding onto furniture

_____ Sits unsupported

_____ Sits down from a standing position

3. What immunizations should the infant receive at this visit if his previous immunizations are current?

4. The nurse is providing teaching to the infant's mother regarding safety. Which of the following statements by the mother indicates an understanding of safety for the infant?

   A. "My baby loved to play with his crib gym, but I took it away from him."

   B. "I just bought a soft mattress so my baby will sleep better."

   C. "My baby really likes riding in the car now that he can sit facing forward."

   D. "I just bought a child-safety gate that folds like an accordion."

CHAPTER 18: INFANT (BIRTH TO 1 YEAR)

 Application Exercises Answer Key

Scenario: A 6-month-old infant is brought to the provider for a well-infant check. The infant weighed 3.2 kg (7 lb) at birth. Currently, he weighs 7.7 kg (17 lb).

1. Is the infant's weight appropriate for this age?

> **Yes. The infant should gain 0.7 kg (1.5 lb) per month in the first 6 months. The infant has gained the appropriate amount of weight.**

 NCLEX® Connection: Safety and Infection Control, Developmental Stages and Transitions

2. The nurse is providing teaching to the infant's mother about gross motor development. Which of the following gross motor skills are expected findings in the next 3 months? (Select all that apply.)

> __X__ **Rolls from back to front**
>
> __X__ **Bears weight on legs**
>
> _____ Walks holding onto furniture
>
> __X__ **Sits unsupported**
>
> _____ Sits down from a standing position

> **The infant should be able to roll from back to front by 6 months, bear weight on legs by 7 months, and sit unsupported by 8 months. The infant is not expected to walk holding onto furniture until 11 months and sit down from a standing position until 12 months.**

 NCLEX® Connection: Safety and Infection Control, Developmental Stages and Transitions

3. What immunizations should the infant receive at this visit if his previous immunizations are current?

> **Hepatitis B (6 to 12 months of age), RV, DTaP, PCV, IPV (6 to 18 months of age); in addition, the infant should receive the annual influenza vaccine at 6 to 12 months of age.**

 NCLEX® Connection: Health Promotion and Maintenance, Health Promotion/Disease Prevention

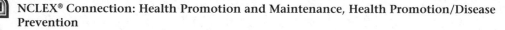

4. The nurse is providing teaching to the infant's mother regarding safety. Which of the following statements by the mother indicates an understanding of safety for the infant?

   A. "My baby loved to play with his crib gym but I took it away from him."

   B. "I just bought a soft mattress so my baby will sleep better."

   C. "My baby really likes riding in the car now that he can sit facing forward."

   D. "I just bought a child-safety gate that folds like an accordion."

   Crib gyms and mobiles should be removed by 4 months, as injury can occur from choking or strangulation. The infant's crib mattress should be firm and fit tightly to prevent suffocation. The infant needs to remain in the backwards facing position until 1 year of age and a weight of 20 lb. Child-safety gates should expand by a horizontal mechanism and not like an accordion to prevent injury to hands and arms.

   NCLEX® Connection: Safety and Infection Control, Accident/Injury Prevention

Expected Growth and Development

- Physical Development

    o The toddler's anterior fontanel closes by 18 months of age.

    o Weight: At 24 months, the toddler should weigh four times his birth weight.

    o Height: The toddler grows by 7.5 cm (3 in) per year.

    o Fine and gross motor skills

AGE	GROSS MOTOR SKILLS	FINE MOTOR SKILLS
15 months	Walks without help. Creeps up stairs.	Uses cup well. Builds tower of two blocks.
18 months	Assumes standing position. Jumps in place with both feet.	Manages spoon without rotation. Turns pages in book two or three at a time.
2 years	Walks up and down stairs.	Builds a tower with six or seven blocks.
2.5 years	Jumps with both feet. Stands on one foot momentarily.	Draws circles. Has good hand-finger coordination.

- Cognitive Development

    o Piaget – Sensorimotor transitions to preoperational.

        ▪ The concept of object permanence is developed fully.

        ▪ Toddlers have and demonstrate memories of events that relate to them.

        ▪ Domestic mimicry is evident (playing house).

        ▪ Preoperational thought does not allow toddlers to understand other viewpoints, but it does allow them to symbolize objects and people in order to imitate activities seen previously.

    o Language Development

        ▪ Language increases to about 400 words with toddlers speaking in two- to three-word phrases.

- Psychosocial Development

  o A toddler's stage of psychosocial development, according to Erikson, is autonomy vs shame and doubt.

    ▪ Independence is paramount for the toddler who is attempting to do everything for himself.

    ▪ Separation anxiety continues to occur when a parent leaves the child.

  o Moral Development

    ▪ Moral development is closely associated with cognitive development.

    ▪ Egocentric – Toddlers are unable to see another's perspective; they can only view things from their point of view.

    ▪ The toddler's punishment and obedience orientation begins with a sense that good behavior is rewarded and bad behavior is punished.

  o Self-Concept Development

    ▪ Toddlers progressively see themselves as separate from their parents and increase their explorations away from them.

  o Body-Image Changes

    ▪ The toddler appreciates the usefulness of various body parts.

    ▪ Toddlers develop gender identity by age 3.

- Age-Appropriate Activities

  o Solitary play evolves into parallel play where the toddler observes other children and then may engage in activities nearby.

  o Appropriate activities include:

    ▪ Filling and emptying containers

    ▪ Playing with blocks

    ▪ Looking at books

    ▪ Playing with toys that can be pushed and pulled

    ▪ Tossing a ball

  o Temper tantrums result when the toddler is frustrated with restrictions on independence. Providing consistent, age-appropriate expectations helps the toddler work through his frustration.

  o Toilet training can begin when it is recognized that the child has the sensation of needing to urinate or defecate. Parents should demonstrate patience and consistency in toilet training their child. Nighttime control may develop last of all.

  o Discipline should be consistent with well-defined boundaries that are established to develop appropriate social behavior.

Health Promotion

- Immunizations

  o Centers for Disease Control and Prevention (CDC) immunization recommendations (http://www.cdc.gov) for healthy toddlers 12 months to 3 years of age include:

    - 12 to 15 months – Inactivated poliovirus (IPV) (6 to 18 months); *Haemophilus influenzae* type B (Hib); pneumococcal vaccine (PCV); measles, mumps, and rubella (MMR); and varicella.

    - 12 to 23 months – Hepatitis A (Hep A), given in two doses, at least 6 months apart.

    - 15 to 18 months – Diphtheria and tetanus toxoids and pertussis (DTaP).

    - 12 to 36 months – Yearly seasonal trivalent inactivated influenza vaccine (TIV). At age 2, toddlers can receive the live, attenuated influenza vaccine (LAIV) by nasal spray.

- Nutrition

  o Toddlers are picky eaters with repeated requests for favorite foods.

  o A toddler should consume 24 to 30 oz of milk per day and may switch from drinking whole milk to drinking low-fat (2% fat) milk at 2 years of age.

  o Limit juice to 4 to 6 oz a day.

  o Food serving size is 1 tbsp for each year of age.

  o Exposure to a new food may need to occur 8 to 15 times before the child develops an acceptance of it.

  o If there is a family history of allergy, then cow's milk, chocolate, citrus fruits, egg white, seafood, and nut butters may be gradually introduced while monitoring the child for reactions.

  o Toddlers prefer finger foods because of their increasing autonomy.

  o Regular meal times and nutritious snacks best meet nutrient needs.

  o Snacks or desserts that are high in sugar, fat, or sodium should be avoided.

  o Avoid foods that are potential choking hazards (nuts, grapes, hot dogs, peanut butter, raw carrots, tough meats, and popcorn).

  o Always provide adult supervision during snack and mealtimes.

  o During food preparation, cut small bite-sized pieces to make them easier to swallow and to prevent choking.

  o Do not allow the child to engage in drinking or eating during play activities or while lying down.

  o Suggest parents follow U.S. Department of Agriculture nutrition recommendations. (http://www.mypyramid.gov)

- Injury Prevention
  - Aspiration of Foreign Objects
    - Avoid small objects, such as grapes, coins, and candy that can become lodged in the throat.
    - Keep toys with small parts out of reach.
    - Provide age-appropriate toys.
    - Check clothing for safety hazards such as loose buttons.
    - Keep balloons away from toddlers.
  - Bodily Harm
    - Keep sharp objects out of the toddler's reach.
    - Keep firearms in a locked box or cabinet.
    - Do not leave toddlers unattended with animals present.
    - Teach stranger safety.
  - Burns
    - Check the temperature of bath water.
    - Turn down the thermostat on the hot water heater.
    - Have working smoke detectors in the home.
    - Turn pot handles toward the back of the stove.
    - Cover electrical outlets.
    - Use sunscreen when outside.
  - Drowning
    - Do not leave the toddler unattended in the bathtub.
    - Keep toilet lids closed.
    - Closely supervise the child at the pool or any other body of water.
    - Teach children to swim.
  - Falls
    - Keep doors and windows locked.
    - Keep the crib mattress in the lowest position with the rails all the way up.
    - Use safety gates across stairs.
  - Motor-vehicle injuries
    - Use an approved car seat in the back seat, away from air bags.
    - The toddler should be in a rear-facing car seat until he weighs 9.1 kg (20 lb) and is 1 year old. The toddler can then sit in an approved forward-facing car seat in the back seat. Usually the toddler can use this car seat until 4 years and/or 40 lb.

- Children who meet the weight requirement but are not 1 year of age should still remain rear facing. In addition, a five-point harness or T-shield should be part of the convertible restraint.

- Poisoning

  - Avoid exposure to lead paint.

  - Place safety locks on cabinets with cleaners and other chemicals.

  - Keep plants out of reach.

  - Keep the poison control number near the phone.

  - Keep medications in childproof containers out of the child's reach.

  - Have a working carbon monoxide detector in the home.

- Suffocation

  - Avoid plastic bags.

  - Be sure the crib mattress fits tightly.

  - Ensure crib slats are no further apart than 6 cm (2.4 in).

  - Keep pillows out of the crib.

  - Remove drawstrings from jackets and other clothing.

CHAPTER 19: TODDLER (1 TO 3 YEARS)

 Application Exercises

1. A nurse is teaching a class on accident prevention to a group of parents with toddlers. Which of the following accident-prevention strategies should the nurse teach the parents to implement? (Select all that apply.)

_____ Keep toxic agents in locked cabinets.

_____ Keep toilet seats up.

_____ Turn pot handles toward the back of the stove.

_____ Place safety gates across stairways.

_____ Raise the setting on the hot water heater.

_____ Place fences around swimming pools.

2. Match the appropriate immunizations with the age of administration.

_____ *Haemophilus influenzae* type B (Hib); pneumococcal vaccine (PCV); inactivated poliovirus (IPV) (6 to 18 months); measles, mumps, and rubella (MMR); and varicella.

A. 15 to 18 months

_____ Hepatitis A (Hep A), given in two doses, at least 6 months apart.

B. 12 to 36 months

_____ Diphtheria and tetanus toxoids and pertussis (DTaP).

C. 12 to 15 months

_____ Yearly trivalent inactivated influenza vaccine (TIV).

D. 12 to 23 months

3. Which of the following are appropriate play activities for a toddler? (Select all that apply.)

_____ Building simple models

_____ Playing on an organized sport team

_____ Filling and emptying containers

_____ Playing with blocks

_____ Looking at books

4. A nurse is providing teaching to the parents of toddler. Which of the following should the nurse include regarding discipline?

A. Establish consistent boundaries.

B. Place the child in a room with the door closed.

C. Have the child learn by trial and error.

D. Use favorite snacks as rewards.

5. A mother tells the nurse that her 2-year-old child has temper tantrums. The child says "no" every time the mother tries to help her get dressed. The nurse explains that, developmentally, the toddler is

    A. trying to increase her independence.

    B. developing a sense of trust.

    C. manifesting an anger management problem.

    D. attempting to finish a project she started.

CHAPTER 19: TODDLER (1 TO 3 YEARS)

 Application Exercises Answer Key

1. A nurse is teaching a class on accident prevention to a group of parents with toddlers. Which of the following accident-prevention strategies should the nurse teach the parents to implement? (Select all that apply.)

__X__	**Keep toxic agents in locked cabinets.**
_____	Keep toilet seats up.
__X__	**Turn pot handles toward the back of the stove.**
__X__	**Place safety gates across stairways.**
_____	Raise the setting on the hot water heater.
__X__	**Place fences around swimming pools.**

Keeping toxic agents out of reach, turning pot handles to the back of the stove, and placing safety gates across stairways and fences around pools are ways to prevent accidents. Toilet seats should be kept down to prevent drowning, and the temperature on the hot water heater should be lowered to prevent burns.

(N) NCLEX® Connection: Safety and Infection Control, Accident/Injury Prevention

2. Match the appropriate immunizations with the age of administration.

__C__	Haemophilus influenzae type B (Hib); pneumococcal vaccine (PCV); inactivated poliovirus (IPV) (6 to 18 months); measles, mumps, and rubella (MMR); and varicella.	A. 15 to 18 months
__D__	Hepatitis A (Hep A), given in two doses, at least 6 months apart.	B. 12 to 36 months
__A__	Diphtheria and tetanus toxoids and pertussis (DTaP).	C. 12 to 15 months
__B__	Yearly trivalent inactivated influenza vaccine (TIV).	D. 12 to 23 months

(N) NCLEX® Connection: Health Promotion and Maintenance, Health Promotion/Disease Prevention

3. Which of the following are appropriate play activities for a toddler? (Select all that apply.)

_____   Building simple models

_____   Playing on an organized sport team

__X__   **Filling and emptying containers**

__X__   **Playing with blocks**

__X__   **Looking at books**

Filling and emptying containers, playing with blocks, and looking at books are appropriate play activities for a toddler. Building simple models and playing on an organized sport team are more appropriate for a school-age child.

 NCLEX® Connection: Health Promotion and Maintenance, Developmental Stages and Transitions

4. A nurse is providing teaching to the parents of toddler. Which of the following should the nurse include regarding discipline?

    A. Establish consistent boundaries.

    B. Place the child in a room with the door closed.

    C. Have the child learn by trial and error.

    D. Use favorite snacks as rewards.

Toddlers need to have consistent boundaries established for discipline to be effective. Placing the child in a room with the door closed may cause anxiety and fear to develop. Trial and error lacks consistent boundaries and may allow the toddler to experience unhealthy consequences. Using favorite foods as rewards may promote unhealthy eating habits.

 NCLEX® Connection: Health Promotion and Maintenance, Developmental Stages and Transitions

5. A mother tells the nurse that her 2-year-old child has temper tantrums. The child says "no" every time the mother tries to help her get dressed. The nurse explains that, developmentally, the toddler is

    A. trying to increase her independence.

    B. developing a sense of trust.

    C. manifesting an anger management problem.

    D. attempting to finish a project she started.

Toddlers express a drive for independence by opposing the desires of those in authority and attempting to do everything themselves. Developing trust is a developmental task for infants, and finishing a project is a developmental task of school-age children. This behavior is normal for a 2-year-old child and is not indicative of an anger management problem.

 NCLEX® Connection: Health Promotion and Maintenance, Developmental Stages and Transitions

UNIT 2	HEALTH PROMOTION
Section	Nursing Throughout the Lifespan
Chapter 20	Preschooler (3 to 6 Years)

Expected Growth and Development

- Physical Development

  o Weight: The preschooler should gain about 2 to 3 kg (4.5 to 6.5 lb) per year.

  o Height: The preschooler should grow about 6.2 to 7.5 cm (2.5 to 3 inches) per year.

    ▪ The preschooler's body evolves away from the characteristically unsteady wide stance and protruding abdomen of the toddler to the more graceful, posturally erect, and sturdy physicality of this age group.

  o Fine and gross motor skills

    ▪ Preschoolers should show an improvement in fine motor skills, such as copying figures on paper and dressing themselves.

AGE	GROSS MOTOR SKILLS
3 years old	• Rides a tricycle • Jumps off bottom step • Stands on one foot for a few seconds
4 years old	• Skips and hops on one foot • Throws ball overhead
5 years old	• Jumps rope • Is capable of walking backward with heel to toe • Moves up and down stairs easily

- Cognitive Development

  o Piaget – Preschoolers are still in the preoperational phase of cognitive development. They participate in preconceptual thought (from 2 to 4 years of age) and intuitive thought (from 4 to 7 years of age).

- Preconceptual thought – Preschoolers make judgments based on visual appearances. Misconceptions in thinking during this stage include:

  □ Artificialism – Everything is made by humans.

  □ Animism – Inanimate objects are alive.

  □ Imminent justice – A universal code exists that determines law and order.

- Intuitive thought – Preschoolers can classify information and become aware of cause-and-effect relationships.

  o Time – The preschooler begins to understand the concepts of the past, present, and future. By the end of the preschool years, the child may comprehend days of the week.

  o Language – The preschooler's vocabulary continues to increase. The preschooler can now speak in sentences, is able to identify colors, and enjoys talking.

- Psychosocial Development

  o The preschooler's stage of psychosocial development, according to Erikson, is initiative vs. guilt.

    - The preschooler may take on many new experiences despite not having all of the physical abilities necessary to be successful at everything. Guilt may occur when children are unable to accomplish a task and believe they have misbehaved. Guiding preschoolers to attempt activities within their capabilities while setting limits is appropriate.

  o Moral Development

    - Preschoolers continue in the good-bad orientation of the toddler years but begin to understand behaviors in terms of what is socially acceptable.

  o Self-Concept Development

    - The preschooler feels good about himself with regard to mastering skills, such as dressing and feeding, that allow independence. During stress, insecurity, or illness, a preschooler may regress to previous immature behaviors or develop habits such as nose picking, bed wetting, or thumb sucking.

  o Body-Image Changes

    - Mistaken perceptions of reality coupled with misconceptions in thinking lead to active fantasies and fears. The greatest fear is that of bodily harm, thus fear of the dark and of animals.

    - Sex-role identification is occurring.

  o Social Development

    - During the preschool time period, children generally do not exhibit stranger anxiety and have less separation anxiety. However, prolonged separation, such as during hospitalization, can provoke anxiety. Favorite toys and play should be used to help ease a preschooler's fears.

    - Pretend play is healthy and allows children to determine the difference between reality and fantasy.

- Sleep disturbances frequently occur during early childhood, and problems range from difficulties going to bed to night terrors. Advise parents to:

  □ Assess whether or not the bedtime is too early if the child is still taking a nap. The average preschooler needs about 12 hr of sleep a day. Some preschoolers still require a daytime nap.

  □ Keep a consistent bedtime routine.

  □ Use a night-light.

  □ Reassure the child who has been frightened, but avoid having the child sleep with them.

- Age-Appropriate Activities

  ○ Parallel play shifts to associative play during the preschool years. Play is not highly organized, but cooperation does exist between children. Appropriate activities include:

    - Playing ball.

    - Putting puzzles together.

    - Riding tricycles.

    - Pretend and dress-up activities.

    - Role play.

    - Painting.

    - Sewing cards and beads.

    - Reading books.

Health Promotion

- Immunizations

  ○ Centers for Disease Control (CDC) immunization recommendations (http://www.cdc.gov) for healthy preschool children 3 to 6 years of age include:

    - 4 to 6 years – diphtheria and tetanus toxoids and pertussis (DTaP); measles, mumps, and rubella (MMR); varicella; and inactivated poliovirus (IPV).

    - Yearly seasonal influenza vaccine: trivalent inactivated influenza vaccine (TIV) or live, attenuated influenza vaccine (LAIV) by nasal spray.

- Health Screenings

  ○ Vision screening is routinely done in the preschool population as part of the prekindergarten physical exam. Visual impairments such as myopia and amblyopia can be detected and treated before poor visual acuity impairs the learning environment.

- Nutrition

  ○ A preschooler consumes about half the amount of energy that an adult does (1,800 kcal).

- o Picky eating remains a problem for some preschoolers, but often by age 5 they become a bit more willing to sample different foods.

- o Preschoolers need 13 to 19 g/day of complete protein in addition to adequate calcium, iron, folate, and vitamins A and C.

- o Parents need to ensure that their child is receiving a balance of nutrients. Healthy food recommendations can be found at the U.S. Department of Agriculture Web site (http://www.mypyramid.gov).

- • Injury Prevention

  - o Bodily harm

    - ▪ Keep firearms in a locked cabinet or container.

    - ▪ Teach stranger safety.

    - ▪ Wear helmets when riding a bicycle or tricycle.

      - □ Wear protective equipment when participating in physical activity (helmet and pads).

  - o Burns

    - ▪ Turn down the thermostat on the hot water heater.

    - ▪ Have working smoke detectors in the home.

    - ▪ Use sunscreen when outside.

  - o Drowning

    - ▪ Do not leave the child unattended in the bathtub.

    - ▪ Closely supervise the child at the pool or any other body of water.

    - ▪ Teach children to swim.

  - o Motor-vehicle Injuries

    - ▪ The preschooler should sit in an approved forward-facing car seat in the back seat, away from airbags. Usually preschoolers can remain in this car seat until 4 years of age and/or 40 lbs. When the preschooler has outgrown this car seat, a booster seat should be used in the back seat. The child should be restrained in a car seat or booster chair until adult seat belts fit correctly. Laws may vary from state to state and requirements may be up to a weight of 80 lb and a height of 4 feet 9 inches, which is when adult seat belts will most likely fit correctly.

  - o Poisoning

    - ▪ Avoid exposure to lead paint.

    - ▪ Keep plants out of reach.

    - ▪ Place safety locks on cabinets with cleaners and other chemicals.

    - ▪ Keep the poison control number near the phone.

    - ▪ Keep medications in childproof containers out of the child's reach.

    - ▪ Have a working carbon monoxide detector in the home.

CHAPTER 20: PRESCHOOLER (3 TO 6 YEARS)

Ⓐ Application Exercises

Scenario: A nurse is caring for a 4-year-old child who is brought to the clinic by her father. The father states that the child is put to bed at 8:30 p.m. every night and wakes up at about 7:30 a.m. every morning, but she often lays in bed talking to herself or gets up a couple times before falling asleep 40 min later. The child attends a preschool, where each afternoon the children take a 2-hr afternoon nap.

1. Which of the following recommendations should the nurse make to improve the child's sleep behavior?

    A. Offer the child a snack of her favorite treat right before bedtime.

    B. Allow the child to watch an extra 30 min of TV in the evening.

    C. Change the child's bedtime to 9 p.m. on days she takes an afternoon nap.

    D. Request the preschool to limit her nap time to 1 hr.

2. The father tells the nurse that he is concerned that his child may not be ready for kindergarten. What developmental tasks should the child currently be doing to indicate that her growth and development is appropriate for her age? (Select all that apply.)

    _____ Demonstrates a good understanding of time

    _____ Able to skip

    _____ Able to ride a tricycle

    _____ Demonstrates good coordination

    _____ Draws copies of shapes on paper

    _____ Speaks in sentences

3. Which of the following developmental tasks should the nurse tell the father is appropriate to be achieved during the preschool years?

    A. Using a knife to cut meat at mealtime

    B. Dressing independently

    C. Following several directions at once

    D. Comprehending satire

4. Which of the following immunizations should this child receive at this health visit if her immunizations are up-to-date? (Select all that apply.)

    _____ Hepatitis A (Hep A), given in two doses, at least 6 months apart

    _____ Diphtheria and tetanus toxoids and pertussis (DTaP)

    _____ Inactivated poliovirus (IPV)

    _____ Measles, mumps, and rubella (MMR)

    _____ Varicella

    _____ Trivalent inactivated influenza vaccine (TIV)

CHAPTER 20: PRESCHOOLER (3 TO 6 YEARS)

(A) Application Exercises Answer Key

Scenario: A nurse is caring for a 4-year-old child who is brought to the clinic by her father. The father states that the child is put to bed at 8:30 p.m. every night and wakes up at about 7:30 a.m. every morning, but she often lays in bed talking to herself or gets up a couple times before falling asleep 40 min later. The child attends a preschool, where each afternoon the children take a 2-hr afternoon nap.

1. Which of the following recommendations should the nurse make to improve the child's sleep behavior?

   A. Offer the child a snack of her favorite treat right before bedtime.

   B. Allow the child to watch an extra 30 min of TV in the evening.

   C. Change the child's bedtime to 9 p.m. on days she takes an afternoon nap.

   D. Request the preschool to limit her nap time to 1 hr.

   A preschool-age child may start to need less sleep, so putting the child to bed 30 min later will be the least disruptive way to improve the child's sleep behavior. Eating a snack, especially one with a high sugar content, and watching TV will provide stimulation that will make it more difficult for the child to fall asleep. It is impractical to ask the preschool to limit the child's nap as this may be disruptive as all of the children are probably required to nap for that amount of time. Also, if the child is napping for that amount of time, it is most likely the child needs that rest during the day.

    NCLEX® Connection: Health Promotion and Maintenance, Aging Process

2. The father tells the nurse that he is concerned that his child may not be ready for kindergarten. What developmental tasks should the child currently be doing to indicate that her growth and development is appropriate for her age? (Select all that apply.)

	Demonstrates a good understanding of time
X	**Able to skip**
X	**Able to ride a tricycle**
	Demonstrates good coordination
X	**Draws copies of shapes on paper**
X	**Speaks in sentences**

   Able to skip, able to ride a tricycle, draws copies of shapes, and speaks in sentences are appropriate developmental tasks. A good understanding of time and good coordination are usually achieved during the school-age years.

   (N) **NCLEX® Connection: Health Promotion and Maintenance, Developmental Stages and Transitions**

3. Which of the following developmental tasks should the nurse tell the father is appropriate to be achieved during the preschool years?

> A. Using a knife to cut meat at mealtime
>
> **B. Dressing independently**
>
> C. Following several directions at once
>
> D. Comprehending satire

> Preschoolers should be able to dress themselves with occasional help in tying shoes or fastening complex buckles or closures. Using a knife to cut meat at mealtime, following several directions at once, and comprehending satire are developmental tasks of school-age children.

 NCLEX® Connection: Health Promotion and Maintenance, Developmental Stages and Transitions

4. Which of the following immunizations should this child receive at this health visit if her immunizations are up-to-date? (Select all that apply.)

> _____ Hepatitis A (Hep A), given in two doses, at least 6 months apart
>
> __X__ **Diphtheria and tetanus toxoids and pertussis (DTaP)**
>
> __X__ **Inactivated poliovirus (IPV)**
>
> __X__ **Measles, mumps, and rubella (MMR)**
>
> __X__ **Varicella**
>
> __X__ **Trivalent inactivated influenza vaccine (TIV)**

> Diphtheria and tetanus toxoids and pertussis (DTaP); inactivated poliovirus (IPV); measles, mumps, and rubella (MMR); varicella; and a yearly trivalent inactivated influenza vaccine (TIV) or live, attenuated influenza vaccine (LAIV) by nasal spray should be given between 4 and 6 years of age. Hepatitis A (Hep A) is given in two doses at 12 to 23 months, at least 6 months apart.

 NCLEX® Connection: Health Promotion and Maintenance, Health Promotion/Disease Prevention

UNIT 2	HEALTH PROMOTION
Section	Nursing Throughout the Lifespan

Chapter 21   School-Age Child (6 to 12 Years)

Expected Growth and Development

- Physical Development

  o Weight: The school-age child will gain about 2 to 4 kg (4.4 to 8.8 lb) per year.

    ▪ Weight gain typically occurs between 9 to 12 years of age (girls 9 to 12 years of ages, boys 10 to 12 years of age).

  o Height: The school-age child will grow by about 5 cm (2 inches) per year.

    ▪ Changes in height usually occur after 10 to 12 years of age for girls and 12 to 14 years of age for boys (after the period of weight gain).

  o Changes related to puberty begin to appear in females. These changes include:

    ▪ Budding of breasts.

    ▪ Appearance of pubic hair.

    ▪ Menarche.

  o Changes related to puberty begin to appear in males. These changes include:

    ▪ Enlargement of testicles with changes in the scrotum, such as increased looseness.

    ▪ Appearance of pubic hair.

  o Permanent teeth erupt.

  o Visual acuity improves to 20/20.

  o Auditory acuity and sense of touch is fully developed.

  o Fine and gross motor development

    ▪ During the school-age years, coordination continues to improve.

- Cognitive Development

  o Piaget – Described as concrete operations.

    ▪ Sees weight and volume as unchanging

    ▪ Understands simple analogies

    ▪ Understands time (days, seasons)

    ▪ Classifies more complex information

- Understands various emotions people experience
- Becomes self-motivated
- Is able to solve problems
    - Language – Defines many words and understands rules of grammar.
        - Understands that a word may have multiple meanings
- Psychosocial Development
    - The school-age child's stage of psychosocial development, according to Erikson, is industry vs. inferiority.
        - A sense of industry is achieved through advances in learning.
        - Motivated by tasks that increase self-worth.
        - Fears of ridicule by peers and teachers over school-related issues are common. Some children manifest nervous behaviors to deal with the stress, such as nail biting.
    - Moral Development
        - Early on, the school-age child may not understand the reasoning behind many rules and may try to find ways around them. Instrumental exchange is in place ("I'll help you if you help me."). The child wants to make the best deal, and she does not really consider elements of loyalty, gratitude, or justice as she makes her decisions.
        - In the latter part of the school years, the child moves into a law-and-order orientation with more emphasis placed on justice being administered.
    - Self-Concept Development
        - School-age children strive to develop healthy self-respect by finding out in what areas they excel.
        - School-age children need parents to encourage them regarding educational or extracurricular successes.
    - Body-Image Changes
        - This is the age at which solidification of body image occurs.
        - Curiosity about sexuality should be addressed with education regarding sexual development and the reproductive process.
        - School-age children are more modest than preschoolers and place more emphasis on privacy issues.
    - Social Development
        - Peer groups play an important part in social development. However, peer pressure begins to take effect.
        - Friendships begin to form between same-gender peers. This is the time period when clubs and best friends are popular.
        - Children at this age prefer the company of same-gender companions.

- Most relationships come from school associations.
- Children at this age may rival the same-sex parent.
- Conformity becomes evident.

- Age-Appropriate Activities

  o Competitive and cooperative play is predominant.

  o 6 to 9 year olds:

    - Play simple board and number games.
    - Play hopscotch.
    - Jump rope.
    - Collect rocks, stamps, cards, coins, or stuffed animals.
    - Ride bicycles.
    - Build simple models.
    - Join organized sports – skill building.

  o 9 to 12 year olds:

    - Make crafts.
    - Build models.
    - Collect/engage in hobbies.
    - Solve jigsaw puzzles.
    - Play board and card games.
    - Join organized competitive sports.

Health Promotion

- Immunizations

  o Centers for Disease Control and Prevention (CDC) immunization recommendations (http://www.cdc.gov) for healthy school-age children 6 to 12 years of age include:

    - If not given between ages 4 to 5, then by age 6: diphtheria and tetanus toxoids and pertussis (DTaP); inactivated poliovirus (IPV); measles, mumps, and rubella (MMR); and varicella.
    - Yearly seasonal influenza vaccine: trivalent inactivated influenza vaccine (TIV) or live, attenuated influenza vaccine (LAIV) by nasal spray.
    - 11 to 12 years – Tetanus and diphtheria toxoids and pertussis vaccine (Tdap); meningococcal vaccine (MCV4); and human papillomavirus vaccine (HPV2) in 3 doses for females; HVP4 may be given to males.

- Health Screenings

  o Scoliosis – School-age children should be screened for scoliosis by examining for a lateral curvature of the spine before and during growth spurts. Screening may take place at schools or at a provider's office.

- Nutrition

  o By the end of the school-age years, the child is eating an adult proportion of food. The child needs quality nutritious snacks.

  o Obesity is an increasing concern of this age group that predisposes them to low self-esteem, diabetes, heart disease, and high blood pressure. Advise parents to:

    ■ Not use food as a reward.

    ■ Emphasize physical activity.

    ■ Make sure a balanced diet is consumed. Healthy recommendations may be found at the U.S. Department of Agriculture's Web site (http://www.mypyramid.gov).

    ■ Teach children to make healthy food selections for meals and snacks.

    ■ Avoid frequent meals eaten at fast-food restaurants.

    ■ Avoid skipping meals.

  o Dental health should be encouraged, including:

    ■ Brushing daily.

    ■ Flossing daily.

    ■ Having regular check-ups.

    ■ Having regular fluoride treatments.

- Injury Prevention

  o Bodily Harm

    ■ Keep firearms in a locked cabinet or box.

    ■ Assist with identifying "safe" play areas.

    ■ Teach stranger safety.

    ■ Teach children to wear helmets and/or pads when rollerblading, skateboarding, bicycling, riding scooters, skiing, and snowboarding.

  o Burns

    ■ Teach fire safety and potential burn hazards.

    ■ Have working smoke and carbon monoxide detectors in the home.

    ■ Use sunscreen when outside.

  o Drowning

    ■ Provide supervision for children when swimming or near a body of water.

      □ Teach children to swim.

- o Motor-vehicle Injuries
  - The child should be restrained in a car seat or booster chair until adult seat belts fit correctly.
  - Laws may vary from state to state and requirements may be up to 36.3 kg (80 lb) and a height of 4 feet 9 inches.
  - Children younger than 13 years of age are safest in the back seat.
- o Substance Abuse/Poisoning
  - Keep cleaners or chemicals in locked cabinet or out of reach of children.
  - Teach children to say "no" to illegal drugs and alcohol.

CHAPTER 21: SCHOOL-AGE CHILD (6 TO 12 YEARS)

 Application Exercises

1. Which of the following developmental tasks should a school-age child be expected to accomplish?

   A. Trust vs. mistrust

   B. Autonomy vs. shame

   C. Initiative vs. guilt

   D. Industry vs. inferiority

2. When caring for a school-age child, which of the following cognitive abilities should a nurse expect? (Select all that apply.)

   _____ Will not understand another person's point of view

   _____ Believes everything is made by humans

   _____ Understands simple analogies

   _____ Demonstrates an understanding of days and weeks

   _____ Identifies inanimate objects as living

3. Which of the following is an age-appropriate activity for a 7-year-old child? (Select all that apply.)

   _____ Playing a card game

   _____ Assuming responsibility for a pet

   _____ Collecting coins

   _____ Participating on a soccer team

   _____ Solving a puzzle

4. A nurse at an elementary school is planning a health promotion and primary prevention class. Which of the following is an appropriate topic to include for the parents of school-age children? (Select all that apply.)

   _____ Obesity

   _____ Substance abuse

   _____ Scoliosis

   _____ Pregnancy prevention

   _____ Stranger awareness

CHAPTER 21: SCHOOL-AGE CHILD (6 TO 12 YEARS)

 Application Exercises Answer Key

1. Which of the following developmental tasks should a school-age child be expected to accomplish?

   A. Trust vs mistrust

   B. Autonomy vs shame

   C. Initiative vs guilt

   D. Industry vs inferiority

   The developmental task of industry should be accomplished during the school-age years. The developmental task of trust should be accomplished during infancy, autonomy should be accomplished during the toddler years, and initiative should be accomplished during the preschool years.

    NCLEX® Connection: Health Promotion and Maintenance: Developmental Stages and Transitions

2. When caring for a school-age child, which of the following cognitive abilities should a nurse expect?

   _____ Will not understand another person's point of view

   _____ Believes everything is made by humans

   __**X**__ **Understands simple analogies**

   __**X**__ **Demonstrates an understanding of days and weeks**

   _____ Identifies inanimate objects as living

   A school-age child should understand simple analogies and demonstrate an understanding of days and weeks. A toddler is unable to see another person's point of view. A preschool child believes everything is made by humans and that inanimate objects are alive.

    NCLEX® Connection: Health Promotion and Maintenance: Developmental Stages and Transitions

3. Which of the following is an age-appropriate activity for a 7-year-old child? (Select all that apply.)

   __**X**__ **Playing a card game**

   _____ Assuming responsibility for a pet

   __**X**__ **Collecting coins**

   __**X**__ **Participating on a soccer team**

   __**X**__ **Solving a puzzle**

   Playing cards, collecting coins, participating on a soccer team, and solving a puzzle are all appropriate activities for a 7-year-old child. Assuming responsibility for a pet is an appropriate activity for an adolescent.

    NCLEX® Connection: Health Promotion and Maintenance: Developmental Stages and Transitions

4. A nurse at an elementary school is planning a health promotion and primary prevention class. Which of the following is an appropriate topic to include for the parents of school-age children? (Select all that apply.)

   __X__   **Obesity**

   __X__   **Substance abuse**

   __X__   **Scoliosis**

   _____   Pregnancy prevention

   __X__   **Stranger awareness**

Obesity, substance abuse prevention, scoliosis, and stranger awareness are all topics that are pertinent to the parents of school-aged children. Pregnancy prevention is appropriate to include in a class for parents of an adolescent.

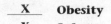 NCLEX® Connection: Health Promotion and Maintenance: Health and Wellness

UNIT 2	HEALTH PROMOTION
Section	Nursing Throughout the Lifespan
Chapter 22	Adolescent (12 to 20 Years)

Expected Growth and Development

- Physical Development

  o The final 20% to 25% of height is achieved during puberty.

  o Acne may appear during adolescence.

  o Girls may cease to grow at about 2 to 2.5 years after the onset of menarche. Girls grow 5 to 20 cm (2 to 8 inches), and 7 to 25 kg (15.5 to 55 pounds).

  o Boys tend to stop growing at around 18 to 20 years of age.

  o In girls, sexual maturation occurs in the following order:

    ■ Appearance of breast buds.

    ■ Growth of pubic hair (although some girls may have hair growth prior to breast bud development).

    ■ Onset of menstruation.

  o In males, sexual maturation occurs in the following order:

    ■ Increase in the size of the testes and scrotum.

    ■ Appearance of pubic hair.

    ■ Rapid growth of genitalia.

    ■ Growth of axillary hair.

    ■ Appearance of downy hair on upper lip.

    ■ Change in voice.

  o Sleep habits change with puberty due to increased metabolism and rapid growth during the adolescent years. Changes are characterized by staying up late, sleeping later in the morning, and perhaps sleeping longer than they did during the school-age years.

- Cognitive Development

  o Piaget – Formal operations.

    ■ Is capable of thinking at an adult level.

    ■ Is able to think abstractly and can deal with principles.

    ■ Is able to evaluate the quality of his own thinking.

- Has a longer attention span.

- Is highly imaginative and idealistic.

- Makes decisions through logical operations.

- Is future-oriented.

- Is capable of deductive reasoning.

- Understands how actions of an individual influence others.

  o Language – Adolescents develop jargon within the peer group. They are able to communicate one way with the peer group and another way with adults or teachers. Development of communication skills is essential for an adolescent.

- Psychosocial Development

  o The adolescent's stage of psychosocial development, according to Erikson, is identity vs. role confusion.

    - The adolescent develops a sense of personal identity that is influenced by expectations of the family.

      □ Group identity – The adolescent may become part of a peer group that greatly influences behavior.

  o Vocationally – Work habits begin to solidify. Plan for future college and career.

  o Sexually – There is increased interest in the opposite gender.

  o Health perceptions – Adolescents may view themselves as invincible to bad outcomes of risky behaviors.

  o Moral Development

    - Conventional law and order – Rules are not seen as absolutes. Each situation needs to be looked at, and perhaps the rules will need to be adjusted. Not all adolescents attain this level of moral development during these years.

  o Self-Concept Development

    - A healthy self-concept is developed by having healthy relationships with peers, family, and teachers. Identifying a skill or talent helps maintain a healthy self-concept. Participation in sports, hobbies, or the community can have a positive outcome.

  o Body-Image Changes

    - Adolescents seem particularly concerned with the body images portrayed by the media. Changes that occur during puberty result in comparisons between the adolescent and the surrounding peer group. Parents also give their input as to hair styles, dress, and activity. Adolescents may require help if depression or eating disorders result due to poor body image.

  o Social Development

    - Peer relationships develop. These relationships act as a support system for the adolescent.

- Best-friend relationships are more stable and long-lasting than they were in previous years.

- Parent-child relationships change to allow a greater sense of independence.

- Age-Appropriate Activities

    o Nonviolent video games

    o Nonviolent music

    o Sports

    o Caring for a pet

    o Career-training programs

    o Reading

    o Social events (going to the movies or school dances)

Health Promotion

- Immunizations

    o Centers for Disease Control (CDC) recommendations, (http://www.cdc.gov), for the healthy adolescent 12 to 20 years include the following vaccines if not given at age 11 to 12: tetanus and diphtheria toxoids and pertussis vaccine (Tdap); meningococcal (MCV4); human papillomavirus vaccine: HPV2 series for females and HPV4 series for males; and yearly seasonal influenza vaccine: trivalent inactivated influenza vaccine (TIV) or live, attenuated influenza vaccine (LAIV) by nasal spray.

- Health Screenings

    o Scoliosis – Screening for scoliosis should continue during the adolescent years by examining for a lateral curvature of the spine before and during growth spurts. Screening may take place at school or at a provider's office.

- Nutrition

    o Rapid growth and high metabolism require increases in quality nutrients. Nutrients that tend to be deficient during this stage of life are iron, calcium, and vitamins A and C.

    o Eating disorders commonly develop during adolescence (more prevalent in girls than in boys) due to a fear of being overweight, fad diets, and/or as a mechanism of maintaining control over some aspect of life. These include:

        - Anorexia nervosa

        - Bulimia nervosa

        - Obesity

    o Advise parents to:

        - Not use food as a reward.

        - Emphasize physical activity.

- Make sure a balanced diet is consumed. Recommendations may be found at the U.S. Department of Agriculture's Web site (http://www.mypyramid.gov).

- Teach children to make healthy food selections for meals and snacks.

  o Dental health should be encouraged including:

    - Brushing daily.

    - Flossing daily.

    - Having regular check-ups.

    - Having regular fluoride treatments.

- Injury Prevention

  o Bodily harm

    - Keep firearms in a locked cabinet or box.

    - Teach proper use of sporting equipment prior to use.

    - Insist on helmet use and/or pads when rollerblading, skateboarding, bicycling, riding scooters, skiing, and snowboarding.

    - Avoid trampolines.

    - Be aware of changes in mood and monitor for self-harm in at-risk adolescents. Watch for:

      □ Poor school performance

      □ Lack of interest in things that had been of interest to the adolescent in the past.

      □ Social isolation

      □ Disturbances in sleep or appetite

      □ Expression of suicidal thoughts

  o Burns

    - Teach fire safety.

    - Use sunscreen when outside.

  o Drowning

    - Teach the adolescent to swim.

    - Teach the adolescent not to swim alone.

  o Motor-vehicle Injury

    - Encourage attendance at drivers' education courses.

    - Emphasize the need for adherence to seat belt use.

    - Discourage use of cell phones while driving.

    - Teach the dangers of combining substance abuse with driving.

- o Substance abuse
  - Monitor for signs of substance abuse in at-risk adolescents
  - Teach adolescents to say "no" to illegal drugs and alcohol.
  - Present a no-tolerance attitude.
- o Sexually transmitted diseases (STDs)
  - Provide education and resources for treatment.
- o Pregnancy prevention
  - Provide education.

CHAPTER 22: ADOLESCENT (12 TO 20 YEARS)

 Application Exercises

1. Place the following male puberty changes in the correct sequence.

_____ Appearance of pubic hair

_____ Change in voice

_____ Growth of axillary hair

_____ Increase in size of testes

_____ Appearance of downy hair on upper lip

_____ Rapid growth of genitalia

2. Which of the following interventions are appropriate for an adolescent male who is hospitalized with a fractured femur? (Select all that apply.)

_____ Suggest that his parents room in with him.

_____ Provide a television and DVDs for him to watch.

_____ Restrict visitors.

_____ Encourage him to get enough rest.

_____ Allow him to perform his own morning care.

3. Which of the following developmental tasks should adolescents be expected to accomplish?

A. Identity vs. role confusion

B. Autonomy vs. shame

C. Initiative vs. guilt

D. Industry vs. inferiority

CHAPTER 22: ADOLESCENT (12 TO 20 YEARS)

 Application Exercises Answer Key

1. Place the following male puberty changes in the correct sequence.

2	Appearance of pubic hair
6	Change in voice
4	Growth of axillary hair
1	Increase in size of testes
5	Appearance of downy hair on upper lip
3	Rapid growth of genitalia

 NCLEX® Connection: Reduction of Risk Potential, System Specific Assessment

2. Which of the following interventions are appropriate for an adolescent male who is hospitalized with a fractured femur? (Select all that apply.)

_____	Suggest that his parents room in with him.
X	**Provide a television and DVDs for him to watch.**
_____	Restrict visitors.
X	**Encourage him to get enough rest.**
X	**Allow him to perform his own morning care.**

DVDs are appropriate diversional activities for an adolescent. It is important for him to get adequate rest, and allowing him to perform his own morning care will provide a sense of independence. Rooming in is most appropriate for an infant, toddler, preschooler, and school-age child. There is no reason to restrict visitors, and allowing his friends to visit can prevent feelings of isolation.

 NCLEX® Connection: Health Promotion and Maintenance, Developmental Stages and Transitions

3. Which of the following developmental tasks should adolescents be expected to accomplish?

A. Identity vs. role confusion

B. Autonomy vs. shame

C. Initiative vs. guilt

D. Industry vs. inferiority

The developmental task of achieving identity vs. role confusion should be accomplished by an adolescent. The developmental task of autonomy vs. shame should be accomplished during the toddler years. The developmental task of initiative vs. guilt should be accomplished during the preschool years. The developmental task of industry vs. inferiority should be accomplished during the school-age years.

 NCLEX® Connection: Health Promotion and Maintenance, Developmental Stages and Transitions

UNIT 2	HEALTH PROMOTION
Section	Nursing Throughout the Lifespan
Chapter 23	Young Adult (20 to 35 Years)

Expected Growth and Development

- Physical Development

  o Growth has concluded around age 20.

  o Physical senses peak.

  o Cardiac output and efficiency peak.

  o Muscles function optimally at ages 25 to 30.

  o Metabolic rate decreases 2% to 4% every decade after age 20.

  o Libido is high for men.

  o Libido for women peaks during the later part of this stage.

  o Time for childbearing is optimal.

  o Pregnancy-related changes occur.

- Cognitive Development

  o Piaget – Formal operations

    ▪ The young adult years are an optimal time for education – both formal and informal. In young adults:

      ◻ Critical thinking skills improve.

      ◻ Memory peaks in the 20s.

      ◻ There is an increased ability for creative thought.

      ◻ The values/norms of friends (social groups) are relevant.

- Psychosocial Development

  o Young adults may pass through two stages of development according to Erikson, intimacy vs. isolation.

  o Young adults may take on more adult commitments and responsibilities.

- o Young adults may make occupational choices characterized by:
  - ■ High goals/dreams
  - ■ Exploration/experimentation
- o Moral Development
  - ■ Young adults may personalize values and beliefs.
  - ■ Reasoning may be based on ethical fairness principles, such as the principle of justice.
- o Self-Concept Development
  - ■ The formation of a healthy self-concept during the young adult years is influenced by:
    - □ Avoidance of substance abuse
    - □ Late formation of a family
    - □ Frequent interactions with family and friends
    - □ Choosing to behave in an ethical manner
- o Body-Image Changes
  - ■ Body-image changes are greatly influenced by what young adults eat and how much exercise they get.
  - ■ Pregnancy-related body image changes may also occur.
- o Social Development
  - ■ Young adults may:
    - □ Leave home and establish independent living situation.
    - □ Establish close friendships (intimacy).
    - □ Transition from being single to being member of new family.
    - □ Question their ability to parent.
    - □ Experience increased anxiety and/or depression, especially after the birth of a child.

Health Promotion

- • Young adults are especially at risk for alterations in health from:
  - o Substance abuse
  - o Periodontal disease due to poor oral hygiene
  - o Unplanned pregnancies – a source of high stress
  - o Sexually transmitted diseases
  - o Infertility
  - o Work-related injuries or exposures

- Immunizations

  - The 2010 Centers for Disease Control (CDC) recommendations (See http://www.cdc.gov for updates) for healthy young adults include:

    - Tetanus diphtheria (Td) booster – Give every 10 years; for adults who did not receive one dose of tetanus, diphtheria, pertussis (Tdap) previously, substitute one dose with Tdap.

    - Measles, mumps and rubella vaccine (MMR) – One dose at ages 19 to 49, with a second dose 4 weeks later if adult is a student in a postsecondary educational institution, works in a health care facility, or plans to travel abroad.

    - Varicella vaccine – Two doses should be given to adults who do not have evidence of previous infection. A second dose should be given 4-8 weeks after the first dose to adults who had only one previous dose.

    - Meningococcal conjugate vaccine (MCV) – Students entering college and living in college dormitories if not previously immunized.

    - Human papilloma virus vaccine (HPV2 or HPV4) – Three doses, recommended for females up to age 26 who were not vaccinated as a child. HPV4: May be given to males up to age 26.

- Health Screenings

  - Young adults should follow age-related guidelines for screening.

- Nutrition

  - Monitor for adequate nutrition and proper physical activity.

  - Women – Monitor calcium intake.

- Routine health care visits should include obtaining height, weight, and vital signs; screening for stress; education related to STDs, substance abuse, and contraception; and encouragement of good nutrition and regular physical activity.

- Injury prevention for young adults includes:

  - Avoiding drugs, including alcohol, that can lead to substance abuse.

  - Avoiding taking drugs and drinking alcohol while driving a vehicle.

  - Wearing a seat belt when operating a vehicle.

  - Wearing a helmet while bike riding, skiing, or snowboarding.

  - Installing smoke and carbon monoxide detectors in the home.

  - Securing firearms in a safe location.

CHAPTER 23: YOUNG ADULT (20 TO 35 YEARS)

 Application Exercises

1. The formal operations stage of development is described by which of the following theorists?

    A. Piaget

    B. Erikson

    C. Freud

    D. Kohlberg

2. Which of the following statements indicates that a client understands health teaching about health promotion and illness prevention?

    A. "I am young, so it does not matter what I eat and whether or not I exercise."

    B. "It is important to schedule routine health care visits even if I am feeling well."

    C. "If I am having any discomfort, I will wait as long as possible before calling the doctor."

    D. "If I am feeling stressed, I will just have a glass of wine to forget my troubles."

3. Which of the following behaviors by a young adult demonstrates appropriate psychosocial development?

    A. Taking active involvement in providing guidance to the next generation

    B. Adjusting to major changes in roles and relationships due to losses

    C. Devoting a great deal of time to establishing an occupation

    D. Finding oneself "sandwiched" in between and being responsible for two generations

CHAPTER 23: YOUNG ADULT (20 TO 35 YEARS)

 Application Exercises Answer Key

1. The formal operations stage of development is described by which of the following theorists?

A. Piaget

B. Erikson

C. Freud

D. Kohlberg

Piaget describes formal operations as the phase of his cognitive development theory that is applicable to adolescents and young adults. Erikson describes intimacy vs. isolation (age 18 to 25) and generativity vs. stagnation (age 25 to 65) as the phases of his psychosocial development theory that are applicable to young adults. Freud describes genital as the stage of his psychosocial development theory that is applicable to young adults. Kohlberg describes law-and-order orientation as the stage of his moral development theory that is applicable to young adults.

 NCLEX® Connection: Health Promotion and Maintenance: Developmental Stages and Transitions

2. Which of the following statements indicates that a client understands health teaching about health promotion and illness prevention?

A. "I am young, so it does not matter what I eat and whether or not I exercise."

B. "It is important to schedule routine health care visits even if I am feeling well."

C. "If I am having any discomfort, I will wait as long as possible before calling the doctor."

D. "If I am feeling stressed, I will just have a glass of wine to forget my troubles."

Young adulthood is a time of relative health, but routine screenings and health care visits are still important. Good nutrition and physical activity should be lifelong habits. It is important that the client not wait too long to seek medical care, as an illness/condition may be prevented or may be easier to manage by early detection. Using substances to manage stress can lead to substance abuse. Clients experiencing stress should seek professional assistance.

 NCLEX® Connection: Health Promotion and Maintenance: Health Promotion/Disease Prevention

3. Which of the following behaviors by a young adult demonstrates appropriate psychosocial development?

    A. Taking active involvement in providing guidance to the next generation

    B. Adjusting to major changes in roles and relationships due to losses

    C. Devoting a great deal of time to establishing an occupation

    D. Finding oneself "sandwiched" in between and being responsible for two generations

Exploring career options and then establishing oneself in a given occupation is a major developmental task for a young adult. Active involvement in the next generation and being responsible for two generations are developmental tasks for the middle adult. Adjusting to major role changes is a developmental task for an older adult.

(N) NCLEX® Connection: Health Promotion and Maintenance: Developmental Stages and Transitions

UNIT 2	HEALTH PROMOTION
Section	Nursing Throughout the Lifespan
Chapter 24	Middle Adult (35 to 65 years)

Expected Growth and Development

- Physical Development

  - Middle adults typically experience decreases in:

    - Skin turgor and moisture

    - Subcutaneous fat

    - Melanin in hair (graying)

    - Hair

    - Visual acuity

    - Auditory acuity

    - Sense of taste

    - Skeletal muscle mass

    - Height

    - Calcium/bone density

    - Blood vessel elasticity

    - Respiratory vital capacity

    - Large intestine muscle tone

    - Gastric secretions

    - Estrogen/testosterone

    - Glucose tolerance

- Cognitive Development

  - Piaget – Formal operations

    - Reaction time/speed of performance slows slightly.

    - Memory is intact.

    - Crystallized intelligence remains (stored knowledge).

    - Fluid intelligence (how one learns and processes new information) declines slightly.

- Psychosocial Development
  - The middle adult's stage of psychosocial development, according to Erikson, is generativity vs. stagnation.
    - Middle adults may strive for generativity.
      - Use life as an opportunity for creativity and productivity.
      - Have concern for others.
      - Consider parenting an important task.
      - Contribute to the well-being of the next generation.
      - Strive to do well in one's own environment.
      - Adjust to changes in physical appearance and abilities.
  - Moral Development
    - Religious maturity
      - Spiritual beliefs and religion may take on added importance.
      - Middle adults may become more secure in their convictions.
      - Middle adults often have advanced moral development.
  - Self-Concept Development
    - Middle adults may experience issues related to:
      - Menopause
      - Sexuality
      - Depression
      - Irritability
      - Difficulty with sexual identity
      - Job performance and ability to provide support
      - Marital changes with the death of a spouse or divorce
  - Body-Image Changes
    - Women – Symptoms of menopause may represent a:
      - Loss of the reproductive role or femininity
      - New interest in intimacy
    - Men – Decreasing strength may be frustrating or frightening.
    - Decreased sex drive may occur as a result of declining hormones, chronic diseases, or medications.
    - Changes in physical appearance may raise concerns about desirability.

- o Social Development
  - ■ Need to maintain and strengthen intimacy.
    - □ Provide assistance to aging parents, adult children, and grandchildren.

Health Promotion

- Middle adults are especially at risk for alterations in health from:
  - o Obesity and type 2 diabetes mellitus
  - o Cardiovascular disease
  - o Cancer
  - o Substance abuse (alcoholism)
  - o Psychosocial stressors
- Immunizations
  - o 2010 Centers for Disease Control and Prevention (CDC) (See http://www.cdc.gov) immunization recommendations for healthy middle adults include:
    - ■ Tetanus diphtheria (Td) booster – Give every 10 years; for adults 35 to 64 years of age who did not receive one dose of tetanus, diphtheria, pertussis (Tdap) previously, substitute one dose with Tdap.
    - ■ Measles, mumps and rubella vaccine (MMR) – One dose at ages 19 to 49, with a second dose 4 weeks later if a student is attending a postsecondary educational institution, works in a health care facility, or plans to travel abroad.
    - ■ Varicella vaccine – Two doses should be given to adults who do not have evidence of previous infection. A second dose should be given 4-8 weeks after the first dose to adults who had only one previous dose.
    - ■ Pneumococcal polysaccharide vaccine (PPV) – If not previously vaccinated, vaccinate once at age 65.
    - ■ Seasonal influenza vaccine – One dose annually recommended for all adults over age 50, for health care providers including those who care for young children, for individuals with chronic medical conditions such as cerebral palsy, asthma, and diabetes mellitus, for individuals who are immunocompromised and for individuals living in long-term care settings. Note that live, attenuated vaccine (LAIV), given as a nasal spray is only indicated for adults under age 50 who are not pregnant or immunocompromised.
    - ■ Herpes Zoster vaccine – One dose recommended for all adults over age 60.

- Health Screenings

  o Middle adults should follow age-related guidelines for screening.

  o Other screenings include:

    ▪ Dual-energy x-ray absorptiometry (DEXA) screening for osteoporosis

    ▪ Eye examination for glaucoma and other disorders every 2 to 3 years or annually depending on provider.

    ▪ Mental health screening for depression

- Nutrition

  o Nutrition counseling for middle adults includes:

    ▪ Obtaining an adequate intake of protein.

    ▪ Increasing the consumption of whole grains.

    ▪ Increasing the consumption of fresh fruits and vegetables.

    ▪ Limiting fat and cholesterol.

    ▪ Increasing vitamin D and calcium supplementation (especially for women).

- Injury Prevention

  o Avoid drugs, including alcohol, that can lead to substance abuse.

  o Avoid taking drugs and drinking alcohol while driving a vehicle.

  o Wear a seat belt when operating a vehicle.

  o Wear a helmet while bike riding, skiing, or snowboarding.

  o Install smoke and carbon monoxide detectors in the home.

  o Secure firearms in a safe location.

CHAPTER 24: MIDDLE ADULT (35 TO 65 YEARS)

Ⓐ Application Exercises

1. According to Erikson's developmental theory, which of the following client activities is an indicator that the client is meeting the tasks expected in middle adulthood?

    A. The client evaluates his behavior after a social interaction.

    B. The client states he is learning to trust others.

    C. The client wishes to find meaningful friendships.

    D. The client expresses concerns about the next generation.

2. When performing a psychosocial assessment, a nurse should expect a healthy middle adult to

    A. develop an acceptance of diminished strength and increased dependence on others.

    B. feel frustrated that time is too short for attempting to start another life.

    C. accept one's life as creative and productive.

    D. find someone to share one's life with.

3. A nurse is collecting data from a client who is 50 years old. Which of the following are expected findings? (Select all that apply.)

    _____ Decreased muscle tone in the large intestine

    _____ Decreased ability to hear high-pitched sounds

    _____ Reduced gastric secretion

    _____ Reduced central vision

    _____ Decrease in subcutaneous fat

CHAPTER 24: MIDDLE ADULT (35 TO 65 YEARS)

 Application Exercises Answer Key

1. According to Erikson's developmental theory, which of the following client activities is an indicator that the client is meeting the tasks expected in middle adulthood?

A. The client evaluates his behavior after a social interaction.

B. The client states he is learning to trust others.

C. The client wishes to find meaningful friendships.

D. The client expresses concerns about the next generation.

The task for a middle age adult is generativity versus stagnation. Concern for the next generation is a positive sign that the middle age adult is meeting the task. The other client activities are expected to occur in earlier developmental stages.

NCLEX® Connection: Health Promotion and Maintenance: Developmental Stages and Transitions

2. When performing a psychosocial assessment, a nurse should expect a healthy middle adult to

A. develop an acceptance of diminished strength and increased dependence on others.

B. feel frustrated that time is too short for attempting to start another life.

C. accept one's life as creative and productive.

D. find someone to share one's life with.

Healthy middle adults accept the life they have created for themselves and have a sense of social responsibility. Acceptance of diminished strength and increased dependence on others is true of older adults. Feeling frustrated that time is too short is true of adults who are having difficulties with the developmental tasks of middle age. Finding someone to share life with is applicable to young adults.

NCLEX® Connection: Health Promotion and Maintenance: Developmental Stages and Transitions

FUNDAMENTALS FOR NURSING

3. A nurse is collecting data from a client who is 50 years old. Which of the following are expected findings? (Select all that apply.)

   __X__   **Decreased muscle tone in the large intestine**

   __X__   **Decreased ability to hear high-pitched sounds**

   __X__   **Reduced gastric secretion**

   _____   Reduced central vision

   __X__   **Decrease in subcutaneous fat**

Decreased muscle tone of the large intestine, a decrease in the ability to hear high-pitched sounds, and a decrease in gastric secretions are expected findings. Reduced central vision may be due to macular degeneration and is not an expected finding. A decrease in subcutaneous fat is an expected finding in an older adult.

Ⓝ NCLEX® Connection: Reduction of Risk Potential: System Specific Assessment

UNIT 2	HEALTH PROMOTION
Section	Nursing Throughout the Lifespan
Chapter 25	Older Adult (65 Years and Older)

Expected Growth and Development

- Physical Development

  - Physical changes related to older adults include:

    - A decrease in both skin turgor and subcutaneous fat, which leads to wrinkles and dry skin

    - A loss of subcutaneous fat makes it more difficult for older adults to adjust to cold temperatures

    - Thinning and graying of the hair, as well as a more sparse distribution

    - Thickening of the fingernails and toenails

    - A decrease in chest wall movement, vital capacity, and cilia, which increases the risk for respiratory infections

    - A slower reaction time

    - A decrease in touch, smell, and taste sensations

    - A decrease in the production of saliva

    - A decline in visual acuity

    - A decreased ability for the eyes to adjust from light to dark can lead to night blindness, which is especially dangerous when driving

    - An inability to hear high-pitched sounds (presbycusis)

    - A decrease in height due to intervertebral disk changes

    - A decrease in muscle strength and tone

    - A decrease in digestive enzymes

    - A decrease in intestinal motility, which can lead to an increased risk of constipation

    - An increase in dental problems

    - Decalcification of bones

    - Degeneration of joints

    - A decrease in bladder capacity

FUNDAMENTALS FOR NURSING

- Prostate hypertrophy in men

- A decline in estrogen/testosterone production

- A decline in tri-iodothyronine T3 production, yet overall function remains effective

- Decreased sensitivity of tissue cells to insulin

- Atrophy of breast tissue in women

- Cognitive Development

  o Piaget – Formal operations

  o Many older adults maintain their cognitive function. There is some decline in speed of the cognitive function versus cognitive ability.

  o A number of factors influence older adults' abilities to function, such as overall health, the number of stressors present at a given point in time, and the client's life-long mental well-being.

  o Slowed neurotransmission, impaired vascular circulation, disease states, poor nutrition, and structural brain changes can result in the following cognitive disorders:

    - Delirium – Acute, temporary, and usually related to other physiologic problems. Delirium is often the first symptom of infection (urinary tract infection) in older adults.

    - Dementia – Chronic, progressive, and possibly with an unknown cause (Alzheimer's disease).

    - Depression – Chronic, acute, or gradual onset (present for at least 6 weeks).

- Psychosocial Development

  o Older adults' stage of psychosocial development, according to Erikson, is integrity vs. despair.

  o Older adults may need to:

    - Adjust to lifestyle changes related to retirement (decreased income, living situation, loss of work role).

    - Adapt to changes in family structure (may be role reversal in later years).

    - Deal with multiple losses (death of a spouse, friends, siblings).

    - Face death.

  o Self-Concept Development

    - Older adults face difficulties in the area of self-concept, which include:

      □ Seeing oneself as an aging person.

      □ Finding ways to maintain a good quality of life.

      □ Becoming more dependent on others for activities of daily living.

- o   Body-Image Changes
    - ▪   Adjustments to decreases in physical strength and endurance may be difficult, especially for older adults who are cognitively active and engaged. Many older adults feel frustrated that their bodies are limiting what they desire to do.
- o   Social Development
    - ▪   Find ways to remain socially active and to overcome loneliness.
    - ▪   Maintain sexual health.

Health Promotion

- •   Health Risks
    - o   Cardiovascular diseases that can affect older adults include:
        - ▪   Coronary artery disease
        - ▪   Hypertension
        - ▪   Stroke
    - o   Factors affecting mobility of older adults include:
        - ▪   Arthritis
        - ▪   Osteoporosis
        - ▪   Falls
    - o   Mental health disorders that can affect older adults include:
        - ▪   Depression
        - ▪   Dementia
        - ▪   Suicide
    - o   Other disorders that can affect older adults include:
        - ▪   Diabetes mellitus
        - ▪   Cancers
        - ▪   Incontinence
        - ▪   Abuse and neglect
        - ▪   Cataracts
        - ▪   Alcoholism
        - ▪   Pain

- Immunizations

  - 2010 Centers for Disease Control and Prevention (CDC) (http://www.cdc.gov) immunization recommendations for healthy older adults include:

    - Tetanus diphtheria (Td) booster – Give at least one dose every 10 years.

    - Varicella vaccine – Two doses should be given to adults who do not have evidence of previous infection. A second dose should be given 4 to 8 weeks after the first dose to adults who had only one previous dose.

    - Pneumococcal polysaccharide vaccine (PPV) – If not previously vaccinated, vaccinate once at age 65.

    - Seasonal influenza vaccine – Give one dose annually.

    - Herpes zoster vaccine – One dose is recommended for all adults over age 60.

- Health Screenings

  - Older adults should follow age-related guidelines for screening.

  - Other screenings include:

    - Dual-energy x-ray absorptiometry (DEXA) screening for osteoporosis

    - Eye examination for glaucoma and other disorders every 2 to 3 years or annually as prescribed

    - Mental health screening for depression

- Nutrition

  - In addition to gastrointestinal alterations, other factors that influence nutrition in older adults include:

    - Difficulty getting to and from the supermarket to shop for food

    - A low income

    - Impaired mobility

    - Depression or dementia

    - Social isolation (preparing a meal for one person and eating alone)

    - Medications that alter taste or appetite

    - Prescribed diets that are unappealing

    - Incontinence that may cause the person to limit fluid intake

    - Constipation

  - Metabolic rates and activity decline as individuals age; therefore, total caloric intake should decrease to maintain a healthy weight. With the reduction of total calorie intake, it becomes even more important that the calories consumed be of good nutritional value.

- o Nutritional recommendations for older adults include:

  - Increasing the intake of vitamins D, B6, and calcium.

  - Increasing fluid intake to minimize the risk of dehydration and prevent constipation.

  - Taking a low-dose multivitamin along with mineral supplementation.

  - Following provider's recommendation for sodium intake.

- Psychosocial interventions to improve self-concept and alleviate social isolation for older adults include:

  - o Therapeutic communication

  - o Touch

  - o Reality orientation

  - o Validation therapy

  - o Reminiscence therapy

  - o Attending to physical appearance

  - o Assistive devices (canes, walkers, hearing aids)

- Injury Prevention

  - o Install bath rails, grab bars, and handrails on stairways.

  - o Remove throw rugs.

  - o Eliminate clutter from walkways/hallways.

  - o Remove extension and phone cords from walkways/hallways.

  - o Instruct in the proper use of ambulation-assistive devices (walkers, canes).

  - o Ensure adequate lighting.

  - o Remind clients to wear eyeglasses and hearing aids.

  - o Avoid drugs, including alcohol. Prevent substance abuse.

  - o Avoid taking drugs and/or drinking alcohol while driving a vehicle.

  - o Wear a seat belt when operating a vehicle.

  - o Wear a helmet while bike riding, skiing, or snowboarding.

  - o Install smoke and carbon monoxide detectors in the home.

  - o Secure firearms in a safe location.

CHAPTER 25: OLDER ADULT (65 YEARS AND OLDER)

Ⓐ Application Exercises

1. Which of the following are expected findings in regard to changes associated with aging? (Select all that apply.)

   _____ Increased insulin resistance

   _____ Increased constipation

   _____ Increased saliva production

   _____ Decrease in subcutaneous fat

   _____ Increase in bladder capacity

2. A nurse is caring for an older adult client who is admitted to the hospital and has lost 4.5 kg (9.9 lb) since his last admission 6 months ago. Which of the following assessment questions should the nurse ask to investigate the source of his weight loss? (Select all that apply.)

   _____ "Do you eat alone or with someone?"

   _____ "Do you watch television while eating your meals?"

   _____ "Have you started any new medications in the past 6 months?"

   _____ "What foods have you eaten within the past 24 hr?"

   _____ "Are you on a fixed income?"

CHAPTER 25: OLDER ADULT (65 YEARS AND OLDER)

 Application Exercises Answer Key

1. Which of the following are expected findings in regard to changes associated with aging? (Select all that apply.)

__X__ **Increased insulin resistance**

__X__ **Increased constipation**

_____ Increased saliva production

__X__ **Decrease in subcutaneous fat**

_____ Increase in bladder capacity

Aging leads to an increase in insulin resistance. A decrease in gastrointestinal motility can lead to constipation. A decrease in subcutaneous fat occurs with aging. Saliva production is decreased with aging. The capacity of the bladder decreases with aging.

 NCLEX® Connection: Reduction of Risk Potential: System Specific Assessment

2. A nurse is caring for an older adult client who is admitted to the hospital and has lost 4.5 kg (9.9 lb) since his last admission 6 months ago. Which of the following assessment questions should the nurse ask to investigate the source of his weight loss? (Select all that apply.)

__X__ **"Do you eat alone or with someone?"**

_____ "Do you watch television while eating your meals?"

__X__ **"Have you started any new medications in the past 6 months?"**

__X__ **"What foods have you eaten within the past 24 hr?"**

__X__ **"Are you on a fixed income?"**

Clients who eat alone are more likely to skip or skimp on meals. Many medications affect the senses of taste and smell, as well as the ability to absorb nutrients. Asking about food eaten within the last 24 hr will provide a basis to determine what the client typically eats in a 24-hr period. Clients who are on a fixed income may not have enough money to buy food. Determining if the client watches television while eating is not relevant in this situation.

 NCLEX® Connection: Health Promotion and Maintenance: Developmental Stages and Transitions

UNIT 2: HEALTH PROMOTION

Section: Health Assessment

- Data Collection and General Survey
- Vital Signs
- Head and Neck
- Thorax, Heart, and Abdomen
- Integumentary and Peripheral Vascular Systems
- Musculoskeletal and Neurosensory Systems

NCLEX® CONNECTIONS

When reviewing the chapters in this section, keep in mind the relevant sections of the NCLEX® outline, in particular:

CLIENT NEEDS: HEALTH PROMOTION AND MAINTENANCE

Relevant topics/tasks include:
- Aging Process
  - Provide care and education that meets the special needs of the adult client ages 19 to 64 years.
- Developmental Stages and Transitions
  - Compare the client's development to expected age/developmental stage and report any deviations.
- Health and Wellness
  - Encourage the client's participation in appropriate behavior modification programs related to health and wellness.

CLIENT NEEDS: MANAGEMENT OF CARE

Relevant topics/tasks include:
- Confidentiality/Information Security
  - Maintain the client's confidentiality/privacy.

CLIENT NEEDS: REDUCTION OF RISK POTENTIAL

Relevant topics/tasks include:
- System Specific Assessment
  - Perform a focused assessment and reassessment.

UNIT 2	HEALTH PROMOTION
Section	Health Assessment
Chapter 26	Data Collection and General Survey

Overview

- Data collection includes obtaining subjective and objective information from clients.

- The health history provides subjective data and is usually obtained during a client interview.

- The physical assessment and diagnostic tests provide objective data.

- Comprehensive health histories are part of the health assessment process.

Interviewing Techniques

- Nurses use a standardized format as a framework for obtaining client information.

- Therapeutic techniques for health assessment are meant to foster communication and create an environment conducive for an optimal health assessment experience for the client.

- Therapeutic communication helps nurses develop a rapport with clients. The techniques encourage a trusting relationship, whereby clients feel comfortable telling their stories. Nurses introduce the purpose of the interview, gather information, and then conclude the interview by summarizing the findings.

  ○ Introduces yourself and the various parts of the assessment to each client.

  ○ Determine what the client wishes to be called.

  ○ Allow more time for responses from older adult clients.

  ○ When possible, start by asking for the health history, performing the general survey, and measuring vital signs to build a rapport with the client prior to moving on to more sensitive parts of the examination.

  ○ Reduce environmental noises (TV, radio, visitors talking) to enhance communication and eliminate distractions.

  ○ Ensure understanding by obtaining interpretive services if indicated.

- Use therapeutic communication techniques including:
    - Active listening – Shows clients that they have your undivided attention.
    - Open-ended questions – Used initially to encourage clients to tell their story in their own way. Ask questions in a language the client can understand.
    - Clarifying – Questioning clients about specific details in greater depth or directing them toward relevant parts of the history.
    - Summarizing – Validates the accuracy of the story.
- Avoid using medical jargon, giving advice, ignoring feelings, and offering false reassurance.

Components of the Health History

- The health history provides subjective data relevant to health status.

HEALTH HISTORY	

Demographic information	• Identifying data includes:
	  ○ Name, address, and phone number
	  ○ Birth date and age
	  ○ Gender
	  ○ Race and ethnic origin
	  ○ Marital status
	  ○ Occupation and working status
	  ○ Insurance
	  ○ Family/significant others living at home

Source of history	• Usually comes from the client, but family members, other medical records, and other providers can provide useful information. • Note the reliability of the historian.
Chief concern	• A brief statement in the client's own words of why he is seeking care
History of present illness	• A detailed, chronological description of why the client seeks care ○ The description should start at the farthest point in time and work toward the present. • Details about the symptom(s), such as location, quality, quantity, setting, timing, alleviating or aggravating factors, and associated phenomena are important aspects to explore with the client.
Past health history and current health status	• Childhood illnesses, both communicable and chronic • Medical, surgical, obstetrical, gynecological, and psychiatric history including time frames, diagnoses, hospitalizations, and treatments • Current immunization status and the dates and results of any screening tests • Allergies to medication, environmental, and food • Current medications including prescription, over-the-counter, vitamins, supplements, and time of last dose(s) taken

HEALTH HISTORY	
Family history	• Health information of immediate relatives such as grandparents, parents, siblings, children, and grandchildren • Current ages or age-at-death are recorded, as well as disorders that were or are present in family members
Social history	• Information regarding the relationships important to the client, support systems, concerns regarding living or work situations, financial status, ability to perform activities of daily living, and spiritual health
Health promotion behaviors	• Exercise/activity, diet, sun exposure, wearing of safety equipment, substance use, stress, and related coping measures • Awareness of risks for heart disease, cancer, diabetes, and stroke

Review of Systems

- Review of systems ascertains information about the functioning of all body systems. Related or other health problems may be discovered at this time. This part of the history is usually extensive and can be incorporated into the physical examination of each body system.

SYSTEM	QUESTIONS TO BE ASKED
Integumentary	• Do you have any skin diseases? • Do you have any itching, bruising, lumps, hair loss, nail changes, or sores? • Do you have any allergies? • How do you care for your hair, skin, and nails? • Do you use lotions, soaps, and/or sunscreen or wear protective clothing?
Head and neck	• Do you experience headaches? If so, how often? and where are they located? ○ Do you have any other symptoms related to your headaches, such as nausea and vomiting? What do you do to relieve the pain? • Have you ever had a head injury? • Are you able to move your head and shoulders with ease? • Are any of your lymph nodes swollen? • Have you noticed any unusual facial movements? • Do you have any family history of thyroid disease?

SYSTEM	QUESTIONS TO BE ASKED
Eyes	• How is your vision? • Have you noticed any changes? • Do you ever have discharge from your eyes? • Do you wear glasses or contact lenses? • When was your last eye examination? • Do you have any family history of eye disorders? • Do you have diabetes?
Ears, nose, mouth, and throat	• How well do you hear? • Have you noticed any changes in your hearing? • Have other people commented that you have hearing loss? • Do you wear a hearing aid? • Do you ever experience tinnitus, discharge, vertigo, or pain? • Do you have a history of ear infections? • What method do you use to clean your ears? • Are you having any pain, stuffiness, or discharge from your nose? • Do you ever experience nosebleeds? • Have you noticed any change in your sense of smell or taste? • How often do you go to the dentist? • Do you have dentures? • Do you have any problems with your gums? • Do you have any difficulty swallowing or problems with hoarseness or a sore throat? • Do you have allergies? • Do you use nasal sprays? • Do you snore?
Breasts	• Do you perform breast self-examinations? What time of month do you perform it? • Do you have any tenderness or lumps in your breast(s)? • Do you have any discharge from the nipples? • Is there any history of breast cancer in your family? • Are you aware of breast cancer risks? • If over 40, do you get an annual mammogram?

SYSTEM	QUESTIONS TO BE ASKED
Respiratory	• Do you have any difficulties breathing? • Do you need to sit up to breathe? • Are you ever short of breath? • Have you been around anyone who has a cough, cold, or influenza? • Do you receive a yearly influenza vaccine? • Have you had the pneumonia vaccine? • Do you smoke? If yes, for how long and how much? Are you interested in quitting? • Are you exposed to second-hand smoke? • Do you experience environmental allergies? • Any family history of lung cancer or tuberculosis? • Any known exposure to tuberculosis?
Cardiovascular	• Do you have any problems with your heart? • Do you ever have pain in your chest? Does it radiate? • Do you have high cholesterol or high blood pressure? • Do you have any swelling in your feet and ankles? • Do you cough frequently? • Are you familiar with the risk factors for heart disease?
Gastrointestinal	• Do you have any problems with your stomach, such as nausea, vomiting, or pain? • Do you have any problems with your bowels, such as diarrhea or constipation? • When was your last bowel movement? • Do you ever use laxatives or enemas? • Have you had any black or tarry stools? • Do you use aspirin or ibuprofen? If so, how often? • Do you have any abdominal or lower back pain or tenderness? • Have you had any recent weight changes? • Do you have any food intolerances? • What is your 24-hr food history? • Do you have any swallowing difficulties? • Do you drink alcohol? If so, how much? • If over 50, have you had a colonoscopy? • Do you know the signs and symptoms of colon cancer? • What is your typical day's intake of food and fluid? • Do you have any dietary restrictions or special practices?

SYSTEM	QUESTIONS TO BE ASKED
Genitourinary	• Do you have any difficulties voiding, such as burning, incontinence, urgency, frequency, nocturia, or hesitancy? • Have you noticed any change in the color of your urine? • Have you noticed any changes in your menstrual cycle, such as cramps, discharge, or itching? • Have you experienced painful intercourse? • Have you experienced any sexual dysfunction? • Have you had any pain in your scrotum or testes?
Musculoskeletal	• Have you noticed any pain in your joints or muscles? • Have you experienced any weakness or twitching? • Have you had any recent falls? • Are you able to care for yourself? • Do you exercise or participate in sports? • For postmenopausal women – What is your maximum height? • For postmenopausal women – Do you take calcium supplements?
Neurological	• Have you noticed any change in your vision, speech, ability to think clearly, or loss of or change in memory? • Do you have any problems with dizziness or headaches? • Do you ever have seizures? • Do you ever have any weakness, tremors, numbness, or tingling anywhere? If so, where?
Mental health	• Is there anything stressful going on at work or at home? • Do you feel as though you are having any problems with depression? • Have you experienced any recent losses? • Are you having any problems concentrating?
Endocrine	• Have you noticed any change in urination patterns? • Have you noticed any change in your energy level? • Have you noticed any change in your ability to handle stress? • Have you experienced any change in weight or appetite? • Have you had any visual disturbances? • Have you had any palpitations?
Allergic/ immunologic	• Do you have any allergies to medications, foods, or environmental substances? • Have you ever received a blood transfusion? If so, did you have any adverse reactions?

Documentation

- Tell the client you will take notes.

- To facilitate note taking during the assessment, summarize information for future clarification. Do not rely on total memory recall.

- Document descriptive, concise, complete, and relevant data.

- Ensure confidentiality.

- Use guidelines for appropriate charting.

Physical Assessment Techniques

- During a physical assessment:

  o Ensure adequate lighting.

  o Maintain a quiet and comfortable environment.

  o Provide privacy, using a gown or draping the client with a sheet and visualizing only one section of the body at a time.

  o Explain the various assessment techniques you will use.

  o Look and observe before touching.

  o Keep nails short, and hands and stethoscope warm.

  o Do not feel or listen through clothing. (Clothing can obscure or create sounds.)

  o Have necessary equipment ready.

  o Use standard precautions when in contact with body fluids, wound drainage, and open lesions.

  o Document any values you might forget later.

- Additional guidelines for performing a physical assessment of older adult clients include:

  o Allow enough time for position changes.

  o Perform assessments in several shorter segments to avoid overtiring older adult clients.

  o Have sensory aids available for older adult clients to use, such as eyeglasses or hearing aids.

- Inspect, palpate, percuss, and auscultate in that order. The exception is the abdomen; inspect, auscultate, percuss, and palpate in that order to avoid altering bowel sounds.

- Inspection

  - Inspection, which is the first step in an assessment, begins with the first interaction with the client and continues throughout the examination.

  - A penlight, an otoscope, an ophthalmoscope, or another lighted instrument may enhance the process.

  - Inspection involves using the senses of vision, smell, and hearing to observe and detect any normal or abnormal findings. Inspect areas for size, shape, color, symmetry, and position.

- Palpation is touching to determine the size, consistency, texture, temperature, location, and tenderness of an organ or body part. Palpate tender areas last.

  - Light palpation (less than 1 cm) is required for most body surfaces. Deeper palpation is used to assess abdominal organs or masses.

  - Various parts of the hands are used to detect different sensations.

    - The dorsal surface is the most sensitive to temperature.

    - The ulnar surface and base of the fingers are sensitive to vibration.

    - Fingertips are sensitive to pulsation, position, texture, size, and consistency.

    - The fingers and thumb are used to grab an organ or mass.

  - Starting with light palpation, be systematic, calm, and gentle. Proceed to deep palpation if indicated.

- Percussion involves tapping body parts with fingers, fists, or small instruments to evaluate size, location, tenderness, and presence or absence of fluid or air in body organs, and to detect any abnormalities.

  - Techniques for percussion include:

    - Direct percussion, which involves striking the body to elicit sounds.

    - Indirect percussion, which involves placing a hand flatly on the body, as the striking surface, for sound production.

    - Fist percussion, which is used to assess for tenderness over the kidneys, liver, and gallbladder.

- Auscultation is the technique used to listen to sounds produced by the body. Some sounds are loud enough to be heard unaided, but most sounds require a stethoscope or a Doppler technique (heart sounds, air moving through the respiratory tract, blood moving through blood vessels). The examiner must learn to isolate the various sounds produced by the body to make accurate assessments.

  - The sounds produced are evaluated for amplitude or intensity (loud or soft), pitch or frequency (high or low), duration (time the sound lasts), and quality (what it sounds like).

  - The diaphragm of the stethoscope is used to listen to high-pitched sounds (normal heart sounds, bowel sounds, breath sounds).

    - The diaphragm should be placed firmly on the body part being examined.

  - The bell of the stethoscope is used to listen to low-pitched sounds (abnormal heart sounds, bruits).

    - The bell should be placed lightly on the body part being examined.

Equipment

- Equipment needed for a screening examination includes:

  - Gown

  - Drapes

  - Scale with height measurement

  - Thermometer

  - Stethoscope with diaphragm and bell

  - Sphygmomanometer

  - Reading/eye chart

  - Otoscope, ophthalmoscope, and nasal speculum

  - Penlight (or ophthalmoscope)

  - Cotton balls

  - Sharp and dull objects

  - Tuning fork

  - Glass of water

  - Items to test smell and taste

  - Clean gloves

  - Tongue depressor

- o   Reflex hammer

- o   Marking pen

- o   Measuring tape and clear, flexible ruler with measurements in centimeters

- o   Watch or clock to measure time in seconds

General Survey

- •   The general survey is a written summary of the impressions of the client's overall health. The nurse gathers this information from the first encounter with the client and continues to make observations throughout the assessment process. The nurse will assess:

  - o   Physical appearance

    - ▪   Age

    - ▪   Gender and race

    - ▪   Level of consciousness

    - ▪   Color of skin

    - ▪   Facial features

    - ▪   Signs of distress (pallor, labored breathing, guarding, anxiety)

    - ▪   Signs of possible physical abuse or neglect

    - ▪   Signs of substance abuse

  - o   Body structure

    - ▪   Body build, stature, height, and weight

    - ▪   Nutritional status

    - ▪   Symmetry of body parts

    - ▪   Posture and usual position

    - ▪   Gross abnormalities (skin lesions, amputations)

  - o   Mobility

    - ▪   Gait

    - ▪   Range of motion

    - ▪   Motor activity

  - o   Behavior

    - ▪   Facial expression and mannerisms

    - ▪   Mood and affect

    - ▪   Speech

    - ▪   Dress, hygiene, grooming, and odors (body and breath)

- o Vital signs
  - Temperature
  - Pulse
  - Respiration
  - Blood pressure

Sample Documentation

- Client – 16-year-old male, alert and oriented x 3. No distress noted. Personal hygiene and grooming slightly unkept but appropriate for age. Weight appropriate for height, good posture, and steady gait. Full range of motion. Does not maintain good eye contact. Volunteers no information but answers questions appropriately when asked. No gross abnormalities noted.

CHAPTER 26: DATA COLLECTION AND GENERAL SURVEY

 Application Exercises

1. Which of the following is an effective technique to use when interviewing a client?

    A. Start the interview with nonthreatening topics.

    B. Use only nondirective questions.

    C. Have the client fill out a printed history form.

    D. Ask questions word for word from the history form.

2. A client presents with severe headache pain. Identify what questions to ask to obtain information regarding a symptom analysis.

Location	
Quality	
Quantity	
Timing	
Setting	
Alleviating or aggravating factors	
Associated phenomena	

3. A client expresses concern over the confidentiality of the information she is providing during her health history. The nurse should respond by telling the client

    A. exactly with whom the information will be shared.

    B. that it is required for her to give any information that is requested.

    C. a confidential piece of information about herself.

    D. her family members will be informed of necessary information.

4. Which of the following therapeutic techniques is used to provide a comfortable environment for performing a health assessment? (Select all that apply.)

    _____ Provide privacy.

    _____ Examine sensitive areas first.

    _____ Reduce environmental noises.

    _____ Explain various techniques before performing them.

    _____ Use medical terminology to save time.

5. Identify the location where the following percussion sounds are normally produced in the body.

PERCUSSION SOUND	EXPECTED LOCATION TO BE HEARD
Tympany	
Resonance	
Dull	
Flat	

6. Put an X in the box for the appropriate technique(s) used to assess each of the following. (Select all that apply.)

ASSESSMENT	INSPECTION	PALPATION	PERCUSSION	AUSCULTATION
Pupil size				
Ankle edema				
Skin temperature				
Bowel sounds				
Loose teeth				
Liver size				
External ear				
Kidney tenderness				

7. The nurse should use which part of the hand to assess for vibration?

    A. Ulnar surface

    B. Finger pads

    C. Dorsal surface

    D. Palmar surface

8. The correct order for performing abdominal assessment techniques is

    A. inspection, palpation, percussion, and auscultation.

    B. inspection, auscultation, percussion, and palpation.

    C. auscultation, inspection, percussion, and palpation.

    D. auscultation, palpation, percussion, and inspection.

CHAPTER 26: DATA COLLECTION AND GENERAL SURVEY

 Application Exercises Answer Key

1. Which of the following is an effective technique to use when interviewing a client?

A. Start the interview with nonthreatening topics.

B. Use only nondirective questions.

C. Have the client fill out a printed history form.

D. Ask questions word for word from the history form.

Starting the interview with nonthreatening topics will facilitate establishing rapport and trust between the client and nurse. Using nondirective questions may make the client feel comfortable, but may allow the client to avoid discussing important details. Having the client fill out a history form and asking questions word for word may discourage the establishment of a therapeutic relationship with the client.

(N) **NCLEX® Connection: Health Promotion and Maintenance, Techniques of Physical Assessment**

2. A client presents with severe headache pain. Identify what questions to ask to obtain information regarding a symptom analysis.

Location	Where is your headache? Point to where it hurts.
Quality	What does the pain feel like? Is it dull, stabbing, throbbing, and/or achy?
Quantity	On a scale of 0 to 10, with 0 being no pain and 10 being the worst pain you have ever experienced, how would you rate the pain?
Timing	When did the pain start? How long have you had it? Is it constant or intermittent?
Setting	Where are you when you experience the pain? Does it happen at work? At home?
Alleviating or aggravating factors	What makes the pain better or worse? Have you taken any medications for the pain?
Associated phenomena	Do you have any nausea? Are you dizzy?

(N) **NCLEX® Connection: Health Promotion and Maintenance, Techniques of Physical Assessment**

3. A client expresses concern over the confidentiality of the information she is providing during her health history. The nurse should respond by telling the client

    A. exactly with whom the information will be shared.

    B. that it is required for her to give any information that is requested.

    C. a confidential piece of information about herself.

    D. her family members will be informed of necessary information.

The client has a right to confidentiality and the right to know with whom her information will be shared. The client has the right to refuse to reveal information if she chooses. The nurse telling the client confidential information about herself is not professional. Giving information to family members is a violation of confidentiality.

 NCLEX® Connection: Management of Care, Confidentiality/Information Security

4. Which of the following therapeutic techniques is used to provide a comfortable environment for performing a health assessment? (Select all that apply.)

    __X__   **Provide privacy.**

    _____   Examine sensitive areas first.

    __X__   **Reduce environmental noises.**

    __X__   **Explain various techniques before performing them.**

    _____   Use medical terminology to save time.

Providing for privacy, reducing environmental noises, and explaining techniques to be used will facilitate establishing a trusting relationship and performing a health assessment. Sensitive areas should be examined after the client has developed some trust and feels more comfortable. Medical terminology may confuse the client and lead to misunderstanding of the intended message.

 NCLEX® Connection: Health Promotion and Maintenance, Techniques of Physical Assessment

5. Identify the location where the following percussion sounds are normally produced in the body.

PERCUSSION SOUND	EXPECTED LOCATION
Tympany	Gastric bubble
Resonance	Lungs
Dull	Liver
Flat	Muscles

NCLEX® Connection: Health Promotion and Maintenance, Techniques of Physical Assessment

6. Put an X in the box for the appropriate technique(s) used to assess each of the following. (Select all that apply.)

ASSESSMENT	INSPECTION	PALPATION	PERCUSSION	AUSCULTATION
Pupil size	X			
Ankle edema	X	X		
Skin temperature		X		
Bowel sounds				X
Loose teeth	X	X		
Liver size		X	X	
External ear	X	X		
Kidney tenderness			X	

 NCLEX® Connection: Health Promotion and Maintenance, Techniques of Physical Assessment

7. The nurse should use which part of the hand to assess for vibration?

   A. Ulnar surface

   B. Finger pads

   C. Dorsal surface

   D. Palmar surface

   The ulnar surface of the hand is the most sensitive to vibration.

 NCLEX® Connection: Health Promotion and Maintenance, Techniques of Physical Assessment

8. The correct order for performing abdominal assessment techniques is

   A. inspection, palpation, percussion, and auscultation.

   B. inspection, auscultation, percussion, and palpation.

   C. auscultation, inspection, percussion, and palpation.

   D. auscultation, palpation, percussion, and inspection.

   The abdomen is examined using inspection, auscultation, percussion, and palpation. Percussion and palpation are delayed to avoid changing normally occurring bowel sounds.

 NCLEX® Connection: Health Promotion and Maintenance, Techniques of Physical Assessment

UNIT 2	HEALTH PROMOTION
Section	Health Assessment
Chapter 27	Vital Signs

 Overview

- Vital signs are measurements of the body's most basic functions. They provide health care staff with information about almost every system in the body. The vital signs most often assessed are temperature, pulse, respiration, and blood pressure. In many health care facilities, pain and oxygen saturation are also considered vital signs and may also be measured depending on the reason the client needs health care. Both pain and oxygen saturation are covered in the chapters on pain management and respiratory management in this review module.

  o Temperature, measured in degrees, reflects the balance between heat produced and lost from the body.

  o Pulse is the measurement of heart rate and rhythm. Pulse corresponds to the bounding of blood flowing through various points in the circulatory system.

  o Respiration is the body's mechanism for exchanging oxygen and carbon dioxide between the atmosphere and the cells of the body, which is accomplished through breathing and recorded as the number of breaths per minute.

  o Blood pressure (BP) reflects the force the blood exerts against the walls of the arteries during contraction (systole) and relaxation (diastole) of the heart.

    ■ Systolic BP (SBP) occurs during ventricular systole of the heart, when the ventricles force blood into the aorta, and represents the maximum amount of pressure exerted on the arteries.

    ■ Diastolic BP (DBP) occurs during ventricular diastole of the heart, when the ventricles relax and exert minimal pressure against arterial walls, and represents the minimum amount of pressure exerted on the arteries.

Temperature

- Physiological Responses

  - The neurological and cardiovascular systems work together to keep body temperature within an expected reference range. Disease or trauma of the hypothalamus or spinal cord will alter temperature control.

  - The rectum, tympanic membrane, and urinary bladder are core temperature measurement sites.

  - The skin, mouth, and axillae are surface temperature measurement sites.

- Expected temperature ranges are as follows:

  - An oral temperature range of 36° to 38° C (96.8° to 100.4° F) is acceptable. The average is 37° C (98.6° F).

  - Rectal temperatures are usually 0.5° C (0.9° F) higher than oral temperatures.

  - Axillary and tympanic temperatures are usually 0.5° C (0.9° F) lower than oral temperatures.

  - Temporal temperatures are close to rectal temperatures, but they are nearly 0.5° C (1° F) higher than oral temperatures, and 1° C (2° F) higher than axillary temperatures.

  - The client's usual temperature serves as a baseline for comparison.

- Heat production results from increases in basal metabolic rate, muscle activity, thyroxine output, and sympathetic stimulation, which increases heat production.

- Heat loss from the body occurs through:

  - Conduction – Transfer of heat from the body directly to another surface (when the body is immersed in cold water).

  - Convection – Dispersion of heat by air currents (wind blowing across exposed skin).

  - Evaporation – Dispersion of heat through water vapor (sweating and diaphoresis).

  - Radiation – Transfer of heat from one object to another object without contact between them (heat lost from the body to a cold room).

- Newborns have a large surface-to-mass ratio; therefore, they lose heat rapidly to the environment. Newborns' temperatures should be maintained between 36.5° and 37.5° C (97.7° and 99.5° F).

- Older adult clients experience a loss of subcutaneous fat that results in lower body temperatures and feeling cold. Their average body temperature is 36° C (96.8° F). Older adult clients are more likely to be adversely affected by extremes in environmental temperatures (heat stroke, hypothermia). It also takes longer for body temperature to register on a thermometer due to changes in temperature regulation.

- Hormonal changes may influence temperature. In general, temperature rises slightly with ovulation and menses. With menopause, intermittent body temperature may increase by up to 4° C (7.2° F).

- Exercise, activity, and dehydration can contribute to the development of hyperthermia.

- Illness and injury are often associated with elevations in temperature. Fever is the body's response to infectious and/or inflammatory processes.

- Recent food or fluid intake and smoking can interfere with accurate measurement of body temperature, so it is best to wait 20 to 30 min before measuring temperature.

Nursing Interventions

- Equipment

  o Electronic thermometers use a probe to measure body temperature. A disposable cover is placed on the probe prior to insertion. An audible signal is emitted when temperature assessment is completed, and a digital reading of the temperature appears. Oral, rectal, and axillary temperatures can be assessed using a similar device. Tympanic temperatures are obtained using a device specifically designed to assess temperature at the tympanic membrane (eardrum).

  o Disposable thermometers are designed for oral or axillary use. These thermometers are individually wrapped and discarded after one use. They offer a reduced risk of cross-infection.

  o Glass, mercury-filled thermometers are rarely used due to the risk of mercury exposure. If using a mercury-filled thermometer, shake the mercury level down to 35° C (95° F) prior to use, and follow facility policy for proper disposable. Avoid contact with mercury, washing skin thoroughly if contact occurs.

- Procedure

  o Perform hand hygiene, provide privacy, and apply clean gloves.

TECHNIQUE	DESCRIPTION
Oral	<ul><li>Gently place the thermometer (with an oral probe) under the tongue in the posterior sublingual pocket lateral to the center of the lower jaw.</li><li>Leave it in place until the signal is heard. (Hold a mercury thermometer in place for 3 min.)</li><li>Safety measure – Do not use glass, mercury-filled thermometers for clients who might bite the thermometer (small children, clients who are confused).</li><li>Age-specific – In general, this is the preferred method for individuals who are 4 years of age and older.</li><li>Note – The oral site may not be appropriate for assessing the temperature of clients who breathe through their mouth or have experienced trauma to the face or mouth.</li></ul>

TECHNIQUE	DESCRIPTION
Rectal	• Provide privacy. • Assist the client to Sims' position with the upper leg flexed. Wearing gloves, expose the anal area while keeping other body areas covered. Spread the buttocks to expose the anal opening. • Ask the client to breathe slowly and relax when placing a lubricated thermometer (with a rectal probe) into the anus in the direction of the umbilicus 3.5 cm (1½ in) for an adult. If resistance is encountered, remove it immediately. Once inserted, hold the thermometer in place until the signal is heard. (Hold a mercury thermometer in place for 3 min.) • Clean the anal area to remove feces or lubricant. • Safety measure: Do not use for clients on bleeding precautions or who have rectal disorders. • Age-specific: A rectal measurement of temperature is more accurate than axillary. However, because of the risk of rectal perforation, the American Academy of Pediatrics recommends screening infants 3 months old and younger by measuring axillary temperature initially. • The rectal site can be used to obtain a second measurement if the temperature is above 37.2° C (99° F). • Note: Stool in the rectum can cause inaccurate readings.
Axillary	• Place the thermometer (with an oral probe) in the center of the client's clean, dry axilla. Lower the arm over the probe. • Hold the arm down, keeping the thermometer in position until the signal is heard. (Hold a mercury thermometer in place for 2 min.)
Tympanic	• Pull the ear up and back (for an adult) or down and back (for a child who is younger than 3 years old). • Place the thermometer probe snugly into the client's outer ear canal and press the scan button. • Leave it in place until the signal is heard. • Carefully remove the thermometer from the ear canal and read the temperature. • Age-specific – The American Academy of Pediatrics advises against the use of electronic ear thermometers for infants 3 months old and younger due to the inaccuracy of readings. • Note – Excess earwax can alter the reading. If noted, use the other ear or select another appropriate site for temperature assessment.
Temporal	• Remove the protective cap and wipe the lens of the scanning device with alcohol to make sure it is clean. • While pressing the scan button, hold the probe flat against the forehead while moving it gently across the forehead over the temporal artery, and then touch the skin behind the earlobe. • Release the scan button to display the temperature reading. • Note – Depending on facility policy, either use disposable probe covers or clean the probe with a disinfectant wipe between clients.

      o   Document findings and report abnormal findings to the provider.

Complications and Nursing Interventions

- Fever – Fever is usually not harmful unless it exceeds 39° C (102.2° F).

- Hyperthermia is an abnormally elevated body temperature.

  o Obtain specimens for blood cultures if ordered.

  o Assess/monitor white blood cell counts, sedimentation rates, and electrolytes as ordered.

  o Administer antibiotics as prescribed (after obtaining specimens for blood culture).

  o Provide fluids and rest. Minimize activity.

  o Provide antipyretics (aspirin, acetaminophen [Tylenol], ibuprofen [Advil]). Aspirin use is not recommended for managing fever in children and adolescents who may have a viral illness (influenza, chickenpox) due to the risk of Reye syndrome. Pediatric antipyretic dosages are calculated based on weight.

  o Prevent shivering as this increases energy demand.

  o Offer blankets during chills and remove them when the client feels warm. A cooling blanket may also be used.

  o Provide oral hygiene and dry clothing and linens.

  o Control environmental temperature, maintaining it between 21° and 27° C (70° to 80° F).

- Hypothermia, a body temperature below 35° C (below 95° F), is an abnormally low body temperature.

  o Provide a warm environmental temperature, heated humidified oxygen, a warming blanket, friction to the extremities, and/or warmed oral or intravenous fluids.

  o Keep the head covered.

  o Provide continuous cardiac monitoring.

  o Have emergency resuscitation equipment on standby.

PULSE

- Physiologic Responses

  o The autonomic nervous system controls the heart rate. The parasympathetic nervous system lowers the heart rate, and the sympathetic nervous system raises the heart rate.

- The wave-like sensations or impulses felt in a peripheral arterial vessel or over the apex of the heart are assessed as a gauge of cardiovascular status.

  o Rate – The number of times per minute the pulse is felt or heard.

FUNDAMENTALS FOR NURSING

○ Rhythm – The regularity at which each impulse is felt. A premature or late heartbeat can result in an irregular interval in which impulses are felt or heard and can indicate abnormal electrical activity of the heart. Typically, an impulse should be sensed at regular intervals.

○ Strength (amplitude) – The strength of the impulse should be the same from beat to beat and can be graded on a scale of 0 to 4.

  ▪ This scale is interpreted as follows:

    □ 0 = Absent, unable to palpate

    □ 1+ = Diminished, weaker than expected

    □ 2+ = Brisk, expected

    □ 3+ = Increased

    □ 4+ = Full volume, bounding

○ Equality – Peripheral pulse impulses should be symmetrical in quality and quantity from the right side of the body to the left. Strength and equality are assessed to evaluate the adequacy of the vascular system.

- The expected reference range for a pulse of an adult client is 60 to 100/min at rest.

  ○ Tachycardia – A rate above the expected range or faster than 100/min.

  ○ Bradycardia – A rate below the expected range or slower than 60/min.

- Dysrhythmia – An irregular heart rhythm often noted as an irregular radial pulse.

- A pulse deficit – An apical rate faster than the radial rate. With dysrhythmias, the heart may contract ineffectively, resulting in a beat heard at the apical site with no pulsation felt at the radial pulse point.

- Age – For infants, the expected pulse rate is 120 to 160/min. The rate gradually decreases as the child grows older. The average pulse for a 12- to 14-year-old child is 80 to 90/min. The strength of the pulsation may weaken in older adult clients due to poor circulation or cardiac dysfunction, which makes the peripheral pulses more difficult to palpate.

FACTORS LEADING TO TACHYCARDIA	FACTORS LEADING TO BRADYCARDIA
Exercise	Long-term physical fitness
Fever	Hypothermia
Medications – Epinephrine, levothyroxine (Synthroid), beta$_2$-adrenergic agonists (albuterol [Proventil])	Medications – Digoxin (Lanoxin), beta-blockers (propranolol [Inderal]), calcium channel blockers (verapamil [Calan])
Changing position from lying down to sitting or standing	Changing position from standing or sitting to lying down
Acute pain	Chronic pain
Hyperthyroidism	Hypothyroidism
Anemia, hypoxemia	

FACTORS LEADING TO TACHYCARDIA	FACTORS LEADING TO BRADYCARDIA
Stress, anxiety, and fear	
Hypovolemia, shock, and heart failure	

Nursing Interventions

- Equipment

  - A watch or clock that allows for counting seconds

  - Stethoscope

- Procedure

  - Perform hand hygiene and provide privacy.

  - Radial pulse is located on the radial- or thumb-side of the forearm at the wrist.

    - Place the index and middle finger of one hand gently but firmly over the pulse. Assess the pulsation for rate, rhythm, amplitude, and quality.

    - If the peripheral pulsation is regular, count the rate for 30 sec and multiply by 2. If the pulsation is irregular, count for a full minute and compare the result to the apical pulse rate.

  - Apical pulse is located at the fifth intercostal space at the left midclavicular line. Use this site for assessing the heart rate of an infant, rapid rates (faster than 100/min), irregular rhythms, and rates prior to the administration of cardiac medications.

    - Place the stethoscope on the chest at the fifth intercostal space at the left midclavicular line. Always count an apical pulse rate for 1 min.

  - Document findings and report abnormal findings to the provider.

View Media Supplement:

- Pulse Points (Image)
- Apical Pulse (Image)

Complications and Nursing Interventions

- Tachycardia

  - Assess/monitor for other signs and symptoms (pain, anxiety, restlessness, fatigue, low blood pressure, low oxygen saturation).

  - Assess/monitor for potential side/adverse effects of medications.

  - Prevent injury.

  - Notify the provider.

- Bradycardia

  o Assess/monitor for other signs and symptoms (hypotension, chest pain, syncope, diaphoresis, dyspnea, altered mental status).

  o Assess/monitor for potential side/adverse effects of medications.

  o Prevent injury.

  o Notify the provider.

RESPIRATIONS

- Physiological Responses

  o Chemoreceptors in the carotid arteries and the aorta primarily monitor carbon dioxide (CO_2) levels of the blood. If carbon dioxide rises, the respiratory center of the brain is triggered to increase the respiratory rate. The increased respiratory rate rids the body of excess CO_2. For clients with chronic obstructive pulmonary disease (COPD), a low oxygen level becomes the primary respiratory drive.

- The processes of respiration includes:

  o Ventilation – The exchange of oxygen and carbon dioxide in the lungs. Measure ventilation with the respiratory rate, rhythm, and depth.

  o Diffusion – The exchange of oxygen and carbon dioxide between the alveoli and the red blood cells. Measure diffusion with pulse oximetry.

  o Perfusion – The flow of blood to and from the pulmonary capillaries. Measure perfusion with pulse oximetry.

- Accurate assessment of respiration involves observing the rate, depth, and rhythm of chest-wall movement during inspiration and expiration. Do not inform the client that you are measuring respirations.

  o Rate – The number of full inspirations and expirations in 1 min. Determine this by observing the number of times the client's chest rises and falls. The expected reference range for adults is 12 to 20/min.

  o Depth – The amount of chest wall expansion that occurs with each breath. Altered depths are described as deep or shallow.

  o Rhythm – The observation of breathing intervals. A regular rhythm with an occasional sigh is expected in adults.

- Pulse Oximetry

  o This is a noninvasive, indirect measurement of the oxygen saturation (SaO_2) of the blood. The expected reference range is 95% to 100%, although acceptable levels for some clients range from 91% to 100%. Some illness states may even allow for an SaO_2 of 85% to 89%. Less than 85% is abnormal.

- Age – Respiratory rate decreases with age. Newborns have rates of 30 to 60/min. School-age children have respiratory rates of 20 to 30/min.

- Gender differences are noted when observing respirations. Men are diaphragmatic breathers, and abdominal movements are more noticeable. Women use more thoracic muscles, and chest movements are more pronounced when they breathe.

- Pain in the chest wall area may decrease the depth of respirations. At the onset of acute pain, the respiration rate increases but stabilizes over time.

- Anxiety increases the rate and depth of respirations.

- Smoking causes the resting rate of respirations to increase.

- Body position – Upright positions allow the chest wall to expand more fully.

- Medications such as opioids, sedatives, bronchodilators, and general anesthetics decrease the respiratory rate and depth. Respiratory depression can be a serious adverse effect. Amphetamines and cocaine increase rate and depth.

- Neurological injury to the brainstem decreases respiratory rate and rhythm.

- Illnesses affecting the shape of the chest wall, changing the patency of passages, impairing muscle function, and diminish respiratory effort. With these conditions, the use of accessory muscles and the respiratory rate increase.

- Impaired oxygen-carrying capacity of the blood that occurs with anemia or at high altitudes results in increases in the respiratory rate and alterations in rhythm to compensate.

Nursing Interventions

- Respiratory Rate

  o Equipment

    ▪ A watch or clock that allows for counting seconds.

  o Procedure

    ▪ Perform hand hygiene and provide privacy.

    ▪ Place the client in semi-Fowler's position, being sure the chest is visible.

    ▪ Have the client rest an arm across the abdomen, or place a hand directly on the client's abdomen.

    ▪ Observe one full respiratory cycle, look at the timer, and then begin counting the rate.

    ▪ Count a regular rate for 30 seconds and multiply by 2. Count the rate for 1 min if irregular, faster than 20/min, or slower than 12/min. Note depth (shallow, normal, or deep) and rhythm (regular or irregular).

    ▪ Document findings and report abnormal findings to the provider.

- Oxygen Saturation

  - Equipment

    - Pulse oximeter

  - Procedure

    - When the readout on the pulse oximeter is stable, record this value as the client's oxygen saturation.

    - Report abnormal findings to the provider.

Complications and Nursing Interventions

- Hypoxemia – SaO_2 below 90%

  - Confirm that the sensor probe is properly placed.

  - Correlate the pulse rate on the oximeter with the client's radial or apical pulse.

  - Confirm that the oxygen delivery system is functioning and that the client is receiving the prescribed amount of oxygen.

  - Place the client in semi-Fowler's or Fowler's position to maximize ventilation.

  - Encourage deep breathing.

  - Suction as needed and if ordered.

  - Assess for signs of hypoxemia (tachypnea, tachycardia, restlessness, anxiety, cyanosis).

  - Check for hyperthermia.

  - Assess/monitor vital signs. Report significant findings to the provider.

  - Remain with the client and provide emotional support to decrease anxiety.

BLOOD PRESSURE

- Physiological responses

  - The principal determinants of blood pressure (BP) are cardiac output (CO) and systemic vascular resistance (SVR).

  - BP = CO x SVR.

CO	SVR
CO is determined by: • HR • Contractility • Blood volume • Venous return	• Systemic (peripheral) vascular resistance (SVR) is determined by the amount of constriction or dilation of the arteries.
• Increases in any of these increase CO and BP • Decreases in any of these decrease CO and BP	• Increases in SVR increase BP • Decreases in SVR decrease BP

- Classifications of BP according to the Seventh Report of the Joint National Committee on Prevention, Detection, Evaluation, and Treatment of High Blood Pressure (JNC 7):

BP CLASSIFICATION	SYSTOLIC BP (SBP) IN MM HG	DIASTOLIC BP (DBP) IN MM HG
Normal	< 120	and < 80
Prehypertension	120 to 139	or 80 to 89
Stage 1 hypertension	140 to 159	or 90 to 99
Stage 2 hypertension	≥ 160	or ≥ 100

- Classification is based on the highest reading. A client with a blood pressure of 124/92 mm Hg has stage 1 hypertension because the DBP places the client in that category. A client with a blood pressure of 146/82 mm Hg also has stage 1 hypertension because the SBP places the client in that category.

- If the client has a SBP of > 140 mm Hg and a DBP of > 90 mm Hg when two or more BP measurements are averaged, he should return for two or more visits for additional readings. A diagnosis of hypertension is made if the readings are elevated on at least three separate occasions over several weeks.

- Hypotension is a BP that is below normal (systolic < 90 mm Hg) and can be a result of fluid depletion, heart failure, or vasodilation.

- Pulse pressure is the difference between the systolic and the diastolic pressure readings.

- Postural (orthostatic) hypotension is a BP that falls when a client changes position from lying to sitting or standing, and it may result from various causes (peripheral vasodilation, medication side effects, fluid depletion, anemia, prolonged bedrest).

  o Orthostatic changes are assessed by taking the client's BP and HR in the supine position. Next, have the client change to the sitting or standing position, wait 1 to 5 min, and reassess the BP and HR. The client is experiencing orthostatic hypotension if the SBP decreases more than 20 mm Hg and/or the DBP decreases more than 10 mm Hg with a 10% to 20% increase in the heart rate (HR).

- Age

  o Infants have a low BP that gradually increases with age.

  o Older children and adolescents have varying BP based on body size. Larger children have a higher BP.

  o Adults' BP tends to increase with age.

  o Older adult clients may have a slightly elevated systolic pressure due to decreased elasticity of blood vessels.

- Circadian (diurnal) rhythms affect BP, with BP usually lowest in the early morning hours and peaking during the later part of the afternoon or evening.

- Stress associated with fear, emotional strain, and acute pain can increase BP.

- Ethnicity – African Americans have a higher incidence of hypertension in general and at earlier ages.

- Gender – Adolescent to middle-age men have higher BPs than their female counterparts. Postmenopausal women have higher BPs than their male counterparts.

- Medications such as opiates, antihypertensives, and cardiac medications can lower BP. Cocaine, smoking, cold medications, oral contraceptives, and antidepressants can raise BP.

- Exercise can cause a decrease in BP for several hours afterwards.

- Obesity is a contributing factor to hypertension.

Nursing Interventions

- Equipment

  ○ The ausculatory method uses a:

    ▪ Sphygmomanometer with a pressure manometer (aneroid or mercury) and an appropriately sized cuff. The width of the cuff should be 40% of the arm circumference at the point where the cuff is wrapped. The bladder (inside the cuff) should surround 80% of the arm circumference of an adult and the whole arm for a child. Cuffs that are too large give a falsely low reading, and cuffs that are too small give a falsely high reading.

    ▪ Stethoscope

  ○ Automatic BP devices may be used when available for monitoring clients who require frequent evaluation. A BP should be obtained first using the ausculatory method to make sure the automatic device readings are valid.

- Procedure (Ausculatory Method)

  ○ Perform hand hygiene and provide privacy.

  ○ Initially measure BP in both arms. If the difference is more than 10 mm Hg, use the arm with the higher reading for subsequent measurements. In addition, this difference may indicate a vascular problem and should be reported to the provider.

THE CLIENT SHOULD	THE NURSE SHOULD
• Not smoke or drink any caffeine for 30 min prior to measurement. • Rest for 5 min before measurement.	• Use the ausculatory method with a properly calibrated and validated instrument. • Use an appropriate cuff size. • Not measure BP in an arm with an IV infusion in progress or on the side where a mastectomy was performed or an arteriovenous shunt or fistula is present.

THE CLIENT SHOULD	THE NURSE SHOULD
• Sit in a chair, with the feet flat on floor, the back and arm supported, and the arm at heart level.	• Average two or more readings, taken at least 2 min apart. (If they differ by more than 5 mm Hg, obtain additional readings and average them.) • After initial readings, measure BP and pulse with the client standing.

○ Apply the BP cuff 2 cm above the antecubital space with the brachial artery in line with the marking on the cuff.

○ Use lower extremity if the brachial artery is not accessible.

○ Estimate systolic pressure by palpating the radial pulse and inflating the cuff until the pulse disappears. Inflate the cuff another 30 mm Hg, and slowly release the pressure to note when the pulse is palpable again (the estimated systolic pressure).

○ Deflate the cuff and wait 1 min.

○ Position the stethoscope over the brachial artery.

○ Close the pressure bulb by turning the valve clockwise until tight.

○ Quickly inflate the cuff to 30 mm Hg above the palpated systolic pressure.

○ Release the pressure no faster than 2 to 3 mm Hg per second.

○ The level at which the first clear sounds are heard is the systolic pressure.

○ Continue to deflate the cuff until the sounds muffle and disappear and note the diastolic pressure.

○ Record the systolic over the diastolic pressure(110/70 mm Hg).

• Unexpected BP Readings

○ It is helpful to measure the BP again near the end of an encounter with the client. Earlier pressures may be higher due to the stress of the clinical setting.

○ Recheck BPs measured by assistive personnel or when an automatic device is used.

○ The cuff must be completely deflated between attempts. Wait at least 1 full min before reinflating the cuff. Air trapped in the bladder can cause a falsely high reading.

○ Notify the provider if the BP is above or below the client's usual value.

Complications and Nursing Interventions

• Orthostatic (Postural) Hypotension

○ Assess/monitor the client's BP.

○ Assess for other related symptoms such as dizziness, weakness, and fainting.

○ Instruct the client to activate the call light and not to get out of bed without assistance.

- o Have the client sit at the edge of the bed for at least 1 min before standing up.

- o Assist with ambulation.

- o Home care instructions include:

  - ▪ Warning the client that lightheadedness and dizziness can occur.

  - ▪ Advising the client to sit or lie down if these symptoms occur.

  - ▪ Suggesting that the client get up slowly when lying or sitting and avoid sudden changes in position.

- • Hypertension

  - o Assess/monitor the client for other signs and symptoms (tachycardia, bradycardia, pain, anxiety). Primary hypertension is usually asymptomatic.

  - o Assess for identifiable causes of hypertension (renal disease, thyroid disease, medication).

  - o Administer pharmacological therapy as prescribed.

  - o Assess for risk factors.

  - o Encourage lifestyle modifications, which include:

    - ▪ Smoking cessation

    - ▪ Dietary modifications – DASH (Dietary Approaches to Stop Hypertension) diet

      - □ Restrict sodium intake.

      - □ Consume adequate potassium, calcium, and magnesium. These minerals help lower BP.

      - □ Restrict cholesterol and saturated fat intake.

    - ▪ Weight control

    - ▪ Modification of alcohol intake

    - ▪ Physical activity

    - ▪ Stress reduction

  - o Encourage the client to follow up with the provider.

CHAPTER 27: VITAL SIGNS

 Application Exercises

1. An 82-year-old man arrives at the emergency department with an oral body temperature of 38.3° C (101° F), a pulse rate of 114/min, and respiratory rate of 22/min. He is restless and his skin is warm to the touch. Which of the following are appropriate nursing interventions for this client? (Select all that apply.)

_____ Obtain culture specimens before initiating prescribed antimicrobials.

_____ Restrict fluids.

_____ Allow for adequate rest.

_____ Provide oral care.

_____ Only change bed linens when the client requests it.

_____ Apply an additional blanket if the client feels chilled.

2. Based on the data provided, select the appropriate temperature-assessment site and note the rationale for the selection. Some clients may have more than one option available to them.

CLIENT ASSESSMENT	SITE SELECTION	RATIONALE
A newborn		
A 6-month-old infant		
A healthy 60-year-old woman		
An 82-year-old man with confusion		
A client with hemorrhoids		
A client with a stuffy nose		
A client with a low platelet count due to chemotherapy		
A client immediately following mandibular surgery		

3. Determine whether each of the following factors increases or decreases the pulse rate. Check the appropriate box.

FACTOR	INCREASES	DECREASES
Hyperthyroidism		
Calcium channel blockers		
Hypothermia		
Acute pain		
Blood loss		
Anxiety		
Walking on the treadmill		

4. Indicate the appropriate pulse measurement site for each of the following situations. Choices may be used more than once.

_____ A 2-month-old infant during a routine checkup

_____ A 76-year-old client showing tachycardia and an irregular rhythm on the cardiac monitor

_____ A 56-year-old client with an order to receive a stat dose of digoxin (Lanoxin)

_____ A 20-year-old client in the emergency department with a hand laceration to be sutured

_____ A 16-year-old client who has been stable for 3 hr following an appendectomy

A. Apical

B. Radial

C. Simultaneous check of apical and radial

5. A nurse is checking the vital signs of a 92-year-old client. The client's radial pulse has an irregular beat about every fifth or sixth beat. The rate is 92/min. The client is asymptomatic. The nurse should do which of the following?

A. Report the findings to the provider immediately.

B. Place the client on telemetry.

C. Obtain an electrocardiogram.

D. Check an apical pulse for 60 seconds and note any pulse deficits.

6. Which of the following interventions are appropriate when assessing a client's respirations? (Select all that apply.)

_____ Count the respiratory rate for 1 min.

_____ Place the client in semi-Fowler's position.

_____ Count the respiratory rate simultaneously with the pulse.

_____ Position the stethoscope on the anterior chest.

_____ Observe one full respiratory cycle before counting the rate.

7. Determine whether each of the following factors increases or decreases the respiratory rate. Check the appropriate box.

FACTOR	INCREASES	DECREASES
Morphine		
Brisk walk on the treadmill		
Sickle cell disease		
Smoking		
Acute gallbladder attack		
Hiking in the mountains		
General anesthetic during surgery		

8. Determine whether each of the following factors increases or decreases the blood pressure. Check the appropriate box.

FACTOR	INCREASES	DECREASES
Cocaine		
A brisk walk on the treadmill		
Antihypertensives		
Acute gallbladder attack		
Postoperative pain		

9. For each of the following readings, identify the blood pressure classification according to the JNC 7.

_____ 132/94 mm Hg   A. Normal

_____ 108/72 mm Hg   B. Prehypertension

_____ 148/86 mm Hg   C. Stage 1 hypertension

_____ 172/92 mm Hg   D. Stage 2 hypertension

_____ 126/82 mm Hg

10. A nurse is checking the vital signs of a newly admitted client who has a fractured femur. The client's BP is 140/94 mm Hg. The client denies any history of hypertension. The nurse should do which of the following?

    A. Ask the client if she is having pain.

    B. Report the elevated BP to the provider.

    C. Return in 30 min to recheck the BP.

    D. Check the client's orthostatic BP.

CHAPTER 27: VITAL SIGNS

 Application Exercises Answer Key

1. An 82-year-old man arrives at the emergency department with an oral body temperature of 38.3° C (101° F), a pulse rate of 114/min, and respiratory rate of 22/min. He is restless and his skin is warm to the touch. Which of the following are appropriate nursing interventions for this client? (Select all that apply.)

__X__	**Obtain culture specimens before initiating prescribed antimicrobials.**
_____	Restrict fluids.
__X__	**Allow for adequate rest.**
__X__	**Provide oral care.**
_____	Only change bed linens when the client requests it.
__X__	**Apply an additional blanket if the client feels chilled.**

Cultures may be ordered to rule out the presence of infection and the specimens for culture should be obtained prior to the initiation of antibiotic therapy. This prevents the antibiotic from interfering with the detection of the infection. Rest helps conserve energy and decreases metabolic rate. Oral care provides comfort for the client's dry mucous membranes. An additional blanket will keep the client warm if he starts to feel chilled. Fluids should be encouraged for the client because he has a fever. The client is likely to sweat, so bed linens should be changed frequently and as needed.

 NCLEX® Connection: Physiological Adaptation, Alterations in Body Systems

2. Based on the data provided, select the appropriate temperature-assessment site and note the rationale for the selection. Some clients may have more than one option available to them.

CLIENT ASSESSMENT	SITE SELECTION	RATIONALE
A newborn	Axillary initially	Axillary avoids the risk of rectal perforation.
A 6-month-old infant	Tympanic	The child is older than 3 months.
A healthy 60-year-old woman	Oral	This is the preferred method for this age.
An 82-year-old man with confusion	Oral, tympanic, or axillary	Oral is preferred if the client is able to close his mouth around the probe. A glass thermometer is contraindicated.
A client with hemorrhoids	Oral, tympanic, or axillary	Oral is the preferred method. Tympanic and axillary can also be used. The rectal method is contraindicated.

CLIENT ASSESSMENT	SITE SELECTION	RATIONALE
A client with a stuffy nose	**Axillary or tympanic**	**This client is probably breathing through his mouth and will be unable to close his mouth around the probe.**
A client with a low platelet count due to chemotherapy	**Oral, tympanic, or axillary**	**Oral is the preferred method. Tympanic and axillary can also be used. The rectal method is contraindicated.**
A client immediately following mandibular surgery	**Axillary or tympanic**	**The oral route is contraindicated for a client with recent mouth trauma.**

Ⓝ NCLEX® Connection: Health Promotion and Maintenance, Techniques of Physical Assessment

3. Determine whether each of the following factors increases or decreases the pulse rate. Check the appropriate box.

FACTOR	INCREASES	DECREASES
Hyperthyroidism	X	
Calcium channel blockers		X
Hypothermia		X
Acute pain	X	
Blood loss	X	
Anxiety	X	
Walking on the treadmill	X	

Ⓝ NCLEX® Connection: Reduction of Risk Potential, System Specific Assessment

4. Indicate the appropriate pulse measurement site for each of the following situations. Choices may be used more than once.

__A__	A 2-month-old infant during a routine checkup	A. Apical
__C__	A 76-year-old client showing tachycardia and an irregular rhythm on the cardiac monitor	B. Radial
__A__	A 56-year-old client with an order to receive a stat dose of digoxin (Lanoxin)	C. Simultaneous check of apical and radial
__B__	A 20-year-old client in the emergency department with a hand laceration to be sutured	
__B__	A 16-year-old client who has been stable for 3 hr following an appendectomy	

Ⓝ NCLEX® Connection: Health Promotion and Maintenance, Techniques of Physical Assessment

5. A nurse is checking the vital signs of a 92-year-old client. The client's radial pulse has an irregular beat about every fifth or sixth beat. The rate is 92/min. The client is asymptomatic. The nurse should do which of the following?

A. Report the findings to the provider immediately.

B. Place the client on telemetry.

C. Obtain an electrocardiogram.

D. Check an apical pulse for 60 seconds and note any pulse deficits.

This radial pulse does not require immediate medical treatment; therefore, the nurse should next measure the client's apical pulse to assess the client's status further. The nurse should then report the findings to the provider, who will then decide if the client requires telemetry and an electrocardiogram.

Ⓝ NCLEX® Connection: Reduction of Risk Potential, System Specific Assessment

6. Which of the following interventions are appropriate when assessing a client's respirations? (Select all that apply.)

_____	Count the respiratory rate for 1 min.
X	**Place the client in semi-Fowler's position.**
_____	Count the respiratory rate simultaneously with the pulse.
_____	Position the stethoscope on the anterior chest.
X	**Observe one full respiratory cycle before counting the rate.**

The best position for the client during respiratory assessment is semi-Fowler's with the chest visible. Observing for one full respiratory cycle before starting to count assists in obtaining an accurate count. If the rate is regular, count for 30 seconds and multiply by 2. Count the rate for 1 full min if irregular, faster than 20/min, or slower than 12/min. It is difficult to measure either the respiratory rate or the pulse accurately if counted simultaneously. The respiratory rate is not auscultated with a stethoscope.

 NCLEX® Connection: Reduction of Risk Potential, Vital Signs

7. Determine whether each of the following factors increases or decreases the respiratory rate. Check the appropriate box.

FACTOR	INCREASES	DECREASES
Morphine		X
Brisk walk on the treadmill	X	
Sickle cell disease	X	
Smoking	X	
Acute gallbladder attack	X	
Hiking in the mountains	X	
General anesthetic during surgery		X

 NCLEX® Connection: Reduction of Risk Potential, System Specific Assessment

8. Determine whether each of the following factors increases or decreases the blood pressure. Check the appropriate box.

FACTOR	INCREASES	DECREASES
Cocaine	X	
A brisk walk on the treadmill		X
Antihypertensives		X
Acute gallbladder attack	X	
Postoperative pain	X	

 NCLEX® Connection: Reduction of Risk Potential, System Specific Assessment

9. For each of the following readings, identify the blood pressure classification according to the JNC 7.

__C__	132/94 mm Hg	A. Normal
__A__	108/72 mm Hg	B. Prehypertension
__C__	148/86 mm Hg	C. Stage 1 hypertension
__D__	172/92 mm Hg	D. Stage 2 hypertension
__B__	126/82 mm Hg	

(N) **NCLEX® Connection: Reduction of Risk Potential, System Specific Assessment**

10. A nurse is checking the vital signs of a newly admitted client who has a fractured femur. The client's BP is 140/94 mm Hg. The client denies any history of hypertension. The nurse should do which of the following?

A. Ask the client if she is having pain.

B. Report the elevated BP to the provider.

C. Return in 30 min to recheck the BP.

D. Check orthostatic BP.

This client has a broken femur, and her BP may be elevated due to pain. The nurse should ask if she is having pain and continue a full pain assessment. If the client's BP is still elevated after pain interventions, the nurse should report this finding to the provider. This client needs further assessment at this time, so returning in 30 min is not appropriate. There is no indication for orthostatic pressures, and it might be difficult to have the client sit or stand with a fractured femur.

(N) **NCLEX® Connection: Reduction of Risk Potential, Changes/Abnormal Vital Signs**

UNIT 2	HEALTH PROMOTION
Section	Health Assessment
Chapter 28	Head and Neck

Ⓞ Overview

- This examination includes the head and neck, eyes, nose, mouth, and throat.

HEAD AND NECK

Ⓞ Overview

- This examination includes the skull, face, hair, neck, shoulders, lymph nodes, thyroid gland, trachea position, carotid arteries, and jugular veins.

- Use the techniques of inspection, palpation, and auscultation to examine the client's head and neck.

- Abnormal findings may include decreased palpation of a mass, range of motion of the neck, or enlarged lymph nodes.

- Equipment includes a stethoscope.

- Test the following cranial nerves during the head and neck examination:

ASSESSMENT	CRANIAL NERVES
Assess the face for strength and sensation.	CN V (trigeminal)
Assess the face for symmetrical movement.	CN VII (facial)
Assess the shoulders for strength.	CN XI (spinal accessory)

Health History – Review of Systems

- Questions you should ask include:
    - Do you experience headaches? If so, how often, and where are they located? Do you have any other symptoms related to your headaches, such as nausea and vomiting?
    - Have you ever had a head injury?
    - Do you experience any pain in your neck?
    - Are you able to move your head and shoulders with ease?
    - Have you noticed any unusual facial movements?

- o   Are any of your lymph nodes swollen?

- o   Do you have any family history of thyroid disease?

Inspection and Palpation

- Head

  - o   Skull

    - Size (Normal is normocephalic.)

    - Depressions

    - Deformities

    - Masses

    - Tenderness

    - Overall contour and symmetry

  - o   Face

    - Symmetry of facial features

    - Symmetry of expressions

    - Involuntary movements (abnormal)

    - Proportionate features (no thickening as with acromegaly)

    - CN V

      - □   Motor – Test the strength of the muscle contraction by asking the client to clench her teeth while palpating the masseter and temporal muscles, and then the temporomandibular joint. TMJ movement should be smooth.

      - □   Sensory – Test light touch by having the client close her eyes while gently touching her face with a cotton swab and asking her to tell you when she feels the touch.

    - CN VII

      - □   Motor – Test facial movement by having the client smile, frown, puff out cheeks, raise eyebrows, close eyes tightly, and show teeth.

- Neck

  - o   Muscles of the neck should be symmetrical.

    - Shoulders should be equal in height and with normal muscle mass.

    - Range of motion (ROM) – The client should be able to move his head smoothly and without distress in the following directions:

      - □   Chin to chest (flexion).

      - □   Ear to shoulder bilaterally (lateral flexion).

      - □   Chin up (hyperextension).

- CN XI – Place your hands on the client's shoulders and ask the client to shrug the shoulders against resistance.

- Lymph nodes – Chains of lymph nodes extend from the lower half of the head down into the neck and should be palpated for enlargement. Lymph nodes to be palpated include:

LYMPH NODE	LOCATION
Occipital lymph node	Base of the skull
Preauricular lymph node	In front of the ear
Postauricular lymph node	Over the mastoid
Submandibular lymph node	Along the base of the mandible
Tonsillar (retropharyngeal) lymph node	Angle of the mandible
Submental lymph node	Midline under the chin
Anterior cervical lymph nodes	Along the sternocleidomastoid muscle
Posterior cervical lymph nodes	Posterior to the sternocleidomastoid muscle
Supraclavicular nodes	Above the clavicles

  o Lymph nodes should be nonpalpable and nontender. Normal nodes are not visible.

  o Use the pads of the index and middle fingers and move the skin over the underlying tissue in a circular motion. Compare from side to side.

  o If an enlargement is found, the node should be further evaluated for:

    - Location
    - Tenderness
    - Size
    - Shape
    - Consistency
    - Mobility
    - Discreteness
    - Warmth

- The thyroid gland is bilobed. Examine the gland by:

  o First, inspecting the lower half of the client's neck to see if an enlargement of the gland is visible. A normal thyroid gland is not visible.

  o Having the client take a sip of water and watching the thyroid tissue move up.

  o Approaching the client from behind and having the client tip her head forward and to the right. Use the left hand to displace the trachea slightly to the right while placing your right fingers between the sternomastoid muscle and the trachea.

  o Instructing the client to take a sip of water and feeling for the movement of the thyroid gland as it moves up with the trachea and larynx.

    ○   Repeating this procedure for the other side, palpating it for:

        ■   Size

        ■   Masses

        ■   Smoothness

- Trachea – Inspect and palpate the trachea for any deviation. The trachea should be midline.

Auscultation

- If the thyroid is enlarged, auscultate the gland using a stethoscope. The presence of a bruit indicates an abnormal increase in blood flow to the area.

EYES

 ## Overview

- This examination includes the external and internal anatomy of the eye, visual pathways, fields, and reflexes.

- The primary technique for examination of the eyes is inspection. A limited amount of palpation is done wearing gloves.

- Abnormal findings may include loss of visual fields, asymmetric corneal light reflex, periorbital edema, conjunctivitis, and corneal abrasion.

- Perform the eye examination in the following sequence, using the appropriate equipment.

TEST	EQUIPMENT
Visual acuity	• Distant vision – Snellen and Rosenbaum charts, eye cover, and Ishihara test • Near vision – Hand-held card
Extraocular movements (EOMs)	• Penlight or ophthalmoscope light • Eye cover
Visual fields	• Eye cover
External structures	• Penlight or ophthalmoscope light • Gloves
Internal structures	• Ophthalmoscope

- Test cranial nerves during the eye examination.

ASSESSMENT	CRANIAL NERVES (CN)
Visual acuity	CN II (optic)
Extraocular movements	CN III (oculomotor), CN IV (trochlear), CN VI (abducens)
Visual fields	CN II (optic)
Corneal light reflex Pupillary reaction to light	CN II (optic), CN III (oculomotor)

Health History – Review of Systems

- Questions you should ask include:

  - How is your vision? Have you noticed any changes?

  - Do you ever experience double vision? Do you ever see spots or halos?

  - Do you ever experience discharge from your eyes?

  - Do you wear eyeglasses or contact lenses?

  - When was your last eye examination?

  - Do you have any family history of eye disorders?

  - Do you have diabetes?

Inspection

- Visual Acuity – CN II

  - Use the Snellen (E) chart with the client standing 20 ft from the chart. The Snellen chart may be used for clients who are unable to read.

  - Evaluate both eyes and then each eye separately with and without correction.

  - For each eye, the opposite eye is covered.

  - Ask the client to read the smallest line of print visible.

  - The line for which two or fewer letters are missed is recorded as the visual acuity (20/20 is normal).

  - The first number indicates the number of feet from the chart the client is standing, and the second number is the distance at which a normal-sighted person can read the line.

- Screen for myopia (impaired far vision) using the Snellen chart.

- Screen for presbyopia (impaired near vision or farsightedness) using the Rosenbaum eye chart held 14 inches from the client's face. Readings correlate with the Snellen chart.

- Assess for color vision using the Ishihara test. The client should be able to identify the various shaded shapes.

- Extraocular movements (EOMs) – Assess EOMs to determine the coordination of the eye muscles using three different tests (CN III, CN IV, CN VI).

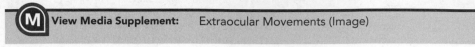
View Media Supplement: Extraocular Movements (Image)

  o Test the corneal light reflex by directing a light onto the client's eyes and looking to see if the reflection is seen symmetrically on the corneas.

  o Screen for strabismus with the cover/uncover test. While covering one eye, the client is asked to look in another direction. The cover is removed and both eyes should be gazing in the same direction.

  o The six cardinal positions of gaze require the client to follow your finger with his eyes without moving his head. Move your finger in a wide "H" pattern about 20 to 25 cm from the client's eyes. Eye movements should be smooth and symmetrical with no jerky or tremor-like movements (nystagmus).

- Evaluate visual fields (CN II) by facing the client at a distance of 60 cm. The client covers one eye while you cover your direct opposite eye (client's right eye and your left eye are covered). Ask the client to look at you and report when she can see the fingers on your outstretched arm coming in from four directions (up, down, temporally, nasally). The expected finding is that the client should see your fingers at the same time you do.

- External Structures

  o Eyes should be parallel to each other without bulging (exophthalmos) or crossing (strabismus).

  o Eyebrows should be symmetrical and evenly distributed from the inner to the outer canthus.

  o Eyelids should close completely and open to allow the lower border and most of the upper portion of the iris to be seen. No ptosis (covering of the pupil by the upper eyelid) should be noted.

  o Eyelashes should curve outward and be evenly distributed with no inflammation around any of the hair follicles.

  o There should be no edema or redness in the area of the lacrimal gland.

  o Conjunctiva

    ▪ Palpebral is pink.

    ▪ Bulbar is transparent.

  o Sclera should be white, light yellow in dark-skinned clients.

  o Corneas are clear.

  o Lenses are clear. Cloudiness occurs with cataracts.

- o PERRLA (CN II, CN III)
  - P – Pupils should be clear.
  - E – Equal in size and between 3 to 5 mm
  - R – Round in shape
  - R – Reactive to light both directly and consensually when a light is directed into one pupil and then the other
  - A – Accommodation of the pupils when they dilate to look at an object far away and then converge and constrict to focus on a near object

- Irises should be round and illuminate fully when a light is shined across from the side. A partially illuminated iris indicates glaucoma. The color of the irises should also be noted.

- Internal Examination Technique and Expected Findings

  - o Darken the surrounding room.

  - o Turn on the ophthalmoscope, and use the lens selector disc to find the large white disc.

  - o The diopter is set at 0. You can change the setting to bring structures into focus during the examination.

  - o Use your right eye to examine the client's right eye and vice versa.

  - o Instruct the client to stare at a point somewhere behind you.

  - o Start slightly lateral and 25 to 30 cm from the client, finding and following the red reflex, to within a distance of 2 to 3 cm of the client's eye.

  - o Expected findings:

    - The optic disc is light pink or more yellow than the surrounding retina.

    - The retina should be without lesions, and color will be dark pink in those with a dark complexion and light pink in fair-skinned clients.

    - The arteries and veins are found in a 2-to-3 ratio and without nicking.

    - The macula may not be readily visible without pupil dilation but may be briefly glimpsed when the client looks directly at the light.

Palpation

- Palpate the lacrimal apparatus to assess for tenderness and to see if any discharge can be expressed from the lacrimal duct. No tenderness and no discharge should be noted. Clear fluid (tears) is an expected finding.

EARS, NOSE, MOUTH, AND THROAT

Overview

- This examination includes the external, middle, and internal ear; evaluation of hearing; the nose and sinuses; and the mouth and throat.

- Use the techniques of inspection and palpation to examine the ears, nose (sinuses), mouth, and throat.

- Abnormal findings include otitis externa, osteoma, polyp, retracted drum, decreased hearing acuity, and lateralization.

- Equipment

  o Otoscope

  o Wristwatch or clock to measure time in seconds

  o Tuning fork

  o Nasal speculum

  o Tongue blade

  o Penlight

  o Gauze square

  o Cotton-tipped applicators

- Test the following cranial nerves during the ears, nose, mouth, and throat examination.

ASSESSMENT	CRANIAL NERVES (CN)
Assess the ears for hearing.	CN VIII (acoustic)
Assess the nose for smell.	CN I (olfactory)
Assess the mouth for taste.	CN VII (facial) and CN IX (glossopharyngeal)
Assess the tongue for movement and strength.	CN XII (hypoglossal)
Assess the mouth for movement of the soft palate and the gag reflex. Assess swallowing and speech.	CN IX (glossopharyngeal) and CN X (vagus)

Health History – Review of Systems

- Questions you should ask include:

  o How well do you hear?

  o Have you noticed any changes in your hearing? Do you wear a hearing aid?

  o Have other people commented that your hearing has diminished?

o   Do you ever experience tinnitus, discharge, vertigo, or pain? Do you have a history of ear infections?

o   What method do you use to clean your ears?

o   Do you ever have pain, stuffiness, or discharge from your nose?

o   Do you ever experience nosebleeds?

o   Have you noticed any change in your senses of smell or taste?

o   Do you use nasal sprays?

o   Do you snore at night?

o   How often do you go to the dentist? Do you have dentures? Do you have any problems with your gums?

o   Do you have any difficulty swallowing or problems with a hoarseness or sore throat?

Inspection and Palpation

● Ears

   o   External ear

      ■   Alignment – The top of the auricles should meet an imaginary horizontal line that extends from the outer canthus of the eye.

      ■   Ear color should be the same as face color.

      ■   Lesions and tenderness in the ears are unexpected findings.

      ■   The ear canal should be free of foreign bodies or discharge.

      ■   Cerumen is an expected finding.

   o   Internal ear

      ■   Straighten the ear canal by pulling the auricle up and back for adults and older children, and down and back for younger children. Using the otoscope, insert the speculum 1 to 1.5 cm following, but not touching, the ear canal to visualize:

         □   Tympanic membranes that are pearly gray and intact, free from tears.

         □   A light reflex that is visible and in a well-defined cone shape.

         □   Umbo and manubrium landmarks that are readily visible.

         □   Ear canals that are pink with fine hairs.

o   Auditory screening tests

TEST	TECHNIQUE	EXPECTED FINDING
Whisper test (CNV III)	• One ear is occluded and the other ear is tested to see if the client can hear whispered sounds without seeing your mouth move. • Repeat with the other ear.	The client can hear you whisper softly 30 to 60 cm away.
Rinne test	• Place a vibrating tuning fork firmly against the mastoid bone and note the time. • Have the client state when he can no longer hear the sound, note the time, and then move the tuning fork in front of the ear canal. When the client can no longer hear the tuning fork, note the time.	Air conduction (AC) greater than bone conduction (BC); 2-to-1 ratio.
Weber test	• Place a vibrating tuning fork on top of the client's head. Ask the client if the sound is heard best in the right ear, left ear, or both ears equally.	Sound is heard equally in both ears (negative Weber test).

 View Media Supplement:

    • Rinne Test (Image)   • Weber Test (Image)

- Nose

  o   The nose should be midline, symmetrical, and the same color as the face.

  o   Each nostril should be patent without excessive flaring. The structure of the nose should be firm and stable.

  o   Examine internal structures using a nasal speculum barely inserted into each nostril as the client tips his head back. Inspection should indicate that the:

    ▪   Septum is midline and intact.

    ▪   Mucosa is deep pink and moist with no discharge or lesions.

  o   Assess smell (CN I) by asking the client to occlude one naris at a time and identifying a familiar smell with the eyes closed.

- Mouth and Throat

  o   Lips are darker pigmented skin than the face, and should be moist, symmetrical, smooth, soft with no lesions, and nontender.

  o   Gums are coral pink and tight against the teeth with no bleeding on gloves when palpated.

- ○ Mucous membranes are without lesions, moist, and pink.

- ○ Tongue – Use a gauze pad to hold the tip and move the tongue from side to side. The dorsal surface is pink, with the presence of papillae, and symmetric. The underside of the tongue should be smooth with a symmetric vascular pattern. Assess taste (CN VII, CN IX) by identification of different foods placed on the tongue with the eyes closed. Ask the client to move his tongue up, down, and side to side. Test strength (CN XII) by applying resistance against each cheek while the client sticks his tongue into each cheek.

  - ▪ The tongue should be midline, moist, free of lesions, and should move freely.

- ○ Assess teeth for malocclusions by asking the client to clench his teeth. Missing or loose teeth, as well as any discoloration, should be noted. Teeth should be shiny, white, and smooth.

- ○ The hard palate is pink, intact, symmetric, firm, and concave.

- ○ The soft palate is lighter pink than the hard palate, intact, symmetric, and moves with vocalization (CN IX, CN X).

- ○ The uvula is pink, midline, intact, and should move with vocalization.

- ○ Tonsils that are visible should be the same color as the surrounding mucosa and graded on a scale of 1 to 4.

  - ▪ +1 – Barely visible

  - ▪ +2 – Halfway to the uvula

  - ▪ +3 – Touching the uvula

  - ▪ +4 – Touching each other or midline

- ○ Elicit the gag reflex by using a tongue blade to stimulate the back of the throat (CN IX, CN X). Explain the procedure to the client prior to performing this assessment.

- ○ Note speech during the course of the examination. Note whether or not the client's speech is clear and articulate.

Palpation of Sinuses

- • Technique

  - ○ Palpate the frontal sinuses by pressing upward with the thumbs from just below the eyebrows on either side of the bridge of the nose.

  - ○ Palpate the maxillary sinuses by pressing upward at the skin crevices that run from the sides of the nose to the corner of the mouth.

- • Expected finding – Nontender, allergies or infection will result in inflamed and/or swollen sinuses.

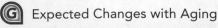 Expected Changes with Aging

AREA OF THE BODY	EXPECTED FINDINGS
Eyes	Decreased visual acuity, decreased peripheral vision, diminishing ability to see close objects or read small print (presbyopia), decreased ability to accommodate extreme changes in light (glare, darkness), difficulty distinguishing colors, intolerance to glare, delayed pupillary reaction to light, yellowing of the lens, thin gray-white ring surrounding the cornea
Ears	Hearing loss, loss of acuity for high-frequency tones (presbycusis), cerumen accumulation in the ear canal, thickening of the tympanic membrane
Mouth	Decreased sense of taste, reduced number of taste buds, tooth loss, and gum disease due to inadequate oral hygiene
Voice	Rise in pitch, loss of power and range
Nose	Decreased sense of smell

Sample Documentation

Client denies any pain in head or neck region.

Skull is normocephalic, symmetrical, and nontender. Client has symmetrical facial features and movements. Trachea is midline. Thyroid lobes are palpable but not enlarged; no nodules noted. Neck is supple with no palpable lymph nodes. Client has full range of motion of the neck.

Visual acuity is 20/30 in the left eye, 20/20 in the right eye, and 20/20 in both eyes without correction. EOMs are symmetrical with no strabismus or nystagmus noted. Peripheral fields are full bilaterally. Eyebrows are evenly distributed. Eyelids close completely with no ptosis. No discharge noted. Bulbar conjunctivae are clear, palpebral conjunctivae are pink, sclerae are white, and irises are blue bilaterally. Corneas and lenses are clear. PERRLA is intact bilaterally. Red reflex is present bilaterally. Retinas are yellowish orange with no nicking or hemorrhaging of vessels.

No lesions or tenderness noted on external ears. Top of ears align with outer canthus of eyes. Tympanic membranes pearly gray and translucent with well-defined cone of light. Light yellow cerumen present in ear canals bilaterally. Auditory acuity intact to whispered voice bilaterally. Negative Weber test and AC > BC bilaterally. Nose is midline and symmetrical. Nares are patent. Nasal mucosa is pink, septum intact and midline, no discharge noted. No sinus tenderness. Lips are darker pink and intact, symmetric. Oral mucosa is pink, no dental caries noted; no missing teeth. Tongue is pink and midline. Papillae present on dorsum, and symmetrical vascular pattern noted on the underside of the tongue. Gums are tight against the teeth with no bleeding noted. Hard and soft palates are intact with no lesions. Uvula is midline. Gag reflex is present. Tonsils are +1 bilaterally. Taste and smell sensations are intact. Speech is clear. CN I through XII intact.

CHAPTER 28: HEAD AND NECK

(A) Application Exercises

1. Match each lymph node of the head and neck with its location for palpation.

_____ Occipital lymph node	A. Along the base of the mandible
_____ Preauricular lymph node	B. Midline under the chin
_____ Postauricular lymph node	C. Base of the skull
_____ Submandibular lymph node	D. Along the sternocleidomastoid muscle
_____ Tonsillar (retropharyngeal) lymph node	E. Posterior to the sternocleidomastoid muscle
_____ Submental lymph node	F. Over the mastoid
_____ Anterior cervical lymph nodes	G. At the angle of the mandible
_____ Posterior cervical lymph nodes	H. In front of the ear

2. Which of the following should be assessed when examining the face? (Select all that apply.)

_____ Lymph nodes

_____ Perception of light touch of the face

_____ Symmetry of facial features

_____ ROM of the neck

_____ Presence of involuntary movements

3. Asking a client to tip her head to one side and slightly forward, palpating either side of the trachea at the lower half of the neck, and then asking the client to swallow is the correct technique for examining

A. lymph nodes.

B. ROM of the neck.

C. symmetry of the skull.

D. the thyroid gland.

4. Match the examination technique or tool needed to screen for the following conditions.

_____ Color blindness	A. Illumination of the iris
_____ Myopia	B. Cover/uncover test
_____ Nystagmus	C. Six cardinal positions of gaze
_____ Presbyopia	D. Snellen chart
_____ Strabismus	E. Rosenbaum chart
_____ Glaucoma	F. Ishihara test

5. A client asks what her Snellen eye test results mean. Her acuity for both eyes together is 20/30. Which of the following is the appropriate response?

    A. "You see at 20 ft what the normal-sighted person sees at 30 ft."

    B. "You see at 30 ft what the normal-sighted person sees at 20 ft."

    C. "You see at 10 ft what the normal-sighted person sees at 50 ft."

    D. "You see at 50 ft what the normal-sighted person sees at 20 ft."

6. A client with nystagmus will demonstrate

    A. one eye gazing in a different direction during the cover/uncover test.

    B. jerky eye movements during the six cardinal positions of gaze test.

    C. droopy eyelids that partially or completely cover the pupil.

    D. nicking of the retinal blood vessels during the internal eye examination.

7. What part of the eye examination should occur first?

    A. Extraocular movements

    B. Internal structures

    C. Visual acuity

    D. Visual fields

8. Match the appropriate technique for each of the following assessments.

    _____ A vibrating tuning fork is placed on the mastoid process and then placed near the ear when the sound is no longer heard.

    _____ A vibrating tuning fork is placed midline on top of the head and the client is asked where the sound is heard best.

    _____ The back of the throat is stimulated with a tongue depressor.

    _____ The client occludes one ear while the nurse whispers in the other ear from 30 cm away.

    A. Whisper test

    B. Weber test

    C. Gag reflex

    D. Rinne test

CHAPTER 28: HEAD AND NECK

 Application Exercises Answer Key

1. Match each lymph node of the head and neck with its location for palpation.

C	Occipital lymph node	A.	Along the base of the mandible
H	Preauricular lymph node	B.	Midline under the chin
F	Postauricular lymph node	C.	Base of the skull
A	Submandibular lymph node	D.	Along the sternocleidomastoid muscle
G	Tonsillar (retropharyngeal) lymph node	E.	Posterior to the sternocleidomastoid muscle
B	Submental lymph node	F.	Over the mastoid
D	Anterior cervical lymph nodes	G.	At the angle of the mandible
E	Posterior cervical lymph nodes	H.	In front of the ear

NCLEX® Connection: Health Promotion and Maintenance, Techniques of Physical Assessment

2. Which of the following should be assessed when examining the face? (Select all that apply.)

_____ Lymph nodes

__X__ **Perception of light touch of the face**

__X__ **Symmetry of facial features**

_____ ROM of the neck

__X__ **Presence of involuntary movements**

Assessment of the perception of light touch to the face indicates that the sensory portion of the trigeminal nerve (CN V) is intact. Symmetry of facial movements and presence of involuntary movements of the face are also assessed. Lymph nodes and ROM of the neck are assessed while examining the neck.

NCLEX® Connection: Health Promotion and Maintenance, Techniques of Physical Assessment

3. Asking a client to tip her head to one side and slightly forward, palpating either side of the trachea at the lower half of the neck, and then asking the client to swallow is the correct technique for examining

    A. lymph nodes.

    B. ROM of the neck.

    C. symmetry of the skull.

    D. the thyroid gland.

    This is the correct technique for examining the thyroid gland.

    (N) NCLEX® Connection: Health Promotion and Maintenance, Techniques of Physical Assessment

4. Match the examination technique or tool needed to screen for the following conditions.

F	Color blindness	A. Illumination of the iris
D	Myopia	B. Cover/uncover test
C	Nystagmus	C. Six cardinal positions of gaze
E	Presbyopia	D. Snellen chart
B	Strabismus	E. Rosenbaum chart
A	Glaucoma	F. Ishihara test

    (N) NCLEX® Connection: Health Promotion and Maintenance, Techniques of Physical Assessment

5. A client asks what her Snellen eye test results mean. Her acuity for both eyes together is 20/30. Which of the following is the appropriate response?

    A. "You see at 20 ft what the normal-sighted person sees at 30 ft."

    B. "You see at 30 ft what the normal-sighted person sees at 20 ft."

    C. "You see at 10 ft what the normal-sighted person sees at 50 ft."

    D. "You see at 50 ft what the normal-sighted person sees at 20 ft."

    The first number indicates the number of feet from the Snellen eye chart that the client is standing, and the second number is the distance at which a normal-sighted person can read the line of the Snellen eye chart.

    (N) NCLEX® Connection: Health Promotion and Maintenance, Techniques of Physical Assessment

6. A client with nystagmus will demonstrate

   A. one eye gazing in a different direction during the cover/uncover test.

   B. jerky eye movements during the six cardinal positions of gaze test.

   C. droopy eyelids that partially or completely cover the pupil.

   D. nicking of the retinal blood vessels during the internal eye examination.

   Nystagmus is demonstrated with jerky eye movements during the six cardinal positions of gaze test. Strabismus is demonstrated by one eye gazing in a different direction than the other eye. Ptosis is demonstrated by droopy eyelids that partially or completely cover the pupil. Nicking of the retinal blood vessels indicates damage to the blood vessels of the eye.

   (N) NCLEX® Connection: Reduction of Risk Potential, System Specific Assessment

7. What part of the eye examination should occur first?

   A. Extraocular movements

   B. Internal structures

   C. Visual acuity

   D. Visual fields

   Visual acuity should be assessed first during an eye examination. Assessing extraocular movements, internal structures, and visual fields may interfere with the ability of the client to read and demonstrate accurate visual acuity.

   (N) NCLEX® Connection: Health Promotion and Maintenance, Techniques of Physical Assessment

8. Match the appropriate technique for each of the following assessments.

   D   A vibrating tuning fork is placed on the mastoid process and then placed near the ear when the sound is no longer heard.

   B   A vibrating tuning fork is placed midline on top of the head and the client is asked where the sound is heard best.

   C   The back of the throat is stimulated with a tongue depressor.

   A   The client occludes one ear while the nurse whispers in the other ear from 30 cm away.

   A. Whisper test
   B. Weber test
   C. Gag reflex
   D. Rinne test

   (N) NCLEX® Connection: Health Promotion and Maintenance, Techniques of Physical Assessment

UNIT 2	HEALTH PROMOTION

Section   Health Assessment

Chapter 29   Thorax, Heart, and Abdomen

Overview

- This examination includes the thorax (breast and lungs), the heart, and the abdomen.

BREASTS

Overview

- Clients who have had a mastectomy, breast augmentation, and/or reconstruction should have the incisional lines palpated. Lymphedema may be noted in clients who have impaired lymphatic drainage on the affected side.

- Breast self-examinations should be addressed with the client during the examination. Ask the client whether or not she performs a monthly self-examination, and if not, instruct the client on the necessity of it and/or how to perform the examination. At home, inspection can be done in front of the mirror, and palpation can be done in the shower. BSE should be performed following the menstrual cycle. If the client is postmenopausal, BSE should be performed on the same day of each month.

- Breast examinations should be performed on both female and male clients.

- Use the techniques of inspection and palpation to examine the breasts.

  - Equipment

    - Gloves

    - Lotion

    - Drape

    - Small pillow or folded towel

- Documentation of nodules should include:

  - Location (quadrant or clock method)

  - Size (actual centimeters)

  - Shape

  - Consistency (soft, firm, or hard)

  - Discreteness (well-defined borders of mass)

- o Tenderness

- o Erythema

- o Dimpling or retraction over the mass

- o Lymphadenopathy

- o Mobility

Health History – Review of Systems

- • Questions the nurse should ask include:

  - o Do you perform breast self-examinations? How often?

  - o Have you noticed any tenderness or lumps? Does this change with your menstrual cycle?

  - o Have you experienced any discharge from the nipples?

  - o If the client is over 40, are you having mammograms performed yearly?

  - o Is there any history of breast cancer in your family?

  - o Are you aware of the risks for breast cancer?

Inspection

FEMALE	MALE
• Four positions (done sitting or standing) o Arms at the side o Arms above the head o Hands on the hips pressing firmly o Leaning forward (arms out in front or can remain on hips)	In sitting or lying position (with arms at the side only)

- • Inspect For:

  - o Size and symmetry (One breast is often slightly larger than the other.)

  - o Shape (convex, conical, pendulous)

  - o Symmetrical venous patterns and consistency of skin color

  - o Absence of lesions, edema, or erythema. (Rashes or ulcerations are abnormal findings.)

  - o Round shape of areola

  - o Darker-pigmented areola and nipple

  - o Direction of nipples (Nipples are usually everted; recent inversion is abnormal.)

  - o For women with large breasts, check for excoriation under the breasts.

Palpation

- Axillary and clavicular lymph nodes are best palpated in the sitting position. Lymph nodes should not be palpable or tender. The following lymph nodes should be assessed:

  - Supraclavicular

  - Axillary

  - Infraclavicular

  - Pectoral

  - Central or deep (may be normal to palpate if smaller than 1 cm and nontender)

  - Lateral

  - Subscapular

  - Epitrochlear

- Breast examination – Wear gloves if skin is not intact. Feel for lumps using the finger pads of four fingers. (Use lotion as a lubricant if needed.) The best position is for the client to be lying down with the arm up by her head and a small pillow or folded towel placed under the shoulder of the side being examined. This position spreads the breast tissue more evenly over the chest wall allowing for easier palpation.

  - Palpate each breast from the sternum to the posterior axillary line, and from the clavicle to the bra line (including the areola, nipple, and tail of Spence) using one of three techniques:

    - Circular pattern

    - Wedge pattern

    - Vertical strip pattern

- Nipples should be carefully compressed between the thumb and index finger to check for discharge. Discharge is not expected in nonlactating women. Note the color, consistency, and odor of any discharge.

- Pendulous breasts require that a bimanual technique be used to support the lower portion of the breast while the tissue is palpated against the supporting hand.

	EXPECTED FINDINGS	ABNORMAL FINDINGS
Female	• Breasts should be firm, elastic, and without lesions or nodules. • Breast tissue may feel granular or lumpy bilaterally in some women.	• Fibrocystic breast disease is characterized by tender cysts that are often more prominent during menstruation.
Male	• No edema, masses, or tenderness should be present. • Areolas are round and darker pigmented.	• Unilateral or bilateral (but asymmetrical) gynecomastia in adolescent boys or bilateral gynecomastia in older adult males may be present.

THORAX AND LUNGS

 Overview

- This examination includes the anterior and posterior thorax and lungs.

- Use the techniques of inspection, palpation, percussion, and auscultation.

- Equipment

  ○ Stethoscope

  ○ Centimeter ruler

  ○ A wristwatch or clock that allows for counting seconds

- Positioning – The posterior thorax is best assessed with the client sitting or standing. The anterior thorax can be assessed with the client sitting, lying, or standing.

- Anatomical reminder: The right lung has three lobes, while the left lung has two lobes. Auscultating the right middle lobe is done using the axillary sites.

- Chest landmarks are used to perform assessments correctly and describe findings. The following vertical landmarks are used:

  ○ The midsternal line is through the center of the sternum.

  ○ The midclavicular line is through the midpoint of the clavicle.

  ○ The anterior axillary line is through the anterior axillary folds.

  ○ The midaxillary line is through the apex of the axillae.

  ○ The posterior axillary line is through the posterior axillary fold.

  ○ The right and left scapular lines are through the inferior angle of the scapula.

  ○ The vertebral line is along the center of the spine.

  (M) View Media Supplement: Lung Landmarks (Animation)

- Percussion and auscultatory sites are in the intercostal spaces. The number of the ICS corresponds to the rib above it.

  ○ Posterior thorax – The sites are between the scapula and the vertebrae on the upper portion of the back. Below the scapula, the sites are along the right and left scapular lines.

  ○ Anterior thorax – The sites are along the midclavicular lines bilaterally, with several sites at the anterior/midaxillary lines bilaterally in the lower portions of the chest wall and on either side of the sternum following along the rib cage.

    ▪ Observe for accessory muscle use.

- o Percussion and auscultation should occur in a systemic pattern so that side-to-side comparisons can be made.

- o Maximize sounds heard by:

    - Having the client take deep breaths with an open mouth each time the stethoscope is moved.

    - Placing the stethoscope directly on the client's skin to prevent muffling or distortion of sounds.

    - Facilitating breathing by medicating for pain, giving clear directions, and assisting the client to a sitting position.

Health History – Review of Systems

- Questions the nurse should ask include:

    - o Do you have any chronic lung conditions such as asthma or emphysema? Do you take any medications for your respiratory condition?

    - o Have you ever had pneumonia? If so, when and how often?

    - o Do you get upper respiratory infections frequently?

    - o Do you have environmental allergies?

    - o Do you ever experience shortness of breath or difficulty breathing with activity?

    - o Do you have a cough? Do you cough up sputum? If so, what does it look like?

    - o Do you currently or have you ever smoked? If you no longer smoke, when did you quit? How long did you smoke? If you do currently smoke, when did you start and how much do you smoke? Are you interested in quitting?

    - o Are you exposed to secondhand smoke?

    - o Is there any family history of lung cancer or tuberculosis? Have you had any exposure to tuberculosis?

    - o Do you receive a yearly influenza vaccine?

Inspection

- Shape – The anteroposterior diameter should be half of the transverse diameter.

- Symmetry – The chest should be symmetric with no deformities of the ribs, sternum, scapula, or vertebrae, with equal movements during respiration.

- ICS – You should not see excessive retractions.

- Respiratory Effort

    - o Rate and pattern – These should be regular with 16 to 20/min.

    - o Character of breathing (diaphragmatic, abdominal, thoracic)

    - o Use of accessory muscles

- ○ Chest wall expansion

- ○ Depth of respirations – Unlabored, quiet breathing is the expected finding.

- • Cough – If productive, note the color/consistency of sputum.

- • Trachea should be midline.

Palpation

- • Surface characteristics include tenderness, lesions, lumps, and deformities. Tenderness is an unexpected finding.

- • Chest Excursion or Expansion of the Posterior Thorax

  - ○ With thumbs aligned parallel along the spine at the level of the tenth rib, and the hands flattened around the client's back, instruct the client to take a deep breath. Thumbs should move outward approximately 5 cm (2 in) when the client takes a deep inspiration.

- • Vocal (Tactile) Fremitus

  - ○ Palpate the chest wall using the ulnar surface of both hands, comparing side to side from top to bottom.

  - ○ Ask the client to say "99" each time the hands are moved.

  - ○ Expected findings – Vibration is symmetric and more pronounced at the top.

Percussion

- • Compare sounds that are produced from side to side.

- • Normal percussion of the thorax should result in resonance.

- • Abnormal Findings and Significance

  - ○ Dullness – Caused by fluid or solid tissue, this can indicate of pneumonia or a tumor.

  - ○ Hyperresonance – Caused by the presence of air, this can indicate pneumothorax or emphysema.

Auscultation

- • Expected Sounds

  - ○ Bronchial – Loud, high-pitched, expiration heard longer than inspiration over the trachea

  - ○ Bronchovesicular – Medium pitch and intensity, equal inspiration and expiration, and heard over the larger airways

  - ○ Vesicular – Soft, low-pitched, inspiration three times longer than expiration heard over most of the peripheral areas of the lungs

- Abnormal or Adventitious Sounds

  o Crackles or rales – Fine to coarse popping heard as air passes through fluid or re-expands collapsed small airways

  o Wheezes – High-pitched whistling, musical sounds heard as air passes through narrowed or obstructed airways, usually louder on expiration

  o Rhonchi – Coarse sounds heard during either inspiration or expiration resulting from fluid or mucus, may clear with coughing

  o Pleural friction rub – Grating sound produced as the inflamed visceral and parietal pleura rub against each other during inspiration or expiration

  o Absence of breath sounds should be noted.

HEART

Overview

- This examination includes measuring heart rate and blood pressure, examining the jugular veins, and auscultating heart sounds.

- Equipment

  o Stethoscope

  o Blood pressure cuff

  o A wristwatch or clock that allows for counting seconds

  o Two rulers

- Cardiac Cycle and Heart Sounds

  o Closure of the mitral and tricuspid valves signals the beginning of ventricular systole (contraction) and produces the S1 sound (lub). This is heard best with the diaphragm of the stethoscope at the apex.

  o Closure of the aortic and pulmonic valves signals the beginning of ventricular diastole (relaxation) and produces the S2 sound (dub). This is heard best with the diaphragm of the stethoscope at the aortic area.

  o An S3 sound (ventricular gallop) is produced by rapid ventricular filling and can be a normal finding in children and young adults. This is heard best with the bell of the stethoscope.

  o An S4 sound is produced by a strong atrial contraction and can be a normal finding in older and athletic adults and children. This is heard best with the bell of the stethoscope.

  o Murmurs are heard when blood volume is increased in the heart, or the flow of blood is impeded or altered. A murmur is heard in the heart as a blowing or swishing sound. This is heard best with the bell of the stethoscope.

    ▪ Systolic murmurs are heard just after S1.

    ▪ Diastolic murmurs are heard just after S2.

- o Thrills are a palpable vibration that may be present with murmurs or cardiac malformation.

- o Bruits are produced by obstructed peripheral blood flow and are heard as a blowing or swishing sound with the bell of the stethoscope.

- Auscultatory Sites for the Heart

(M) View Media Supplement: Cardiac Landmarks (Image)

- o Aortic – Just right of the sternum at the second ICS

- o Pulmonic – Just left of the sternum at the second ICS

- o Erb's point – Just left of the sternum at the third ICS

- o Tricuspid – Just left of the sternum at the fourth ICS

- o Apical/mitral – Left midclavicular line at the fifth ICS

Health History – Review of Systems

- Questions the nurse should ask include:

- o Do you have any problems with your heart? Do you take any medications?

- o Do you have high blood pressure or high cholesterol?

- o Do your feet and ankles ever swell?

- o Do you cough frequently?

- o Do you have chest pain? When? How long does it last? How often does it occur? Describe the pain. Does it radiate to other areas?

- o What are you doing before the pain begins?

- o Are there any other symptoms associated with the pain (nausea, shortness of breath, sweating, dizziness)?

- o What have you tried to relieve the pain? Does it work?

- o Describe your energy level. Are you frequently tired? Do you have unusual fatigue?

- o Do you have fainting spells or dizziness? If so, how often? When was the last time it occurred?

- o Are you familiar with the risk factors for heart disease?

Inspection and Palpation

- Vital signs – Pulse and blood pressure are indicators of cardiovascular status.

- Peripheral Vascular System

  o Inspect jugular veins with the client in bed with the head of the bed at a 30° to 45° angle to assess for right-sided heart failure.

    ▪ Appearance – No neck vein distention should be noted.

    ▪ Jugular venous pressure (JVP) – Should be measured at less than 2.5 cm above the sternal angle using the following technique:

      □ Place one ruler vertically at the sternal angle.

      □ Locate the pulsation in the external jugular vein and place the straight edge of another ruler parallel to the floor at the level of the pulsation.

      □ Line up the two rulers as a T square, keeping the horizontal ruler at the level of pulsation.

      □ The level where the horizontal ruler intersects the vertical ruler is where the JVP is measured.

- Heart

  o Apical pulse or point of maximal impulse (PMI)

    ▪ May be visible just lateral to the left midclavicular line at the fifth ICS. With female clients, displace the breast tissue.

    ▪ Palpate where it was visualized. If not visualized, try to palpate the location and the size.

    ▪ Expected finding – The apical pulse should be just lateral to the left midclavicular line at the fifth ICS and no larger than 2.5 cm in diameter.

  o Heaves (or lifts) are abnormal, visible elevations of the chest wall that are seen with heart failure, and are often located along the left sternal border or at the PMI.

  o Thrills – Use the ulnar surface of the hand to feel for vibrations similar to that of a purring kitten. This is not an expected finding.

Auscultation

- Heart

  o Positioning the client in three different ways allows for optimal assessment of heart sounds, as some extra or abnormal sounds are accentuated by the various positions.

    ▪ Sitting, leaning forward

    ▪ Lying supine

    ▪ Turned toward the left side (best position for picking up extra heart sounds or murmurs)

- o   Use both the diaphragm and the bell of the stethoscope in a systematic manner to listen at all of the auscultatory sites.

- o   To determine the heart rate, listen and count for 1 min. Determine if the rhythm is regular. If a dysrhythmia exists, check for a pulse deficit in which the radial pulse will be slower than the apical pulse.

- Assess the peripheral vascular system for the presence of bruits. Locations to assess for bruits include:

  - o   Carotid arteries – Over the carotid pulses

  - o   Abdominal aorta – Just below the xiphoid process

  - o   Renal arteries – Midclavicular lines above the umbilicus on the abdomen

  - o   Iliac arteries – Midclavicular lines below the umbilicus on the abdomen

  - o   Femoral arteries – Over the femoral pulses

ABDOMEN

Overview

- This examination includes observing the shape of the abdomen, palpating for masses, and auscultating for vascular sounds.

- Use the techniques of inspection, auscultation, percussion, and palpation. The order of assessment techniques changes to allow bowel sounds to be auscultated just after inspection. This change is done to allow the client's bowel sounds to be heard without being disturbed or distorted by percussion or palpation assessments.

- Equipment

  - o   Stethoscope

  - o   Tape measure or ruler

  - o   Marking pen

- Preparing and positioning the client includes having the client void prior to the abdominal examination. Then, position the client lying supine with his arms at his sides and with his knees slightly bent.

- Abdominal landmarks are designated using the umbilicus. Imaginary vertical and horizontal lines through the umbilicus divide the abdomen into four quadrants with the xiphoid process as the upper boundary and the symphysis pubis as the lower boundary:

 View Media Supplement: Abdominal Assessment (Image)

  - o   Right upper quadrant (RUQ)

  - o   Left upper quadrant (LUQ)

- o   Right lower quadrant (RLQ)
- o   Left lower quadrant (LLQ)

Health History – Review of Systems

- Questions the nurse should ask include:
  - o   Do you ever have nausea or vomiting?
  - o   Have you had any change in your appetite? Do you have any food intolerances? Any recent weight changes?
  - o   Do you have any swallowing difficulties?
  - o   Do you have any problems with your bowels? Do you get diarrhea? Constipation? When was your last bowel movement? Do you often use laxatives or enemas?
  - o   Have you had any black or tarry stools?
  - o   Do you frequently use aspirin or ibuprofen?
  - o   Do you ever have heartburn? When? How often?
  - o   Have you had any low abdominal or back pain? Any tenderness in these areas?
  - o   Do you have a family history of colon cancer?
  - o   If over 50, are you getting routine colonoscopies?
  - o   Are you aware of the signs and symptoms of colon cancer?
  - o   Do you drink alcohol? If so, how much?
  - o   What is your typical day's intake of food and fluid?
  - o   Do you have any dietary restrictions or special practices?

Inspection

- Note any guarding or splinting of the abdomen.
- Skin is assessed for:
  - o   Lesions – Note any bruising, rashes, or other primary lesions.
  - o   Scars – Note the location and length.
  - o   Striae or stretch marks that are silver in color – These are considered expected findings.
  - o   Dilated veins – An unexpected finding associated with cirrhosis or inferior vena cava obstruction.
  - o   Jaundice, cyanosis, or ascites – May be associated with cirrhosis.
- Shape or contour can be described as:
  - o   Flat – Lies in a horizontal line from the chest to the symphysis pubis
  - o   Convex – Rounded

     FUNDAMENTALS FOR NURSING

- o Concave – Has a sunken appearance
- o Distended – A large protrusion of the abdomen caused by fat, fluid, or flatus that can be differentiated as follows:
  - ■ Fat – The client has rolls of fat tissue along her sides, and the skin does not look taut.
  - ■ Fluid – The flanks also protrude, and when the client turns onto her side, the protrusion moves to the dependent side.
  - ■ Flatus – The protrusion is mainly midline, and the flanks are unchanged.
  - ■ Hernias – Protrusions through the abdominal muscle wall are visible.
- • Movement of the abdominal wall may be observed as:
  - o Peristalsis – Wave-like movements are visible in thin adults or in clients with intestinal obstructions.
  - o Pulsations – Regular beats of movement seen midline above the umbilicus are expected findings in thin adults, but a pulsating mass would be unexpected.
- • Umbilicus should be inspected for position, shape, color, inflammation, discharge, or masses. No discharge, inflammation, or masses should be noted.

Auscultation

- • Bowel sounds are produced by the movement of air and fluid in the intestines. The most appropriate time to auscultate bowel sounds is in between meals.
  - o Technique – Listen with the diaphragm of the stethoscope in all four quadrants.
  - o Expected sounds – High-pitched clicks and gurgles are heard 5 to 30 times/min. To make the determination of absent bowel sounds, you must listen for a full 5 min without hearing anything.
- • Friction rubs are abnormal sounds caused by the rubbing together of inflamed layers of the peritoneum. The technique is as follows:
  - o Listen with the diaphragm over the liver and spleen.
  - o Ask the client to take a deep breath while you listen for any grating sounds (like sandpaper rubbing together).
- • Vascular Sounds (bruits caused by narrowed vessels disrupting blood flow)
  - o Abdominal aorta – Just below the xiphoid process
  - o Renal arteries – Midclavicular lines above the umbilicus on the abdomen
  - o Iliac arteries – Midclavicular lines below the umbilicus on the abdomen
  - o Femoral arteries – Over the femoral pulses

Percussion

- Tympany is the expected percussion sound heard over most of the abdomen. A lower-pitch tympany over the gastric bubble in the left upper quadrant may be heard.

- Dullness over the liver or a distended bladder may be heard.

- The liver span is a measurement of liver size taken at the right midclavicular line and can be determined using percussion techniques.

    o Establish the lower border of the liver by percussing upward from below the umbilicus at the right midclavicular line until tympany turns to dullness.

    o Make a mark.

    o Establish the upper border by percussing downward, starting at the right midclavicular line over the lung until resonance turns to dullness.

    o Make a mark.

    o Measure the distance between the two marks for the size of the liver span.

    o The expected finding is 6 to 12 cm.

- Kidney tenderness is assessed by fist percussion over the costovertebral angles at the scapular lines on the back. The expected finding is no tenderness.

Palpation

- Tender areas should be palpated last.

- Light

    o Use the finger pads on one hand to palpate to a depth of 1 cm in each quadrant.

    o Expected findings include consistency of softness, no nodules, and no guarding.

    o The bladder may be palpated if full; otherwise, it is nonpalpable.

- Deep

    o Two-handed approach – The top hand depresses the bottom hand 3 to 4 cm in depth. The bottom hand assesses for organ enlargement or masses. The location, consistency, shape, and size of any mass should be documented.

    o Expected findings:

        ▪ The bladder may be palpated if full; otherwise, it is nonpalpable.

        ▪ The stool may be palpated in the descending colon.

- Rebound tenderness (Blumberg's sign) is an indication of irritation or inflammation somewhere in the abdominal cavity. The following technique should be done in all four quadrants.

    o Apply firm pressure for 4 seconds with the hand at a 90° angle and with the fingers extended.

    o After releasing the pressure, observe the client's response to see if pain was elicited once the pressure was released.

    o   Ask about pain/tenderness.

    o   Never deep palpate an abdominal mass, tender organs, or surgical incisions.

Ⓖ Expected Changes with Aging

AREA OF BODY	EXPECTED CHANGES
Breasts	• With menopause, breast tissue atrophies and is replaced with adipose tissue, making it feel softer and more pendulous. The atrophied ducts may feel like thin strands. • Nipples no longer have erectile ability and may invert.
Lungs	• Chest shape changes so that the AP diameter becomes similar to the transverse diameter (barrel chest), resulting in decreased vital capacity. • Chest excursion or expansion diminishes • Cough reflex diminishes • Cilia ineffectively removes dust and irritants from the airways • Alveoli dwindle and there is a greater airway resistance and higher risk of pulmonary infection • Kyphosis, an increased curvature of the thoracic spine due to osteoporosis and weakened cartilage, results in vertebral collapse and impairment of respiratory effort
Cardiovascular system	• Systolic hypertension (widened pulse pressure) is a common finding with atherosclerosis in older adult clients. • The PMI becomes more difficult to palpate because the AP diameter of the chest widens. • Coronary blood vessel walls thicken and become more rigid with a narrowed lumen • Cardiac output decreases and strength of contraction leads to poor activity tolerance • Heart values stiffen due to calcification • The left ventricle thickens • Pulmonary vascular tension increases • Systolic blood pressure rises • Peripheral circulation lessens
Abdomen	• Weaker abdominal muscles declining in tone and more adipose tissue result in a rounder, more protruding abdomen. • Diminished signs and symptoms of peritoneal inflammation, such as less pain, guarding, fever, or rebound tenderness, may alter the demonstration of typical clinical manifestations by older adult clients. • Saliva, gastric secretions, and pancreatic enzymes decrease • Smooth-muscle changes with decreased esophageal peristalsis and small-intestine motility

Sample Documentation

- Breasts are conical, symmetric in size, and without masses or lesions. Nipples and areolae are darker pigmented and symmetric. Everted nipples are without discharge. No palpable axillary or clavicular lymph nodes. Client denies pain or tenderness.

- Respiratory rate is 16/min and regular. Respirations are easy and unlabored. Thorax has a greater transverse than AP diameter. No chest wall deformities noted. Trachea is midline. Movement is symmetrical with 5 cm of expansion. Equal tactile fremitus noted. Resonant sounds percussed throughout. Vesicular sounds heard primarily over the bases bilaterally. No adventitious sounds noted. No cough noted. Client denies any shortness of breath or difficulty breathing.

- Heart rhythm and rate is regular at 72/min on auscultation. Blood pressure is 118/76 mm Hg. No thrills or heaves. PMI is approximately 1 cm at the fifth ICS left midclavicular line. S1 is louder at the apex than S2. S2 is loudest in the pulmonary area on inspiration. No extra heart sounds, murmurs, or bruits heard. JVP is 2 cm bilaterally. Client denies chest pain or discomfort.

- Abdomen is flat with active bowel sounds heard every 10 to 20 seconds in all four quadrants. No bruits or friction rubs heard. Abdomen is soft, nontender, and without masses or enlargement of spleen or liver. Liver span is 8 cm. No rebound or costovertebral tenderness noted. Bladder is not palpable. Client denies pain or discomfort in abdominal region.

CHAPTER 29: THORAX, HEART, AND ABDOMEN

 Application Exercises

1. What information should be documented when describing a breast mass?

2. Which of the following are expected changes of the breast tissue after menopause? (Select all that apply.)

_____ Clear discharge from nipples

_____ More pendulous

_____ Breast tissue replaced by adipose tissue

_____ Firmer

_____ Nodular

3. During palpation of the breast, the client is instructed to extend an arm over her head, and a small pillow or folded towel is placed under her shoulder to

A. spread the tissue more evenly over the chest wall for easier palpation.

B. keep the client from guarding during the exam.

C. expose the tail of Spence for easier inspection.

D. determine whether or not a breast mass is consistently irregular when palpating a nodule.

4. Match each of the following sounds with its correct description.

_____ Bronchial sounds   A. Fine, coarse popping sounds produced by sudden opening of collapsed alveoli

_____ Bronchovesicular sounds   B. High-pitched whistling, musical sounds produced by narrowed airways

_____ Vesicular sounds   C. Grating sound produced by inflamed moving pleura

_____ Crackles/rales   D. The expected percussion sound over the thorax

_____ Pleural friction rub   E. Inspiration > expiration, softer, and lower-pitched

_____ Wheezes   F. Percussion sound heard over air-filled lung tissue

_____ Resonance   G. Expiration = inspiration, medium pitch, and intensity

_____ Hyperresonance   H. Expiration > inspiration, loud and high-pitched, and heard over trachea

5. Which of the following is assessed when performing palpation of the thorax and lungs? (Select all that apply.)

_____ Breath sounds

_____ Respiratory effort

_____ Tactile fremitus

_____ Surface characteristics

_____ Chest excursion

6. When auscultating breath sounds, the nurse should

    A. listen to the top of the anterior chest and then the top of the posterior chest.

    B. compare side to side proceeding from top to bottom.

    C. listen only to the posterior chest.

    D. complete one side of the chest before proceeding to the other side.

7. Match the action within the heart/peripheral vascular system with the sound it produces.

_____	Rapid ventricular filling	A. S1
_____	Closure of the mitral and tricuspid valves	B. S2
_____	Strong atrial contraction	C. Murmur
_____	Obstructed blood flow in peripheral circulation	D. S3
_____	Impeded blood flow in the heart	E. S4
_____	Closure of the aortic and pulmonic valves	F. Bruits

8. The proper placement of the stethoscope for auscultating the aortic valve is the

    A. second ICS just right of the sternum.

    B. second ICS just left of the sternum.

    C. fourth ICS just left of the sternum.

    D. fifth ICS at the left midclavicular line.

9. A nurse should perform the abdominal assessment using which of the following sequences?

    A. Inspection, palpation, percussion, and auscultation

    B. Auscultation, inspection, palpation, and percussion

    C. Percussion, inspection, auscultation, and palpation

    D. Inspection, auscultation, percussion, and palpation

10. When performing percussion, which of the following sounds should be heard over most of the abdomen?

    A. Dullness

    B. Tympany

    C. Grating

    D. Gurgling

CHAPTER 29: THORAX, HEART, AND ABDOMEN

 Application Exercises Answer Key

1. What information should be documented when describing a breast mass?

> **Location, size, shape, consistency, discreteness, tenderness, erythema, dimpling or retraction over the lump, lymphadenopathy, and mobility**

 NCLEX® Connection: Reduction of Risk Potential, System Specific Assessment

2. Which of the following are expected changes of the breast tissue after menopause? (Select all that apply.)

_____	Clear discharge from nipples
__X__	**More pendulous**
__X__	**Breast tissue replaced by adipose tissue**
_____	Firmer
_____	Nodular

> **The breasts become more pendulous, breast tissue is replaced by adipose tissue, and breasts may feel softer. Discharge from the nipples is an abnormal finding.**

 NCLEX® Connection: Reduction of Risk Potential, System Specific Assessment

3. During palpation of the breast, the client is instructed to extend an arm over her head, and a small pillow or folded towel is placed under her shoulder to

> **A. spread the tissue more evenly over the chest wall for easier palpation.**
>
> B. keep the client from guarding during the exam.
>
> C. expose the tail of Spence for easier inspection.
>
> D. determine whether or not a breast mass is consistently irregular when palpating a nodule.

> **This position spreads the tissue more evenly over the chest wall for easier palpation. It does not keep the client from guarding, exposing the tail of Spence, or determining the irregularity of a breast mass.**

 NCLEX® Connection: Health Promotion and Maintenance, Techniques of Physical Assessment

4. Match each of the following sounds with its correct description.

__H__	Bronchial sounds	A. Fine, coarse popping sounds produced by sudden opening of collapsed alveoli
__G__	Bronchovesicular sounds	B. High-pitched whistling, musical sounds produced by narrowed airways
__E__	Vesicular sounds	C. Grating sound produced by inflamed moving pleura
__A__	Crackles/rales	D. The expected percussion sound over the thorax
__C__	Pleural friction rub	E. Inspiration > expiration, softer, and lower-pitched
__B__	Wheezes	F. Percussion sound heard over air-filled lung tissue
__D__	Resonance	G. Expiration = inspiration, medium pitch, and intensity
__F__	Hyperresonance	H. Expiration > inspiration, loud and high-pitched, and heard over trachea

NCLEX® Connection: Health Promotion and Maintenance, Techniques of Physical Assessment

5. Which of the following is assessed when performing palpation of the thorax and lungs? (Select all that apply.)

_____	Breath sounds
_____	Respiratory effort
__X__	**Tactile fremitus**
__X__	**Surface characteristics**
__X__	**Chest excursion**

Tactile fremitus, surface characteristics, and chest excursion are all assessed during palpation. Breath sounds are assessed by auscultation. Respiratory effort is assessed by inspection.

NCLEX® Connection: Health Promotion and Maintenance, Techniques of Physical Assessment

6. When auscultating breath sounds, the nurse should

A. listen to the top of the anterior chest and then the top of the posterior chest.

B. compare side to side proceeding from top to bottom.

C. listen only to the posterior chest.

D. complete one side of the chest before proceeding to the other side.

Comparing side-to-side breath sounds is the correct technique to use. This allows the nurse to make comparisons between right and left lungs in a systematic way. The nurse should listen to the anterior and posterior aspects of the chest in a consistent manner.

NCLEX® Connection: Health Promotion and Maintenance, Techniques of Physical Assessment

7. Match the action within the heart/peripheral vascular system with the sound it produces.

__D__	Rapid ventricular filling	A. S1
__A__	Closure of the mitral and tricuspid valves	B. S2
__E__	Strong atrial contraction	C. Murmur
__F__	Obstructed blood flow in peripheral circulation	D. S3
__C__	Impeded blood flow in the heart	E. S4
__B__	Closure of the aortic and pulmonic valves	F. Bruits

NCLEX® Connection: Health Promotion and Maintenance, Techniques of Physical Assessment

8. The proper placement of the stethoscope for auscultating the aortic valve is the

A. second ICS just right of the sternum.

B. second ICS just left of the sternum.

C. fourth ICS just left of the sternum.

D. fifth ICS at the left midclavicular line.

Auscultate the aortic valve at the second ICS just right of the sternum. Auscultate the pulmonic valve at the second ICS just left of the sternum. Auscultate the tricuspid valve at the fourth ICS just left of the sternum. Auscultate the mitral valve at the fifth ICS at the left midclavicular line.

NCLEX® Connection: Health Promotion and Maintenance, Techniques of Physical Assessment

9. A nurse should perform the abdominal assessment using which of the following sequences?

A. Inspection, palpation, percussion, and auscultation

B. Auscultation, inspection, palpation, and percussion

C. Percussion, inspection, auscultation, and palpation

D. Inspection, auscultation, percussion, and palpation

This sequence allows the client's bowel sounds to be heard without being disturbed or distorted by percussion or palpation assessments.

NCLEX® Connection: Reduction of Risk Potential, System Specific Assessment

10. When performing percussion, which of the following sounds should be heard over most of the abdomen?

  A. Dullness
  B. Tympany
  C. Grating
  D. Gurgling

  The abdomen is primarily filled with air, and tympany is the sound that will predominate. Dullness is heard over the liver or a distended bladder. A grating sound may indicate a friction rub. Gurgling sounds are heard through a stethoscope and indicate peristalsis.

  (N) NCLEX® Connection: Health Promotion and Maintenance, Techniques of Physical Assessment

UNIT 2	HEALTH PROMOTION
Section	Health Assessment
Chapter 30	Integumentary and Peripheral Vascular Systems

Overview

- Assessment of the integumentary and peripheral vascular systems can take place at the same time. Be aware of what aspects of the assessment are being performed.

- For infants, skin assessment can be done all at once. For adults, it is generally easier to complete the skin assessment in segments as other parts of the body are being evaluated. Examine the upper extremities when the client is sitting or recumbent. Remove stockings/socks, and drape the client to expose the entire lower extremity at once.

- Comparisons should be made from side to side to evaluate for any variations.

- Lesions should be examined individually, using appropriate terminology when documenting.

- The Braden scale or a similar assessment tool can be used to predict the risk for pressure ulcer formation.

- Inspection and palpation are typically performed simultaneously.

- Equipment includes:

  - Adequate lighting

  - Gloves used for palpating of open or draining lesions

  - A flexible ruler or tape measure to measure the size and depth of lesions in centimeters

Health History – Review of Systems

- Integumentary and Peripheral Vascular Systems

  - Questions the nurse should ask include:

    - Have you noticed any changes in your skin color? If so, is the change generalized or localized?

    - Do you have a rash? Where is it located? Does it itch? How long have you had it? What have you used to treat the rash?

    - Is your skin excessively dry or oily? Does this change with the seasons? Do you use anything to treat it?

- Have you developed any new moles or lesions? Have any of the moles or lesions changed in any way (color, borders, size)?

- How often are you out in the sun? Do you use sunscreen or wear protective clothing and a hat?

- Do you have any swelling? If in your legs, is it in both legs? Does the swelling cause pain? What do you do to relieve the swelling? Does it occur at any particular time of day?

Inspection and Palpation

- Assess the color of the hair, nails, and skin for uniformity. Hair color may vary due to dyes or from aging changes. Normal skin color varies from ivory to ruddy to deep brown. Color changes are more difficult to notice in dark-skinned clients. Common color variations in the skin can occur as follows:

COLOR CHANGE	DESCRIPTION	INDICATION
Pallor	Loss of color – Best noted in face, conjunctivae, nail beds, palms	Anemia or lack of blood flow
Cyanosis	Bluish – Best noted in nail beds, lips, mouth, skin	Hypoxia or impaired venous return
Jaundice	Yellow – Orange of skin, sclera, and mucous membranes	Liver dysfunction, red blood-cell destruction
Erythema	Redness – Best noted in face, trauma and pressure sore areas	Inflammation

- Note cleanliness of the hair, skin, and nails, as well as any odors. The nail base should be firm when palpated. Note the curvature of the nail plate in relationship to the tissue just before the cuticle. The angles should be < 160°. Clubbing is an abnormal curvature of the nail with an angle > 160°. This can result from chronic low oxygen saturation (emphysema, chronic bronchitis).

- Note hair distribution patterns. If hair loss is present, it should be symmetric as with male pattern baldness. Note any infestations of the hair or skin. Alopecia may be related to certain endocrine disorders. Poor nutrition will also affect the condition of hair.

- Nail beds should be pink and symmetric. Capillary refill assesses circulation to the periphery. Blanching the nail bed with firm pressure and then quick release should result in a brisk return of color. Color should return to normal within 3 seconds.

(M) **View Media Supplement:** Capillary Refill (Video)

- Skin color of the extremities should be symmetric and similar to that of the rest of the body.

  - Brown pigmentation changes with venous insufficiency.

  - Shiny and translucent skin without hair on the toes and foot is seen with arterial insufficiency.

- Palpate the temperature of the skin with the dorsal part of the hand; check for symmetry. The skin should feel warm. Changes may reflect circulation impairment or environmental temperature. Slightly cooler temperatures of the hands or feet are acceptable.

- The texture of the skin should be smooth, soft, and even when palpated. The nails should be firm and smooth. Hair texture should be smooth and coarse or fine. Thicker skin of the palms and soles of the feet is an expected finding.

- Assess skin turgor by lifting and releasing a fold of skin on the forearm or sternum to evaluate that it returns quickly into place. Tenting is a delay in the skin returning to its normal place. Poor turgor may indicate dehydration or be a sign of aging.

 View Media Supplement: Skin Turgor (Video)

- Moisture in the axillae can be a normal finding. Otherwise, the skin should be dry. Diaphoresis, oiliness, or excessive dryness with flaking or scaling should be noted.

- Peripheral Arteries

  - Palpate the peripheral pulses for strength (amplitude) and equality (symmetry).

    - Strength (amplitude) – The strength of the pulse should be the same from beat to beat and can be graded on a scale of 0 to 4.

    - A common scale to use is:

      - 0 = Absent, unable to palpate

      - 1+ = Diminished, weaker than expected

      - 2+ = Brisk, expected

      - 3+ = Increased

      - 4+ = Full volume, bounding

    - Equality – Peripheral pulsations should be symmetric in quality and quantity from the right side of the body to the left.

  - With the exception of the carotid arteries, pulse sites can be palpated bilaterally to make comparisons.

    - Carotid pulse – On either side of the trachea, just medial to the sternocleidomastoid muscle on the neck

    - Radial pulse – On the radial side of each wrist

    - Brachial pulse – In the antecubital fossa above the elbow

- - Femoral pulse – Midway between the symphysis pubis and the anterosuperior iliac spine

  - Popliteal pulse – Behind the knee, deep in the popliteal fossa, just lateral to midline

  - Dorsalis pedis pulse – On the top of the foot, along a line with the groove between the first toe and the extensor tendons of the great toe

  - Posterior tibial pulse – Behind and below the medial malleolus of the ankles

  o Inspect peripheral veins for varicosities, redness, and swelling.

- Edema is the presence of fluid in the tissues causing swollen, tight, and shiny skin surfaces. The swelling should be assessed for discoloration, location, and tenderness. In the extremities, the circumference of the swollen body area should be measured and compared to the other side.

  o Common clinical practice includes grading the level of pitting edema present. The depth of pitting indicates the degree of edema. Use the facility's grading scale. This grading is somewhat subjective as findings may vary from examiner to examiner. Findings are most reliable when performed as serial assessments by the same examiner.

  o Evaluate pitting by compressing the skin for at least 5 seconds over a bony prominence (behind the medial malleolus, the dorsum of foot, or over the shin) and then assess.

FOUR-POINT SCALE	DEGREE	RESPONSE
1+	2 mm – Trace	Rapid
2+	4 mm – Mild	10 to 15 seconds
3+	6 mm – Moderate	1 to 2 min
4+	8 mm – Severe	2 to 5 min

- Examine lesions for size, color, shape, consistency, elevation, location, distribution, configuration, tenderness, and presence of fluid or drainage. Measure the height, width, and depth of lesions. Any change noted should be reported to the provider. Lesions commonly occur in healthy individuals.

  o Primary lesions arise from healthy skin tissue. Common examples include:

LESIONS	DESCRIPTIONS	EXAMPLES
Macule	Nonpalpable, skin color change, < 1 cm	Freckle
Papule	Palpable, circumscribed , < 0.5 cm	Elevated nevus
Nodule/tumor	Palpable, circumscribed, 0.5 cm or >	Wart
Vesicle	Serous fluid-filled, < 1 cm	Blister
Pustule	Pus-filled	Acne

LESIONS	DESCRIPTIONS	EXAMPLES
Wheal	Palpable, irregular borders, edematous	Insect bite

- o Secondary lesions result from a change in a primary lesion. Common examples include:

LESIONS	DESCRIPTIONS	EXAMPLES
Erosion	Lost epidermis, moist surface, no bleeding	Ruptured vesicle
Crust	Dried blood, serum, or pus	Scab
Scale	Flakes of skin that exfoliate	Dandruff or psoriasis
Fissure	Linear crack	Tinea pedis
Ulcer	Loss of epidermis and dermis with possible bleeding and scarring	Venous stasis ulcer or pressure ulcers

- Common examples of skin lesions in various age groups include:

CHILDREN	ADULTS	OLDER ADULTS
<ul><li>Diaper dermatitis</li><li>Intertrigo</li><li>Impetigo</li><li>Atopic dermatitis (eczema)</li></ul>	<ul><li>Primary contact dermatitis</li><li>Tinea pedis (ringworm of the foot)</li><li>Psoriasis</li><li>Labial herpes simplex (cold sores)</li></ul>	<ul><li>Lentigines (liver spots)</li><li>Seborrheic keratosis</li><li>Acrochordons (skin tags)</li><li>Sebaceous hyperplasia</li></ul>

- o Vascular lesions are created with aging changes or when damage occurs to the blood vessels in or near the skin. Common examples include:

LESIONS	DESCRIPTIONS
Spider angioma	Red center with radiating red legs, up to 2 cm, and can be raised
Cherry angioma	Red, 1 to 3 cm, round, and can be raised
Spider vein	Bluish, spider-shaped or may be linear, with up to several inches in size
Petechia/purpura	Deep reddish purple, flat, petechiae = 1 to 3 mm, purpura > 3 mm
Ecchymosis	Purple fading to green or yellow over time, variable in size, and flat
Hematoma	Raised ecchymosis

Ⓖ Expected Changes with Aging

SYSTEM	CHANGES
Integumentary	• Skin looks thin and translucent, dry, flaky, tears easily, loss of elasticity and wrinkling • Thinning of hair • Slow growth of nails with thickening • Decline in glandular structure and function (less oil, moisture, sweat) • Uneven pigmentation • Slow wound healing • Little subcutaneous tissue over bony prominences
Peripheral vascular	• Thicker, more rigid peripheral blood vessel walls with a narrowed lumen leading to poor peripheral circulation • Higher systolic blood pressure

Sample Documentation

Skin is pink, warm, and dry. Turgor is brisk and skin is elastic. Rough, thickened skin over heels, elbows, and knees; otherwise, skin is smooth. A 0.5 cm brown papule on right forearm and a 2.5 cm scar on left knee that is healed. Scalp is dry with slight dandruff noted. Hair is brown, clean, smooth, straight, and evenly distributed on the head. Axillary and pubic hair is evenly distributed with no infestations noted. Nails are short and firm with no clubbing noted. Capillary refill is < 3 seconds. No edema is noted. Pulses palpable and equal bilaterally.

CHAPTER 30: INTEGUMENTARY AND PERIPHERAL VASCULAR SYSTEMS

Ⓐ Application Exercises

1. Match the type of lesion commonly seen on a skin assessment with its correct assessment terminology.

_____	Freckle	A. Wheal
_____	Wart	B. Macule
_____	Blister	C. Nodule
_____	Acne	D. Pustule
_____	Psoriasis	E. Scale
_____	Insect bite	F. Vesicle

2. A nurse is performing a skin assessment on a client. Which of the following should the nurse consider expected findings? (Select all that apply.)

_____ A. No clubbing noted

_____ B. Capillary refill less than 2 seconds

_____ C. 3+ pitting edema in feet bilaterally

_____ D. Numerous light brown macules, < 3 mm in size, located on nose and cheeks

_____ E. Shiny and thin skin without hair on shins

3. When assessing a client's skin temperature, the nurse should use which part of the hand?

A. Fingertips

B. Dorsal surface

C. Palmar surface

D. Base of the hand

4. Assessment of an older adult client reveals significant tenting of the skin over his forearm. Which of the following best explains this finding?

A. Loss of adipose tissue and elasticity

B. Parchment-like skin

C. Significant flaking and dryness

D. Skin tags

5. A nurse is caring for a client following total knee arthroplasty. Which of the following should the nurse examine to assess the peripheral vascular system of the affected extremity? (Select all that apply.)

_____ Range of motion

_____ Skin color

_____ Skin temperature

_____ Presence of skin lesions

_____ Capillary refill

_____ Edema

CHAPTER 30: INTEGUMENTARY AND PERIPHERAL VASCULAR SYSTEMS

 Application Exercises Answer Key

1. Match the type of lesion commonly seen on a skin assessment with its correct assessment terminology.

__B__	Freckle	A.	Wheal
__C__	Wart	B.	Macule
__F__	Blister	C.	Nodule
__D__	Acne	D.	Pustule
__E__	Psoriasis	E.	Scale
__A__	Insect bite	F.	Vesicle

(N) NCLEX® Connection: Reduction of Risk Potential, System Specific Assessment

2. A nurse is performing a skin assessment on a client. Which of the following should the nurse consider expected findings? (Select all that apply.)

__X__ **A. No clubbing noted**

__X__ **B. Capillary refill less than 2 seconds**

_____ C. 3+ pitting edema in feet bilaterally

__X__ **D. Numerous light brown macules, < 3 mm in size, located on nose and cheeks**

_____ E. Shiny and thin skin without hair on shins

Expected skin findings include no clubbing, capillary refill less than 2 seconds, and light brown macules noted on the nose and cheeks. No edema should be present, and the skin should have a dull, opaque appearance with some hair present.

(N) NCLEX® Connection: Reduction of Risk Potential, System Specific Assessment

3. When assessing a client's skin temperature, the nurse should use which part of the hand?

A. Fingertips

B. Dorsal surface

C. Palmar surface

D. Base of the hand

The dorsal surface of the hand is the most sensitive to temperature changes.

(N) NCLEX® Connection: Health Promotion and Maintenance, Techniques of Physical Assessment

4. Assessment of an older adult client reveals significant tenting of the skin over his forearm. Which of the following best explains this finding?

    A. Loss of adipose tissue and elasticity

    B. Parchment-like skin

    C. Significant flaking and dryness

    D. Skin tags

    Tenting is a result of loss of adipose tissue and elasticity of the skin. Thin, parchment-like skin, dryness, and skin tags do not cause tenting.

 NCLEX® Connection: Reduction of Risk Potential, System Specific Assessment

5. A nurse is caring for a client following total knee arthroplasty. Which of the following should the nurse examine to assess the peripheral vascular system of the affected extremity? (Select all that apply.)

    _____ Range of motion

    __**X**__ **Skin color**

    __**X**__ **Skin temperature**

    _____ Presence of skin lesions

    __**X**__ **Capillary refill**

    __**X**__ **Edema**

    Assessment of the peripheral vascular system should include skin color, skin temperature, capillary refill, and edema. Determining range of motion will assess joint function. Inspecting for skin lesions is a routine included in the skin assessment.

 NCLEX® Connection: Reduction of Risk Potential, System Specific Assessment

UNIT 2	HEALTH PROMOTION
Section	Health Assessment
Chapter 31	Musculoskeletal and Neurosensory Systems

Overview

- This examination includes muscles, joints, range of motion, mental status, cranial nerves, and motor and sensory function.

MUSCULOSKELETAL SYSTEM

Overview

- Examination of the musculoskeletal system includes looking at the structure and function of the musculoskeletal system.

- This involves examining each joint and muscle and the surrounding tissues and comparing symmetric parts.

- Use the techniques of inspection and palpation to assess the musculoskeletal system.

- Equipment – A tape measure may be needed to measure joint or limb enlargements and to make bilateral comparisons.

- Assess

  o   Gait

  o   Alignment

  o   Symmetry and muscle mass

  o   Muscle tone

  o   Range of motion (ROM)

  o   Any involuntary movements

  o   Signs of inflammation (redness, swelling, warmth, tenderness, loss of function)

  o   Gross deformities

- Normal Range of Motion of Joint Movement

  o   Flexion – A decrease the angle

  o   Extension – An extension the angle

- o   Hyperextension – An extreme extension

- o   Supination – The ventral surface is facing up

- o   Pronation – The ventral surface is facing down

- o   Abduction – The movement of an extremity away from midline

- o   Adduction – The movement of an extremity toward the midline

- o   Dorsiflexion – The movement toward the dorsum (or top of the wrist or foot)

- o   Plantar flexion – The movement toward the plantar surface (or bottom of the foot)

- o   Eversion – Turning the body part away from midline

- o   Inversion – Turning the body part toward the midline

Health History – Review of Systems

- •   Questions the nurse should ask include:

  - o   Do you have any pain in your joints or muscles?

  - o   Do you have any stiffness, weakness, or twitching?

  - o   Have you fallen recently?

  - o   Are you able to care for yourself?

  - o   Is your activity limited by any physical factors?

  - o   How would you describe your physical activity? Do you exercise on a regular basis?

  - o   Do you exercise or participate in sports?

  - o   For postmenopausal women, how tall are you? Do you take calcium supplements?

Inspection

- •   Height – Measure for comparison over time; gradual height loss is a common finding as a person ages.

- •   Posture – Observe when the client is unaware he is being assessed. Expected finding – The client is standing with head erect. Both shoulders and both hips should be at the same height bilaterally.

- •   Spine – Inspect from the side. The following curvatures may be noted:

  - o   Normal curvatures

    - ▪   Concave cervical spine

    - ▪   Convex thoracic spine

    - ▪   Concave lumbar spine

- o Common abnormalities

  - ▪ Kyphosis – Exaggerated curvature of the thoracic spine, common in older adults

  - ▪ Lordosis – Exaggerated curvature of the lumbar spine (common during the toddler years and pregnancy)

  - ▪ Scoliosis – Exaggerated lateral curvature

Inspection and Palpation

- Range of motion (ROM) should be equal in the joints bilaterally.

  - o Assess passive ROM by moving the client's joints through his full range of movements. Do not move a joint past the point of pain or resistance.

  - o Assess active ROM by having the client repeat the movements demonstrated by the nurse.

  - o Assess joints for abnormalities such as warmth, inflammation, edema, stiffness, crepitus, deformities, tenderness, limitations, or instability. The joints to be assessed include:

    - ▪ Temporomandibular joint (TMJ)

    - ▪ Shoulders

    - ▪ Elbows

    - ▪ Wrists and hands

    - ▪ Spine (scoliosis)

    - ▪ Hips

    - ▪ Knees

    - ▪ Ankles and feet

- Muscles should be firm and symmetric in size and strength. The dominant side is usually slightly larger with a less than 1 cm difference not being significant.

  - o Size variations include:

    - ▪ Hypertrophy – An enlargement of muscle due to strengthening

    - ▪ Atrophy – A decrease in muscle size due to disuse

  - o Assess tone during ROM. Tone is determined by the presence of slight resistance of the muscles during relaxation.

  - o Assess the strength of muscle groups by asking the client to push or pull against resistance. Expected finding – Strength should be equal or slightly stronger on the dominant side of the body.

  - o Assess for muscle tremors.

- Inspect and palpate the spine from the back for any lateral deviations or scoliosis.

  o Instruct the client to bend at the waist with the arms reaching for the toes.

  o Inspect and palpate down the spine using the thumb and forefinger.

  o Inspect and palpate the spine again with the client standing.

  o Expected finding – There is no tenderness with spinal vertebrae that are midline.

NEUROSENSORY SYSTEM

Overview

- A neurological screening examination can evaluate the major indicators of neurological function and assist with recognition of areas of dysfunction.

- Integration of the neurological system with other assessments is recommended.

- The examination is based on the client's level of consciousness and general state of health.

- A neurological screening examination includes:

  o Mental status examination to test cerebral function

  o Assessment of cranial nerves

  o Motor function to test cerebellar function

  o Sensory function

  o Reflexes

- Equipment

  o Snellen and Rosenbaum eye charts

  o Aromatic substances

  o Tongue blades

  o Penlight

  o Sugar and salt

  o Tuning fork

  o Reflex hammer

  o Cotton balls

  o Two test tubes filled with water (one cold, one warm)

  o Pencil

  o Paper clips

  o Key

Health History – Review of Systems

- Questions the nurse should ask include:

    o Do you have any problems with dizziness or headaches? Do you ever have seizures?

    o Do you have a history of head trauma or any loss of consciousness?

    o Have you noticed any change in your vision, speech, ability to think clearly, or loss of or change in memory?

    o Do you have any weakness, numbness, tremors, or tingling? If so, where?

Mental Status

- Levels of consciousness may be described using the following terms. Observed behavior should be included in documentation:

    o Alert – The client is responsive and able to fully respond by opening the eyes and attending to a normal tone of voice and speech. Answers questions spontaneously and appropriately.

    o Lethargy – The client is able to open the eyes and respond, but is drowsy and falls asleep readily.

    o Obtundation – The client needs to be lightly shaken to respond, but may be confused and slow to respond.

    o Stupor – The client requires painful stimuli (pinching a tendon or rubbing the sternum) to achieve a brief response. The client may not be able to respond verbally.

    o Coma – There is no response to repeated painful stimuli. Abnormal posturing in clients who are comatose:

        ▪ Decorticate rigidity – Flexion and internal rotation of upper extremity joints and legs

        ▪ Decerebrate rigidity – Neck and elbow extension, with the wrists and fingers flexed

- Assess appearance by observing hygiene, grooming, and clothing choice. Expected findings – The client is well-kept, clean, and dressed appropriately for the environment or situation.

- Assess mood by inspecting mannerisms and actions during interactions with the client. Expected findings – The client makes eye contact, and emotions correspond to the conversation and situation.

- Assess cognitive and intellectual processes:

    o Memory, both recent and remote, should be assessed.

        ▪ Recent – Ask the client to repeat a series of numbers or a list of objects.

        ▪ Remote – Ask the client to state his birth date or mother's maiden name (verifiable).

- ○ Level and fund of knowledge – Ask the client what he knows about his current hospitalization or illness.

- ○ Ability for calculation – Ask the client to count backward from 100 in serials of 7.

- ○ Abstract thinking – Ask the client the interpretation of a cliché such as, "A bird in the hand is worth two in the bush." This would demonstrate a higher level of thought processes.

- ○ Insight – Objective assessment of the client's perception of illness

- ○ Judgment – Ask the client about the solution to a specific dilemma ("What would you do if you locked your keys in your car?"). The response should be logical.

- ○ Thought process – Processing differences, such as a rapid change of topic (flight of ideas) and use of nonsense words ("hipsnippity").

- ○ Thought content – Presence of delusions, hallucinations, and other ideas the client presents during the interview.

- • Speech and language rate and features, such as quality, quantity, and volume, should be articulate and responses meaningful and appropriate.

- • Standardized Screening Tools

  - ○ Use the Mini-Mental State Examination (MME) to objectively assess cognitive status. The tool evaluates:

    - ▪ Orientation to time and place

    - ▪ Attention and calculation of counting backward by 7s

    - ▪ Registration and recalling of objects

    - ▪ Language, including naming of objects, following of commands, and ability to write

  - ○ Use the Glasgow Coma scale to obtain a baseline assessment of the client's level of consciousness and for ongoing assessment.

    - ▪ This assessment looks at eye, verbal, and motor response, and assigns a number value based on the client's response. The highest value possible is 15, indicating the client is awake and responds appropriately. A score of 3 indicates the client is in a coma.

Cranial Nerve Function

CRANIAL NERVE (CN)	FUNCTION OF THE NERVE	SYSTEM
I (Olfactory)	• Sensory – Smell	Ears, nose, mouth, and throat
II (Optic)	• Sensory – Visual acuity, visual fields	Eyes
III (Oculomotor), IV (Trochlear), and VI (Abducens)	• Motor PERRLA, six cardinal positions of gaze	Eyes
V (Trigeminal)	• Sensory – Light touch sensation to the face (forehead, cheek, jaw) • Motor – Jaw opening, clenching, chewing	Head and neck
VII (Facial)	• Sensory – Taste (salt/sweet) on anterior two thirds of the tongue • Motor – Facial movements	Head and neck
VIII (Auditory)	• Sensory – Hearing and balance	Ears, nose, mouth, and throat
IX (Glossopharyngeal)	• Sensory – Taste (sour/bitter) on posterior third of the tongue • Motor – Swallowing, speech sounds, and gag reflex	Ears, nose, mouth, throat, neurological
X (Vagus)	• Sensory – Gag reflex • Motor – Swallowing, speech sounds	Ears, nose, mouth, and throat
XI (Spinal accessory)	• Motor – Turn head, shrug shoulders	Head and neck
XII (Hypoglossal)	• Motor – Tongue movement	Ears, nose, mouth, and throat

Motor Function

- Assess coordination by asking the client to extend his arms and rapidly touch his finger to his nose, alternating hands, and then doing it with his eyes closed. Expected findings include smooth, coordinated movements.

- Assess gait when the client is unaware of being assessed. Expected finding – Gait is steady, smooth, and coordinated.

- Assess balance using the following tests:

  o Romberg test – Ask the client to stand with his feet at a comfortable distance apart, his arms at his sides, and his eyes closed. Expected finding – The client should be able to stand with minimal swaying for at least 5 seconds.

  o Heel-to-toe walk – Ask the client to place the heel of one foot in front of the toes of the other foot as he walks in a straight line. Expected finding – The client is able to walk in a straight line without losing his balance.

- Muscle Strength

  o Assess the strength of muscle groups by asking the client to push or pull against resistance. Expected finding – Strength should be equal or slightly stronger on the dominant side of the body.

Sensory Function

- Perform tests on all four extremities with the client's eyes closed.

  o Assess pain sensation by alternating sharp and dull objects on the skin and asking the client to report what he feels.

  o Assess temperature by using two test tubes filled with water (one warm and one cold), and ask the client to identify which he feels (usually deferred).

  o Assess light touch by asking the client to report when and where he feels a cotton ball touching his skin.

  o Assess vibration by having the client report when and where he feels the handle of the vibrating tuning fork on his skin.

  o Assess position by repositioning the client's appendages and asking him to report whether each is positioned up or down.

  o Assess discrimination by using one of the following:

    ▪ Two-point discrimination – Use open paper clips to determine the distance at which the two points are felt as one. Compare bilaterally. Minimal distance will vary depending on the body part being evaluated.

    ▪ Stereognosis – Use a familiar object (key, cotton ball) placed in the client's hand, and ask him to identify it.

    ▪ Graphesthesia – Ask the client to identify a number drawn on his palm with the blunt end of a pencil.

Deep tendon reflexes (DTR)

- Using a reflex hammer, assess DTRs bilaterally and compare results for symmetry as follows:

DTR – SPINAL CORD INNERVATION	TECHNIQUE	EXPECTED RESPONSE
Biceps – C_5 and C_6	• Flex arm 45°. • Place the thumb on the tendon in antecubital fossa. • Strike the thumb with a reflex hammer.	Flexion of the elbow
Brachioradialis – C_5 and C_6	• Rest a forearm on the examiner's forearm with the wrist slightly pronated. • Strike the tendon 2.5 to 5 cm above the wrist.	Pronation of the forearm and flexion of the elbow
Triceps – C_7, and C_8	• Support the upper arm with the forearm hanging at a 90°. • Strike the tendon above the elbow.	Extension of the elbow
Patellar – L_2, L_3, and L_4	• With the upper leg supported and the lower leg dangling freely, strike the tendon below the knee.	Extension of the lower leg
Achilles – S_1 and S_2	• Flex the knee, dorsiflex the foot, and strike the tendon above the heel.	Plantar flexion of the foot

- DTR responses are graded on a scale of 0 to 4.

  - 4+ = Very brisk with clonus

  - 3+ = More brisk than average

  - 2+ = Expected

  - 1+ = Diminished

  - 0 = No response

(G) Expected Changes with Aging

SYSTEM	CHANGES
Musculoskeletal	• Reduced muscle mass • Declines in speed, strength, resistance to fatigue, reaction time, coordination • Osteoporosis (fragility of bones, loss of bone mass and height) • Greater risk of fractures and vertebral compression • Degenerative alterations in joints • Limited range of motion • Flexed elbows, hips, and knees • Thinning intervertebral discs, kyphosis (with height loss), wider stance altering posture
Neurological	• Some short-term memory decline • Diminished/slowed reflex and motor responses, impulse transmission, and reaction times • Altered vibration, position, hearing, vision, smell, and deep pain and temperature sensation • Slower fine finger movement (no change in superficial pain and light touch sensation, standing balance) • Decline in mental function is probably related to less cognitive stimulation and solitude. • Fewer brain cells, smaller brain volume, deteriorating nerve cells, fewer neurotransmitters • With infection, delirium is more common than fever. • Greater risk of depression

Sample Documentation

Full range of motion without pain in all joints and spine. No joint deformities, warmth, or swelling. Posture is erect. Spine is midline with expected cervical, thoracic, and lumbar curvatures. No scoliosis noted. Muscle strength is equal and strong bilaterally.

CHAPTER 31: MUSCULOSKELETAL AND NEUROSENSORY SYSTEMS

 Application Exercises

1. Which of the following are normal aging changes of the musculoskeletal system? (Select all that apply.)

_____ Wider stance resulting in posture changes

_____ Loss of height

_____ Increased range of motion

_____ Increased muscle bulk

_____ Thinning intervertebral discs

2. Assessment of the musculoskeletal system should start with

A. measuring limb length.

B. testing range of motion.

C. inspecting for symmetry and posture.

D. assessing muscle strength.

3. During an assessment, the client reports pain on internal rotation of her right shoulder. This will most likely affect which of the following activities?

A. Brushing the back of her hair

B. Fastening her bra behind her back

C. Reaching for something in a cabinet above the sink

D. Mopping the floor

4. Unilateral hypertrophy of the arm muscles is most likely seen in an individual who regularly

A. lifts weights.

B. plays soccer.

C. moves furniture.

D. plays tennis.

5. Dorsiflexion of the feet is assessed by instructing the client to

A. point the toes toward the head.

B. point the toes toward the floor.

C. turn the soles of the feet outward.

D. turn the soles of the feet inward.

6. Which of the following questions should be asked during a health history to assess the client's cerebral function?

    A. "Do your fingers ever feel numb and tingly?"

    B. "Do you have difficulty remembering things?"

    C. "Do you have any problems keeping your balance?"

    D. "Do you have any difficulties with your sense of taste?"

7. Match the following cranial nerves with the appropriate assessment technique.

_____	Olfactory (CN I)	A. Snellen chart
_____	Optic (CN II)	B. Six cardinal positions of gaze
_____	Oculomotor (CN III), Trochlear (CN IV), Abducens (CN VI)	C. Identification of a familiar smell with eyes closed
_____	Facial (CN VII)	D. Smiling, frowning, and raising the eyebrows
_____	Spinal Accessory (CN XI)	E. Shrugging the shoulders against resistance
_____	Hypoglossal (CN XII)	F. Moving the tongue up, down, and side to side

8. When the triceps tendon is hit with a reflex hammer, the expected response is for the elbow to

    A. flex.

    B. extend.

    C. internally rotate.

    D. pronate.

9. To evaluate stereognosis, the nurse should ask the client to close his eyes and to identify

    A. a number drawn in the palm of his hand.

    B. a word whispered 30 cm from his ear.

    C. a familiar object placed in his hand.

    D. the vibration of a tuning fork placed on his foot.

10. Which of the following is included in the assessment of a client's cognitive processes? (Select all that apply.)

    _____ Level of consciousness

    _____ Mood

    _____ Appearance

    _____ Knowledge

    _____ Judgment

CHAPTER 31: MUSCULOSKELETAL AND NEUROSENSORY SYSTEMS

 Application Exercises Answer Key

1. Which of the following are normal aging changes of the musculoskeletal system? (Select all that apply.)

<u> X </u>   **Wider stance resulting in posture changes**

<u> X </u>   **Loss of height**

<u>   </u>   Increased range of motion

<u>   </u>   Increased muscle bulk

<u> X </u>   **Thinning intervertebral discs**

Normal aging changes of the musculoskeletal system include posture changes, loss of height, and thinning intervertebral discs. Range of motion and muscle size also decrease.

 NCLEX® Connection: Health Promotion and Maintenance, Aging Process

2. Assessment of the musculoskeletal system should start with

    A. measuring limb length.

    B. testing range of motion.

    C. inspecting for symmetry and posture.

    D. assessing of muscle strength.

Assessment of the musculoskeletal system should start with inspection of the skeleton. Measuring limb length, testing range of motion and muscle strength are performed after inspection.

 NCLEX® Connection: Health Promotion and Maintenance, Techniques of Physical Assessment

3. During an assessment, the client reports pain on internal rotation of her right shoulder. This will most likely affect which of the following activities?

    A. Brushing the back of her hair

    B. Fastening her bra behind her back

    C. Reaching for something in a cabinet above the sink

    D. Mopping the floor

Fastening a bra from behind requires internal rotation of the shoulder. Brushing the back of the hair and reaching for something up high require external rotation of the shoulder. Mopping the floor requires flexion and extension of the shoulder.

 NCLEX® Connection: Reduction of Risk Potential, System Specific Assessment

4. Unilateral hypertrophy of the arm muscles is most likely seen in an individual who regularly

    A. lifts weights.

    B. plays soccer.

    C. moves furniture.

    D. plays tennis.

A tennis player will use one arm primarily, and unilateral hypertrophy will most likely result. Lifting weights, moving furniture, and playing soccer will most likely result in bilateral muscle hypertrophy.

(N) NCLEX® Connection: Reduction of Risk Potential, System Specific Assessment

5. Dorsiflexion of the feet is assessed by instructing the client to

    A. point the toes toward the head.

    B. point the toes toward the floor.

    C. turn the soles of the feet outward.

    D. turn the soles of the feet inward.

Pointing the toes toward the head results in dorsiflexion. Pointing the toes toward the floor results in plantar flexion. Turning the soles of the feet outward results in eversion, and turning the soles of the feet inward results in inversion.

(N) NCLEX® Connection: Reduction of Risk Potential, System Specific Assessment

6. Which of the following questions should be asked during a health history to assess the client's cerebral function?

    A. "Do your fingers ever feel numb and tingly?"

    B. "Do you have difficulty remembering things?"

    C. "Do you have any problems keeping your balance?"

    D. "Do you have any difficulties with your sense of taste?"

Memory is tested during the mental status examination, which evaluates cerebral function. Numbness and tingling are abnormal findings of the sensory system. Balance is a test for muscle function, and the sense of taste is controlled by cranial nerves VII and IX.

(N) NCLEX® Connection: Physiological Adaptation, Alterations in Body Systems

7. Match the following cranial nerves with the appropriate assessment technique.

C	Olfactory (CN I)	A. Snellen chart
A	Optic (CN II)	B. Six cardinal positions of gaze
B	Oculomotor (CN III), Trochlear (CN IV), Abducens (CN VI)	C. Identification of a familiar smell with eyes closed
D	Facial (CN VII)	D. Smiling, frowning, and raising the eyebrows
E	Spinal Accessory (CN XI)	E. Shrugging the shoulders against resistance
F	Hypoglossal (CN XII)	F. Moving the tongue up, down, and side to side

 NCLEX® Connection: Reduction of Risk Potential, System Specific Assessment

8. When the triceps tendon is hit with a reflex hammer, the expected response is for the elbow to

A. flex.

B. extend.

C. internally rotate.

D. pronate.

Striking the triceps tendon with a hammer results in extension of the elbow. The elbow does not flex, internally rotate, or pronate.

 NCLEX® Connection: Reduction of Risk Potential, System Specific Assessment

9. To evaluate stereognosis, the nurse should ask the client to close his eyes and to identify

A. a number drawn in the palm of his hand.

B. a word whispered 30 cm from his ear.

C. a familiar object placed in his hand.

D. the vibration of a tuning fork placed on his foot.

Identifying a familiar object placed in the hand assesses for stereognosis. Graphesthesia is identifying a number drawn in the palm of the hand. Hearing whispered words tests CN VIII. Identifying a vibrating tuning fork tests the vibratory sense.

 NCLEX® Connection: Reduction of Risk Potential, System Specific Assessment

10. Which of the following is included in the assessment of the client's cognitive processes? (Select all that apply.)

	Level of consciousness
	Mood
	Appearance
X	**Knowledge**
X	**Judgment**

All are components of a mental status examination. Assessment of knowledge and judgment are included in cognitive processes.

Ⓝ **NCLEX® Connection: Reduction of Risk Potential, System Specific Assessment**

UNIT 3: PSYCHOSOCIAL INTEGRITY

- Therapeutic Communication
- Coping
- Self-Concept and Sexuality
- Cultural and Spiritual Nursing Care
- Grief, Loss, and Palliative Care

NCLEX® CONNECTIONS

When reviewing the chapters
in this unit, keep in mind
the relevant sections of the
NCLEX® outline, in particular:

CLIENT NEEDS: PSYCHOSOCIAL INTEGRITY

Relevant topics/tasks include:
- Coping Mechanisms
  - Provide information to the client on stress management techniques.
- Cultural Diversity
  - Incorporate the client's cultural practices and beliefs when planning and providing care.
- End-of-Life Care
  - Identify end-of-life needs of the client.
- Religious and Spiritual Influences on Health
  - Assess and plan interventions that meet the client's emotional and spiritual needs.
- Therapeutic Communication
  - Allow time to communicate with the client.

UNIT 3	PSYCHOSOCIAL INTEGRITY
Chapter 32	Therapeutic Communication

Overview

- Communication is a complex process of sending, receiving, and comprehending messages between two or more people. It is a dynamic and ongoing process that creates a unique experience between the participants.

  ○ Communicating effectively is a skill that can be developed.

  ○ Nurses use communication when providing care to demonstrate caring, establish relationships, obtain information, and assist with changing behavior.

  ○ Therapeutic communication is foundational to the nurse-client relationship.

Basic Communication

- Levels of Basic Communication

  ○ Intrapersonal communication – Communication that occurs within an individual. Also identified as "self-talk." This is the internal discussion that takes place when an individual is thinking but not outwardly verbalizing the thoughts. In nursing, intrapersonal communication allows the nurse to assess clients and/or situations and critically think about the clients/situations before verbally communicating.

  ○ Interpersonal communication – Communication that occurs between two people. This form of communication is the most common in nursing and requires an exchange of information with an individual or small group.

  ○ Public communication – Communication that occurs within large groups of people. In nursing, this commonly occurs during educational endeavors where the nurse is teaching a large group of individuals, such as in a community setting.

  ○ Transpersonal communication – Addresses spiritual needs and provides interventions to meet these needs.

  ○ Small group communication – Communication within a group of people.

- Functional Components of Basic Communication

COMPONENT	DESCRIPTION
Referent	• The incentive or motivation for communication to occur between one person and another
Sender	• The person who initiates the message
Message	• The verbal and/or nonverbal information that is expressed by the sender and intended for the receiver
Channel	• The method of transmitting and receiving a message (received via sight, hearing, and/or touch)
Receiver	• The person to whom the message is aimed at and received by
Environment	• The emotional and physical climate in which the communication takes place
Feedback	• May be verbal and/or nonverbal, positive and/or negative • The message that is returned to the sender by the receiver that indicates that the message was received • An essential component of ongoing communication
Interpersonal variables	• Variables that influence communication between the sender and the receiver

- Verbal Communication

CONTENT OF THE MESSAGE	IMPACT ON THE COMMUNICATION
Vocabulary – These are the words used to communicate either a written or spoken message.	Limited vocabulary or speaking another language may make it difficult for the nurse to communicate with the client. Use of medical jargon may decrease client understanding.
Denotative/connotative meaning – When communicating, participants must share meanings.	Words that have multiple meanings may cause miscommunication if interpreted differently.
Clarity/brevity – The shortest, simplest communication is usually most effective.	Long and complex communication may be difficult to understand.
Timing/relevance – Knowing when to communicate allows the receiver to be more attentive to the message.	Communicating with a client who is in physical discomfort or distracted will make it difficult to convey the message.
Pacing – The rate of speech can communicate a meaning to the receiver.	Speaking rapidly may communicate the impression that the nurse is in a rush and does not have time for the client.
Intonation – The tone of voice can communicate a variety of feelings.	The nurse can communicate feelings such as acceptance, judgment, and dislike through tone of voice.

- Nonverbal Communication

  o Nurses should be aware of how they communicate nonverbally. The nurse should assess the client's nonverbal communication for the meaning being conveyed, remembering that culture impacts interpretation. Attention to the following in both the communicator and the receiver is necessary:

    - Appearance

    - Posture

    - Gait

    - Facial expressions

    - Eye contact

    - Gestures

    - Sounds

    - Territoriality – Space or things that a client considers belonging to self

    - Personal space

    - Silence

Therapeutic Communication

- Therapeutic communication is the purposeful use of communication to build and maintain helping relationships with clients, families, and significant others.

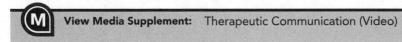

View Media Supplement: Therapeutic Communication (Video)

- The nurse uses interactive, purposeful communication skills to:

    - Elicit and attend to the client's thoughts, feelings, concerns, and needs.

    - Express empathy and genuine concern for the client and family's issues.

    - Obtain information and give feedback about the client's condition.

    - Intervene to promote functional behavior and effective interpersonal relationships.

    - Evaluate the client's progress toward desired goals and outcomes.

- Children and older adults frequently require altered techniques to enhance communication.

- Use of the nursing process depends on therapeutic communication between the nurse, client/family/significant other, and the interdisciplinary health care team.

- Characteristics of Therapeutic Communication

  - Client centered – Not social or reciprocal

  - Purposeful, planned, and goal-directed

- Essential Components of Therapeutic Communication

  - Time – Plan for and allow adequate time to communicate with others.

  - Attending behaviors or active listening – A means of conveying interest in another.

    - Eye contact typically conveys interest and respect but varies with culture and situation.

    - Body language and posture may demonstrate comfort and ease in the situation.

    - Vocal quality enhances rapport and emphasizes particular topics or issues.

    - Verbal tracking provides feedback by restating or summarizing the client's statements.

  - Caring attitude – Show concern and facilitate an emotional connection/support between the nurse and the client/family/significant other.

  - Honesty – Be open, direct, truthful, and sincere.

  - Trust – Demonstrate to the client/family/significant other that they can rely on the nurse without doubt, question, or judgment.

  - Empathy – Convey an objective awareness and understanding of the feelings, emotions, and behaviors of the client/family/significant other, including trying to envision what it must be like to be in the client/family/significant other's position.

  - Nonjudgmental attitude – A display of acceptance of the client/family/significant other will encourage open, honest communication.

Nursing Process

- Assessment/Data Collection

  - Determine verbal and nonverbal communication needs.

  - Consider physical status.

  - Consider the developmental level and alter communication accordingly.

    - Children

      - Use simple, straightforward language.

      - Be aware of nonverbal messages, as children are sensitive to nonverbal communication.

      - Enhance communication by being at the child's eye level.

      - Incorporate play in interactions.

⒢

- Older adult clients
  - Recognize that the client may require amplification.
  - Minimize distractions and face the client when speaking.
  - Allow plenty of time for the client to respond.
  - When impaired communication is assessed, ask for input from caregivers or family to determine the extent of the deficits and how best to communicate.
- Identify any cultural considerations that may impact communication.

- Planning
  - Minimize distractions.
  - Provide privacy.
  - Identify mutually agreed-upon client outcomes.
  - Set priorities according to the client's needs.
  - Plan adequate time for interventions.

- Implementation
  - Establish a trusting nurse-client relationship. The client feels more at ease during the implementation phase when a helping relationship has been established.
  - Provide empathetic responses and explanations to the client by using observations, giving information, conveying hope, and using humor.

Effective Skills and Techniques

EFFECTIVE COMMUNICATION	INFLUENCE ON COMMUNICATION
Silence	Silence allows time for meaningful reflection.
Active listening	The nurse is able to hear, observe, and understand what the client communicates and provide feedback.
Open-ended questions	This technique facilitates spontaneous responses and interactive discussion. Allows the client to explore feelings and thoughts. Avoids yes/no answers.
Clarifying techniques	This technique is used to determine if the message received was accurate: • Restating – Uses the client's exact words • Reflecting – Directs the focus back to the client in order for the client to examine his feelings • Paraphrasing – Restates the client's feelings and thoughts for the client to confirm what has been communicated • Exploring – Allows the nurse to gather more information regarding important topics mentioned by the client

EFFECTIVE COMMUNICATION	INFLUENCE ON COMMUNICATION
Offering general leads, broad opening statements	This encourages the client to start and to continue talking.
Showing acceptance and recognition	This technique acknowledges the nurse's interest and nonjudgmental attitude.
Focusing	This technique helps the client concentrate on what is important.
Asking questions	Asking questions is a way to seek additional information.
Giving information	This technique provides details that the client may need for decision making.
Presenting reality	This technique is used to help the client focus on what is actually happening and to dispel delusions, hallucinations, or faulty beliefs.
Summarizing	This technique emphasizes important points and reviews what has been discussed.
Offering self	This technique demonstrates a willingness to spend time with the client. Limited personal information may be shared, but the focus should return to the client as soon as possible. Relevant self-disclosure by the nurse allows the client to see that his experience is shared by others and understood.
Touch	If appropriate, touch may communicate caring and provide comfort.

Barriers to Effective Communication

- Asking irrelevant personal questions
- Offering personal opinions
- Giving advice
- Giving false reassurance
- Minimizing feelings
- Changing the topic
- Asking "why" questions or asking for explanations
- Offering value judgments
- Excessive questioning
- Responding approvingly or disapprovingly

Client Outcomes

- The client verbalizes concerns to the nurse.
- The client requests assistance from the nurse as appropriate.
- The client communicates needs to the nurse.

CHAPTER 32: THERAPEUTIC COMMUNICATION

(A) Application Exercises

Scenario: The following conversation occurs between a nurse and a client: Nurse: "Do you have any pain from your knee incision this morning?" Client: "No, but my back is really hurting. I think I want a pain pill for it." Nurse: "Is the back pain a new problem or is this something you had before your surgery?" Client: "Oh, I've had back problems for years." Nurse: "I see you have a heating pad behind you. Does the heating pad help your back?" Client: "Yes, it helps relax the muscles."

1. Fill in the following table:

COMMUNICATION COMPONENT	EXAMPLE FROM SCENARIO
Referent	
Sender	
Channels for communication	
Receiver	
Message	
Feedback	

2. A nurse is bathing an older adult client and says to him, "Turn to your side now, honey." The nurse believes she is demonstrating warmth and caring by calling the client "honey." However, the client finds the term offensive. What has caused this miscommunication to occur?

    A. The connotative meaning of the word is different to the client and the nurse.

    B. The client was unable to hear the nurse's message.

    C. The nurse's verbal communication was not congruent with her nonverbal communication.

    D. It is not the appropriate time for performing the client's bath.

3. A nurse recognizes that a helping relationship is established with a client if the communication

    A. is equally reciprocal between the nurse and the client.

    B. encourages the client to express his thoughts and feelings.

    C. has no time limits.

    D. occurs spontaneously throughout the nurse-client relationship.

4. When communicating with a child who is seated, the nurse should

    A. touch the child.

    B. sit at eye level with the child.

    C. stand facing the child.

    D. stand with a relaxed posture.

5. Which of the following are behaviors of active listening? (Select all that apply.)

_____ Maintaining an open posture

_____ Writing down what the client says so that details are not forgotten

_____ Establishing and maintaining eye contact

_____ Nodding in agreement with the client throughout the conversation

_____ Responding positively when giving feedback

CHAPTER 32: THERAPEUTIC COMMUNICATION

Ⓐ Application Exercises Answer Key

Scenario: The following conversation occurs between a nurse and a client: Nurse: "Do you have any pain from your knee incision this morning?" Client: "No, but my back is really hurting. I think I want a pain pill for it." Nurse: "Is the back pain a new problem or is this something you had before your surgery?" Client: "Oh, I've had back problems for years." Nurse: "I see you have a heating pad behind you. Does the heating pad help your back?" Client: "Yes, it helps relax the muscles."

1. Fill in the following table:

COMMUNICATION COMPONENT	EXAMPLE FROM SCENARIO
Referent	The nurse needed to assess the client's pain.
Sender	The nurse
Channels for communication	Verbal communication, hearing
Receiver	The client
Message	"Are you having pain and how are you experiencing it?"
Feedback	"I have chronic pain in my back."

Ⓝ NCLEX® Connection: Psychosocial Integrity, Therapeutic Communications

2. A nurse is bathing an older adult client and says to him, "Turn to your side now, honey." The nurse believes she is demonstrating warmth and caring by calling the client "honey." However, the client finds the term offensive. What has caused this miscommunication to occur?

   A. The connotative meaning of the word is different to the client and the nurse.

   B. The client was unable to hear the nurse's message.

   C. The nurse's verbal communication was not congruent with her nonverbal communication.

   D. It is not the appropriate time for performing the client's bath.

   The nurse believes that the word "honey" communicates warmth and caring. The client interprets the word as being derogatory and perhaps unprofessional. The client did not have any difficulty hearing the message. There is no indication that verbal and nonverbal communication is not congruent, or that it is an inappropriate time for performing the bath.

Ⓝ NCLEX® Connection: Psychosocial Integrity, Therapeutic Communications

3. A nurse recognizes that a helping relationship is established with a client if the communication

    A. is equally reciprocal between the nurse and the client.

    B. encourages the client to express his thoughts and feelings.

    C. has no time limits.

    D. occurs spontaneously throughout the nurse-client relationship.

Therapeutic communication facilitates a helping relationship that maximizes the client's ability to openly express his thoughts and feelings. The communication is not reciprocal but client-focused. Therapeutic communication is limited to the boundaries of the therapeutic relationship. Therapeutic communication is planned by a health care professional.

Ⓝ NCLEX® Connection: Psychosocial Integrity, Therapeutic Communications

4. When communicating with a child who is seated, the nurse should

    A. touch the child.

    B. sit at eye level with the child.

    C. stand facing the child.

    D. stand with a relaxed posture.

The nurse should be at the same eye level as the child to facilitate communication. Touching may intimidate the child and block communication. Standing will prevent the nurse from being at eye level with the child.

Ⓝ NCLEX® Connection: Psychosocial Integrity, Therapeutic Communications

5. Which of the following are behaviors of active listening? (Select all that apply.)

    __X__ **Maintaining an open posture**

    _____ Writing down what the client says so that details are not forgotten

    __X__ **Establishing and maintaining eye contact**

    _____ Nodding in agreement with the client throughout the conversation

    __X__ **Responding positively when giving feedback**

Having an open posture and leaning forward, establishing and maintaining eye contact, and responding positively when giving feedback are ways the nurse can demonstrate active listening. Writing down everything the client says will interfere with the nurse's ability to maintain eye contact and an open posture. Nodding in agreement throughout the conversation may be interpreted as agreement with what the client is saying when it was only intended to indicate attending to what was being said.

Ⓝ NCLEX® Connection: Psychosocial Integrity, Therapeutic Communications

COPING **chapter 33**

UNIT 3	PSYCHOSOCIAL INTEGRITY

Chapter 33   Coping

Overview

- Coping describes how an individual deals with problems, such as illness and stress. Factors involved in coping and adaptation include the client's family dynamics, adherence to treatment regimens, and the role an individual may play in important relationships.

STRESS, ADAPTATION, COPING, AND ADHERENCE

Overview

- Stress

  - Stress describes changes in an individual's state of balance in response to stressors, the internal and external forces that disrupt that state of balance. Any stressor, whether it is perceived as "good" or "bad," produces a similar biological response in the body.

  - Stress may be situational (adjusting to a chronic disease or a stressful job change).

  - Stress may be developmental (varying with life stage). An adult stressor may include losing parents or getting married.

  - Stress may be caused by sociocultural factors, including substance abuse, lack of education, and prolonged poverty.

  - Stress may contribute to illness vulnerability.

- Coping

  - Coping is a term that describes how an individual deals with problems and issues.

  - Factors influencing an individual's ability to cope include the number, duration, and intensity of the stressors; the individual's past experiences; the current support system; and available resources (financial).

  - Caregiver burden results from the accumulated stress that family members experience after caring for a loved one over a period of time. Some responses include fatigue, difficulty sleeping, and illness (increased blood pressure, mental illness).

- Adaptation

  - Coping behavior that describes how an individual handles demands imposed by the environment.

- General Adaptation Syndrome (GAS)

  o Alarm reaction – Body functions are heightened to respond to stressors (elevated blood pressure and heart rate, heightened mental alertness, increased secretion of epinephrine and norepinephrine).

  o Resistance stage – Body functions normalize while responding to the stressor. The body attempts to cope with the stressor.

  o Exhaustion stage – Body functions are no longer able to maintain a response to the stressor.

- Adherence

  o The commitment and ability of the client and family to follow a given treatment regimen.

  o Commitment to the regimens increases adherence.

  o Complicated regimens interfere with adherence.

  o Adverse/side effects of medications diminish adherence.

  o Coping mechanisms, such as denial, can cause nonadherence.

  o Available resources increase adherence.

Assessment/Data Collection

- Ask the client questions related to:

  o Current stress, meaning of stressors, and ability to cope

  o Support systems

  o Adherence to the treatment regimen – How motivated the client is to commit to the regimen.

  o Sleep patterns

  o Altered elimination patterns and change in appetite

- Observe the client's appearance and eye contact.

- Measure vital signs.

- Observe for irritability, anxiety, and tension.

Collaborative Care

- Nursing Care

NURSING INTERVENTIONS FOR STRESS, COPING, AND ADHERENCE	
Stress	• Encourage health promotion strategies including regular exercise, optimal nutrition, and adequate sleep and rest. • Assist with time management and determine priority tasks. • Encourage appropriate relaxation techniques including breathing exercises, massage, imagery, yoga, and meditation. • Listen attentively, and take the time to understand the client's perspective. • Control the environment to reduce the number of external stressors including noise and breaks in the continuity of care. • Identify available support systems. • Use effective communication techniques to foster the expression of feelings.
Coping	• Be empathetic in communication, and encourage the client to verbalize feelings. • Identify the client's and family's strengths and abilities. • Discuss the client's and family's abilities to deal with the current situation. • Encourage the client to describe coping skills used effectively in the past. • Identify available community resources, and refer the client for counseling if needed.
Adherence	• Put instructions in writing. • Allow the client to give input into the treatment regimen. • Simplify treatment regimens as much as possible. • Follow up with the client to address any questions or problems.

Family Systems and Family Dynamics

- Family is defined by the client.
- Consider five realms of processes involved in family function during a family assessment:
  - Interactive
  - Developmental
  - Coping
  - Integrity
  - Health
- Assessment of a family can focus on family as a context, a client, or a system.

- Families and clients are not mutually exclusive; family-centered care creates a holistic approach to nursing care.

- Family dynamics are constantly evolving due to the processes of family life and developmental stages of the family members.

- Current Trends

  o Family Forms

    ▪ Nuclear – Wife, husband, child(ren)

    ▪ Extended – Nuclear plus relative(s) (Aunts, uncles, grandparents, cousins)

    ▪ Blended – Nuclear plus stepchildren; families of divorce with remarriage

    ▪ Alternative – "Grandparents caring for grandchildren, nonfamilies (single adults living alone), cohabiting partners, and same-gender couples

  o Marital roles

    ▪ Single-income families

    ▪ Dual or multiple-income families

  o Fastest growing population – those older than 65 years, leading to caregiver issues

  o Declining economic status of families (increased unemployment)

  o Family violence and its endless cycle

  o Any acute or chronic illness the disrupts the family unit (may include end-of-life care issues)

  o Homelessness – lack of stable environment, financial issues, and inadequate access to health care (The fastest growing homeless population is families with children.)

- Attributes of Families

  o Structure dictates the family's ability to cope.

    ▪ Rigid structure is dictatorial and strict.

    ▪ Open structure includes few or no boundaries, consistent behavior, or consequences.

    ▪ Either structure may provide positive or negative outcomes.

  o Function describes the course of action the family uses to reach its goals, including members' communication skills, problem-solving abilities, and available resources.

Assessment/Data Collection

- Assess all clients within the context of the family.

- Assess a family by looking at its structure and function.

- Identify who is a family member, what role each family member plays, and the dynamic interactions within the family.

- Listen attentively, and use the therapeutic communication techniques of reflection and restatement to clarify the family's concerns.

- Cultural variables – All of which may differ between and within generations

  o Perception of events

  o Rites and rituals

  o Health beliefs

Collaborative Care

- Nursing Care

  o Identify and adapt family strengths to perceived stressor(s).

    ▪ Communication

    ▪ Adaptability

    ▪ Nurturing

    ▪ Crisis as a growth element

    ▪ Parenting skills

    ▪ Resiliency

  o Set realistic goals with the family.

  o Provide information about support networks and community resources.

    ▪ Child and adult day care

    ▪ Caregiver support groups

  o Promote family unity.

  o Ensure safety for families at risk for violence.

  o Encourage conflict resolution when it exists.

  o Minimize family process disruption effects.

  o Remove barriers to health promotion.

  o Increase family members' abilities to participate.

  o Perform interventions that the family cannot perform.

  o Evaluate goals within the context of the family by checking back to ensure that goals were realistic and achievable.

SITUATIONAL ROLE CHANGES

Overview

- A role is the function a person adopts within his life. Seldom is it limited to one role, but rather is multidimensional and is often relative to the role of others.

    o   Grandparent

    o   Parent

    o   Dependent child

    o   Employee/employer

    o   Committee member

    o   Community activist

- Stress affects roles in many ways.

- The presence of stressors delays a client's return to health in the same way that the presence of a foreign body or infection delays the healing of a wound.

- Illness causes role stress by creating a situation where roles may and do change simply due to the impact and progression of the illness.

- Nurses must be aware of a client's roles in life, as well as how the situation of illness might change these roles, either temporarily or permanently.

- A basic assumption is that a client can either advance or regress in the face of a situational role change.

- Types of role problems include:

    o   Role conflict – This develops when a person must assume opposing roles with incompatible expectations. Role conflicts may be interpersonal (when parents expect adolescents to participate in sports and perform household tasks) or inter-role (when a young mother wants to stay at home with her infant, but family finances require her to work)

    o   Sick role – Expectations of others and society regarding how one should behave when sick (caring for self and continuing to provide childcare to grandchildren)

    o   Role ambiguity – Uncertainty about what is expected when assuming a role

    o   Role strain – The frustration and anxiety that occurs when a person feels inadequate for assuming a role

    o   Role overload – More responsibility and roles than are manageable (assuming the role of student, employee, and parent)

- Situational Role Changes

  o Caused by situations other than physical growth and development (marriage, job changes, divorce)

  o Can disrupt one or more of the client's roles in life (with illness or hospitalization)

  o With resolution, can contribute to healing in the physical, mental, and spiritual realms

    ▪ Temporary role changes – The client will resume the role when illness resolves.

    ▪ Permanent role changes – Illness has altered the level of the client's health to a point that previous role(s) are no longer available.

Assessment/Data Collection

- Identify the roles the client perceives as owning.

- Identify the client's roles as perceived by significant others.

- Validate any discrepancies.

- Identify the impact that the loss or addition of a role is having on the client. The client may grieve the loss of a role.

- Identify who will now take on the client's role while the client cannot.

- Questions to Consider in the Assessment Phase of Care

  o Client as primary wage earner in family

    ▪ How does illness influence family finances?

    ▪ Who will ensure the family's fiscal soundness during illness?

    ▪ Should this role be permanently removed from the client, and if so, how will the family meet fiscal needs?

  o Client as caregiver

    ▪ Who will fill this role during the client's illness for the person(s) being cared for?

    ▪ Who will fill this role for the client if the client requires a caregiver?

    ▪ What is happening to those to whom the client gave care now that the client is no longer able to fulfill that role?

Collaborative Care

- Nursing Care

  o Provide short-term care to provide relief for the family caregiver.

  o Provide encouragement during times of stress.

  o Seek congruence among perceived roles.

  o Prepare the client for the anticipated situational crisis.

- o   Anticipate role conflict or overload on the client's part.

- o   Help the client improve relationships by supplementing specific role behaviors.

- o   Explore which roles the client can relinquish.

- o   Help the client improve personal judgment of self-worth given the current situational role change.

- o   Counsel the client about roles that are permanently altered.

- o   Refer the client to community services for outpatient adaptation to lost or new roles.

- o   Refer the client to social services for assistance in some roles.

- o   Evaluate the client after acceptance of the role change(s) to assess adaptation.

CHAPTER 33: COPING

 Application Exercises

1. A nurse is caring for a client whose partner passed away 4 months ago and who has been recently diagnosed with diabetes mellitus. He is tearful and states, "How could you possibly understand what I am going through?" Which of the following would be an appropriate response by the nurse?

    A. "It takes time to get over the loss of a loved one."

    B. "You are right; I cannot really understand. Perhaps you'd like to tell me more about what you're feeling."

    C. "Why don't you try something to take your mind off your troubles, like watching a funny movie."

    D. "I might not share your exact situation, but I do know what people go through when they deal with a loss."

2. Which of the following types of stress is being experienced by a middle adult client who is stressed by the concerns of caring for young adults still in the home and her aging parents?

    A. Developmental

    B. Situational

    C. Social

    D. Cultural

3. A home health nurse performs a 3-day postpartum visit for a first-time mother. The household includes her husband, her mother, and her father. Which type of family form is represented here?

    A. Nuclear

    B. Extended

    C. Blended

    D. Alternative

4. Which of the following is the priority nursing intervention for a family with a history of violence?

    A. Educating the family about anger management

    B. Viewing the family in context

    C. Refining the family's communication skills

    D. Using the family's strengths to define them

5. Which of the following approaches should the nurse use when working with a family using an open structure for coping with crisis?

    A. Prescribing tasks unilaterally

    B. Delegating care to one member

    C. Speaking to the primary client privately

    D. Convening a family meeting

6. Which of the following is considered a situational role change?

    A. A toddler learning to control elimination

    B. An adolescent experiencing puberty

    C. A young adult getting married for the first time

    D. A middle adult experiencing menopause

7. Once a nurse has counseled a client about her situational role changes and she has accepted them, what is the next step in her recovery?

    A. Adaptation

    B. Resentment

    C. Tension

    D. Apprehension

CHAPTER 33: COPING

 Application Exercises Answer Key

1. A nurse is caring for a client whose partner passed away 4 months ago and who has been recently diagnosed with diabetes mellitus. He is tearful and states, "How could you possibly understand what I am going through?" Which of the following would be an appropriate response by the nurse?

> A. "It takes time to get over the loss of a loved one."
>
> **B. "You are right; I cannot really understand. Perhaps you'd like to tell me more about what you're feeling."**
>
> C. "Why don't you try something to take your mind off your troubles, like watching a funny movie."
>
> D. "I might not share your exact situation, but I do know what people go through when they deal with a loss."

> **By stating that she is not in his situation, the nurse is using the therapeutic communication technique of validation, whereby she shows sensitivity to the meaning behind his behavior. She is also creating a supportive and nonjudgmental environment, and inviting him to express his frustrations. Telling the client it will take more time to heal belittles the client's feelings and gives false reassurance. Telling the client to try a distraction dismisses the client's feelings and gives common advice instead of expert advice. Saying she knows what clients feel is presumptive and inappropriate.**

> **NCLEX® Connection: Psychosocial Integrity, Therapeutic Communications**

2. Which of the following types of stress is being experienced by a middle adult client who is stressed by the concerns of caring for young adults still in the home and her aging parents?

> **A. Developmental**
>
> B. Situational
>
> C. Social
>
> D. Cultural

> **Developmental stress is related to the stages of life. Situational stress is an unexpected, sudden stressor, such as a job loss. Social and cultural stresses are widespread problems, such as poverty that affect a community as a whole.**

> **NCLEX® Connection: Psychosocial Integrity, Coping Mechanisms**

3. A home health nurse performs a 3-day postpartum visit for a first-time mother. The household includes her husband, her mother, and her father. Which type of family form is represented here?

    A. Nuclear

    B. Extended

    C. Blended

    D. Alternative

This is an extended family because, in addition to the nuclear family unit (husband, wife, and child), grandparents live in the same household. A blended family combines the nuclear unit plus stepchildren. An alternative family can be "skipped" generation households, nonfamilies (single adults living alone), cohabiting partners, or same-gender couples.

 NCLEX® Connection: Psychosocial Integrity, Family Dynamics

4. Which of the following is the priority nursing intervention for a family with a history of violence?

    A. Educating the family about anger management

    B. Viewing the family in context

    C. Refining the family's communication skills

    D. Using the family's strengths to define them

The priority intervention is to collect more data to determine which family member(s) is a victim of abuse and needs assistance to be protected. Teaching anger management is a good strategy, but first there must be a family assessment to determine if there are anger and safety issues. Refining communication skills and using family strengths are not the priorities if the safety of a family member is in jeopardy.

 NCLEX® Connection: Psychosocial Integrity, Family Dynamics

5. Which of the following approaches should the nurse use when working with a family using an open structure for coping with crisis?

    A. Prescribing tasks unilaterally

    B. Delegating care to one member

    C. Speaking to the primary client privately

    D. Convening a family meeting

An open structure is loose, and convening a family meeting would give all family members input and an opportunity to express their feelings. Prescribing tasks and delegating care are too rigid for acceptance by a family with an open structure. Speaking to the primary client privately excludes the family.

 NCLEX® Connection: Psychosocial Integrity, Family Dynamics

6. Which of the following is considered a situational role change?

   A. A toddler learning to control elimination

   B. An adolescent experiencing puberty

   C. A young adult getting married for the first time

   D. A middle adult experiencing menopause

   Marriage adds the role of spouse. Puberty, menopause, and elimination control are expected physiologic growth and development phenomena and are not considered situational role changes.

   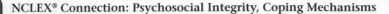 NCLEX® Connection: Psychosocial Integrity, Coping Mechanisms

7. Once a nurse has counseled a client about her situational role changes and she has accepted them, what is the next step in her recovery?

   A. Adaptation

   B. Resentment

   C. Tension

   D. Apprehension

   A client who has accepted role changes will demonstrate adaptation. Resentment, tension, and apprehension are not behaviors or emotions consistent with acceptance.

   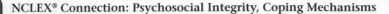 NCLEX® Connection: Psychosocial Integrity, Coping Mechanisms

| UNIT 3 | PSYCHOSOCIAL INTEGRITY |
| Chapter 34 | Self-Concept and Sexuality |

Overview

- Self-concept is the way individuals feel and view themselves. This involves conscious and unconscious thoughts, attitudes, beliefs, and perceptions.

  ○ Body image, a component of self-concept, refers to the way individuals perceive their appearance, size, and body structure/function.

- Sexuality and sexual orientation are integrated into individuals' personalities as well as their general health. Sexuality encompasses their sense of maleness and/or femaleness and their physical and emotional connections with others.

- Individuals' sexuality and sexual health are influenced by self-concept, body image, gender identity, and sexual orientation.

- Nurses should assess their own comfort levels with issues related to sexuality, as clients can usually sense any discomfort nurses have about these issues.

  ○ Some of the skills that nurses use in dealing with clients' sexuality issues are a knowledge of sexual growth and development, and an understanding of how health problems and treatments affect sexuality.

Self-Concept

- Self-concept is subjective and includes self-identity, body image, role performance, and self-esteem.

  ○ Individuals with high self-esteem are better equipped to cope successfully with life's stressors.

  ○ Stressors that affect self-concept include unrealistic expectations, surgery, chronic illness, and changes in role performance.

- Individuals with positive self-concepts tend to feel good about themselves.

- Individuals' self-concepts can be adversely affected by physical, spiritual, emotional, sexual, familial, and sociocultural stressors.

- Body Image

o Body image changes with growth and development. During adolescence, hormonal changes, including the development of secondary sex characteristics, influence body image. Among older adults, changes in mobility, thinning and graying of hair, and decreased visual and hearing acuity are just a few factors that affect body image.

o Stressors that affect body image include a loss of body parts due to an amputation, mastectomy, or hysterectomy; a loss of body function due to arthritis, a spinal cord injury, or a stroke; and an unattainable body ideal.

o External influences (movies, books, magazines) can affect body image.

Sexuality

- Sexuality and sexual health are vital components of general health, and part of a nursing assessment.

- Aspects of sexual health include a knowledge of sexual behavior, an understanding of expected growth and development, and the access to appropriate health care resources for preventing and treating problems related to sexual health.

- Sexuality is affected by one's developmental stage. For example, during adolescence, primary and secondary sex characteristics develop, menarche occurs, relationships involving sexual activity may develop, and masturbation is common.

- Sexuality is influenced by culture. Various cultures view premarital sex, homosexuality, and polygamy differently.

- Sexuality affects health status. Certain conditions may alter sexual expression. For example, the presence of a sexually transmitted disease may cause fear of transmission to a partner, leading to a decrease in sexual desire.

- Some prescription medications affect sexual functioning (Diuretics decrease vaginal lubrication, cause erectile dysfunction, and reduce sexual desire.) Erectile dysfunction can also be caused by antidepressant medications.

Assessment/Data Collection

SUBJECTIVE DATA	OBJECTIVE DATA
• Cultural background • Quality of relationships • Feelings related to recent body image changes, self-concept, or issues of sexuality • Coping mechanisms used in the past • Expectations	• Posture • Appearance • Demeanor • Eye contact • Grooming • Unusual behavior

Collaborative Care

Self-concept	• Suggest a healthier lifestyle (exercise, diet, stress management). • Encourage the client to verbalize fears or anxieties. • Use therapeutic communication skills to assist the client with self-awareness. • Encourage the use of effective coping skills. • Reinforce successes and strengths.
Body image	• Establish a therapeutic relationship with the client. A caring and nonjudgmental manner puts the client at ease and fosters meaningful communication. • Ensure privacy and confidentiality. Let the client know that sensitive issues are safe to discuss. • Identify individuals who may be at risk for body image disturbances. • Acknowledge anger, depression, and denial as feelings to be expected when adjusting to body changes. • Encourage the client to participate in the plan of care. • Arrange for a visit from a volunteer who has experienced a similar body image change.
Sexuality	• Allow the client to discuss issues and concerns related to sexuality. • Be straightforward with questions. ("Are you, or have you been, concerned about sexual functioning since your surgery?") • Health promotion: Determine the client's current knowledge base regarding sexuality and provide education as needed. • Acute care: Increase awareness by introducing or clarifying information, and referring the client for counseling if necessary. • Inform the client of available resources and support groups. • Discuss alternative means of sexual expression if the client experiences a change in body functioning or structure (hugging, cuddling).

CHAPTER 34: SELF-CONCEPT AND SEXUALITY

 Application Exercises

1. A nurse in an ambulatory care clinic is caring for a client who had a mastectomy 6 months ago. The client tells the nurse that she has not had much desire for sexual relations since her surgery, stating, "My body is so different now." Which of the following is an appropriate response by the nurse?

    A. "Really, you look just fine to me. There's no need to feel undesirable."

    B. "I'm interested in finding out more about how your body feels to you."

    C. "Consider an afternoon at a spa. A facial will make you feel more attractive."

    D. "It's still too soon to expect to feel normal. Give it a little more time."

2. Which of the following factors positively affect self-concept? (Select all that apply.)

    _____ Diabetes mellitus

    _____ Parental approval

    _____ Success at school

    _____ Receiving a promotion at work

    _____ Excessive use of alcohol

CHAPTER 34: SELF-CONCEPT AND SEXUALITY

 Application Exercises Answer Key

1. A nurse in an ambulatory care clinic is caring for a client who had a mastectomy 6 months ago. The client tells the nurse that she has not had much desire for sexual relations since her surgery, stating, "My body is so different now." Which of the following is an appropriate response by the nurse?

    A. "Really, you look just fine to me. There's no need to feel undesirable."

    B. "I'm interested in finding out more about how your body feels to you."

    C. "Consider an afternoon at a spa. A facial will make you feel more attractive."

    D. "It's still too soon to expect to feel normal. Give it a little more time."

Showing interest in the client is applying the therapeutic communication technique of offering self; asking more about how the client feels is applying the therapeutic communication technique of encouraging a description of perception. Telling the client she looks fine is using the nontherapeutic communication technique of giving an opinion; assuming she feels undesirable is using the nontherapeutic communication technique of interpreting. Suggesting a facial is using the nontherapeutic communication technique of giving advice. Telling her it is too soon to feel normal and to give it more time is belittling the client's feelings and giving false reassurance.

Ⓝ NCLEX® Connection: Psychosocial Integrity, Coping Mechanisms

2. Which of the following factors positively affect self-concept? (Select all that apply.)

    _____ Diabetes mellitus

    __X__ **Parental approval**

    __X__ **Success at school**

    __X__ **Receiving a promotion at work**

    _____ Excessive use of alcohol

Parental approval, success at school, and receiving a promotion at work all have a positive impact on the individual's self-concept, as these situations promote good feelings about self-concept. A chronic illness usually has a negative impact on self-concept, as the client is required to adapt to the changes. Excessive use of alcohol is a symptom of a poor self-concept.

Ⓝ NCLEX® Connection: Psychosocial Integrity, Coping Mechanisms

| UNIT 3 | PSYCHOSOCIAL INTEGRITY |
| Chapter 35 | Cultural and Spiritual Nursing Care |

Overview

- Clients vary widely in their cultural and spiritual backgrounds and belief systems.

- Nurses must examine their own beliefs before providing optimal cultural and spiritual care to their clients.

Culture

- Culture is a collection of learned, adaptive, and socially and intergenerationally transmitted behaviors, values, beliefs, and customs that form the context from which a group interprets the human experience. Culture includes language, communication style, traditions, religions, art, music, dress, health beliefs, and health practices. These components can be shared by members of an ethnic, racial, social, or religious group.

  o Ethnicity, the bond or kinship people feel with their country of birth or place of ancestral origin, affects culture. Ethnicity exists whether or not a person has ever lived outside the United States.

  o Cultural nursing care involves the delivery of care that transcends cultural boundaries and considers a client's culture as it affects health, illness, and lifestyle. Communication, dietary preferences, and dress are influenced by culture.

  o Within the context of cultural nursing care is terminology that describes how nurses approach clients' culture. Culturally sensitive means that nurses are knowledgeable about the cultures prevalent in their area of practice. Culturally appropriate means that nurses apply their knowledge of a client's culture to their care delivery. Culturally competent means that nurses understand and address the entire cultural context of each client within the realm of the care they deliver.

  o Culture influences health beliefs, health practices, and the manifestations of, responses to, and treatment of illness or injury. Culture evolves over time and is shared by a group who has similar needs and life experiences.

  o Cultural nursing care improves communication, fosters mutual respect, promotes sensitive and effective care, and increases adherence with the treatment plan as clients' and families' needs are met.

  o Many cultures consider the mind-body-spirit to be a single entity; therefore, no distinction is made between physical and mental illness.

- o Differences in language, habits, customs, attitudes, and beliefs can lead to clients' feelings of isolation and loneliness. This is especially true for children who cannot resolve their illness-related grief issues because of cultural barriers, which can lead to posttraumatic stress disorder or depression.

- o A key prerequisite to the delivery of cultural nursing care is the nurses' understanding and awareness of their own culture and any cultural biases that might affect care delivery.

- o Nurses should accommodate each client's cultural beliefs and values whenever possible, unless they are in direct conflict with essential health practices.

- o Barriers to providing cultural nursing care include:

    - Language and communication differences

    - Culturally inappropriate tests and tools that lead to misdiagnosis

    - Ethnic variations in drug metabolism related to genetics

- o When a culturally motivated behavior conflicts with client care, the behavior must be repatterned.

- o Ethnocentrism is the belief that one's culture is superior to others. Ethnocentric ideas interfere with the provision of cultural nursing care.

- o Acculturation occurs when a client is living in a new dominant culture and adopts those patterns of behavior.

- o The predominant culture in the United States is anglicized or English-based, with a general cultural tendency to:

    - Express positive and negative feelings freely

    - Prefer direct eye contact when communicating

    - Address people in a casual manner

    - Prefer a strong handshake as a way of greeting

- o Culture evolves as:

    - Knowledge

    - Values

        □ Values are a set of rules by which individuals in a culture live.

        □ Values guide decision-making and behavior. For example, if health promotion and maintenance are valued, monthly self-breast examinations are done.

        □ Values develop unconsciously during childhood.

    - Beliefs

    - Art

    - Morals and law

    - Customs and habits

- While everyone within a culture shares cultural values, diversity exists, forming subcultures, and is based on:

  - Age

  - Gender

  - Sexual orientation

  - Marital status

  - Family structure

  - Income

  - Education level

  - Religious views

  - Life experiences

Spirituality

- Spirituality can also play an important role in clients' abilities to achieve balance in life, to maintain health, to seek health care, and to deal with illness and injury. Hope, faith, and transcendence are integral components of spirituality.

  - Spiritual distress is a challenge to belief systems or spiritual well being. It often arises as a result of catastrophic events.

  - When faced with health care issues such as acute, chronic, or life-limiting illness, clients often find ways to cope through the use of spiritual practices. Clients who begin to question their belief systems and are unable to find support from those belief systems may experience spiritual distress.

  - Nursing interventions are directed at identification, restoration, and/or reconnection of clients and families to spiritual strength.

  - Spirituality implies connectedness.

    - Intrapersonal – Within one's self

    - Interpersonal – With others and the environment

    - Transpersonal – With an unseen higher power

  - Faith is a belief in something or a relationship with a higher power

    - Faith can be defined by a culture or a religion.

  - Hope is a concept that includes anticipation and optimism and provides comfort during times of crisis.

  - Religion is a system of beliefs practiced outwardly to express one's spirituality.

- Spiritual rituals and observances include:

RELIGION	BIRTH RITUALS AND HEALTH CARE DECISIONS	DIETARY RITUALS	DEATH RITUALS
Hinduism	Those practicing Hinduism do not prolong life.	• Some are vegetarians.	• Clients may want to lie on the floor while dying. • A thread is placed around the neck/wrist. • The family pours water into the mouth. • The family bathes the body. • Clients may want to be cremated.
Buddhism	Buddhists may refuse care on holy days.	• Some are vegetarians. • Those practicing Buddhism avoid alcohol and tobacco. • Clients may fast on holy days.	• Clients may request a priest to deliver last rites. • Chanting is common.
Islam	At birth, a prayer is said into the infant's ear.	• Those practicing Islam avoid alcohol and pork. • Clients may fast during Ramadan.	• Dying clients confess their sins. • The body faces Mecca. • The body is washed and enveloped in a white cloth. • A prayer is said.
Judaism	On the eighth day after birth, males are circumcised.	• Some may practice a Kosher diet.	• Someone stays with the body. • A burial society prepares the body.
Christianity	Some baptize infants at birth.	• Some avoid alcohol, tobacco, and caffeine. • Clients may fast during Lent.	• Some give last rites.

RELIGION	BIRTH RITUALS AND HEALTH CARE DECISIONS	DIETARY RITUALS	DEATH RITUALS
Mormonism	Children are baptized at age 8 by immersion.	• Those practicing Mormonism avoid alcohol, tobacco, and caffeine.	• Last rites are given. • Communion is offered. • Burial is preferred.
Jehovah's Witnesses	Jehovah's Witnesses do not accept blood transfusions.	• Clients avoid foods having or prepared with blood.	• Clients can choose burial or cremation.

Assessment/Data Collection

- To meet a client's cultural needs, a nurse must first perform a cultural assessment to identify those needs.

- Perform the cultural assessment in a language that is common to both nurse and client, or use a facility-approved medical interpreter.

- Inform the interpreter of questions that may be asked, including:

    o What do you call the problem you are having now?

    o When did the problem start?

    o What do you think caused the problem?

    o What does the illness do to you? How does it work?

    o What makes it better or worse?

    o How severe is the illness?

    o What treatments have you tried? How do you think it should be treated?

    o What are the chief problems the illness has caused you?

    o What do you fear most about the illness?

- Assess the client's gestures, vocal tones, and inflections.

DATA TO BE COLLECTED	EXAMPLE
Cultural background and the client's acculturation	The client was born in Central America and has been a resident of New York for 2 years.
Health and wellness beliefs/practices	The client relies on folk medicine to treat or prevent illness.
Family patterns	The client is from a patriarchal culture where the oldest male family member makes decisions for all family members.
Verbal and nonverbal communication	Within the client's culture, it is disrespectful to make direct eye contact.

DATA TO BE COLLECTED	EXAMPLE
Space and time orientation	Within the client's culture, little importance is placed on how past behavior affects future health.
Nutritional patterns	The client believes that some foods have healing properties.
Meaning of pain	Within the client's culture, pain is viewed as a punishment for misbehavior or sin.
Death rituals	Within the client's culture, suicide is acceptable.

- o Nonverbal Behavior
  - ■ Culturally competent nurses must understand how nonverbal behaviors vary among cultures.

NONVERBAL BEHAVIOR	CULTURE	VARIATION
Tone of voice	• Asian	• Many Asians use a soft tone of voice to convey respect.
	• Italian and Middle Eastern	• Many Italian and Middle Eastern individuals use a loud tone of voice.
Eye contact	• American	• Americans use direct eye contact. Lack of direct eye contact implies deception or embarrassment.
	• Middle Eastern	• Middle Eastern individuals usually avoid making direct eye contact with nonrelated members of the opposite gender. Direct eye contact may be seen as rude, hostile, or sexually aggressive.
	• Asian	• Asians may believe that direct eye contact is disrespectful.
	• Native American	• Native Americans may believe that direct eye contact leads to soul loss or soul theft.

NONVERBAL BEHAVIOR	CULTURE	VARIATION
Touch	• American	• Americans may use touch during conversations between intimate partners or family members.
	• Italian and Latin American	• Italian and Latin American individuals may view frequent touch as a sign of concern, interest, and warmth.
Use of space	• Anglo-American/North Europeans (English, Swiss, Scandinavian, German)	• Anglo-American/North Europeans tend to keep their distance during communication except in intimate or family relationships.
	• Italian, French, Spanish, Russian, Latin American, Middle Eastern	• These cultures prefer closer personal contact and less distance between individuals during communication.

- Methods for assessing culture include:
  - Observation
    - Study the client and his environment for examples of cultural relevance.
  - Interview
    - Establish a therapeutic relationship with the client. This may be hindered by misinterpretations of communication.
    - Use focused, open-ended, and nonjudgmental questions.
  - Participation
    - Become involved in culturally related activities outside of the health care setting.
    - Awareness of population demographics includes:
      - Number of members in a practice area
      - Average educational and economic levels
      - Typical occupations
      - Commonly practiced religious spiritual beliefs
      - Prevalence of illnesses/health issues
      - Most commonly held health, wellness, illness, and death beliefs
      - Social organization
- A spiritual assessment includes several components:
  - Primary – Self-reflection (nurses) on personal beliefs and spirituality

- o Initial – Identifying the client's religion, if any
- o Focused – Ongoing, as nurses identify the clients at risk for spiritual distress
- o Spirituality is a highly subjective area requiring the development of rapport and trust among the client, family, and health care provider.
- o Assessment of the client includes:
  - Faith/beliefs
  - Perception of life and self-responsibility
  - Satisfaction with life
  - Culture
  - Fellowship and the client's perceived place in the community
  - Rituals and practices
  - Incorporation of spirituality within profession or work place
  - The client's expectations for health care in relation to spirituality (traditional vs. alternative paths, such as shamans, priests, prayer)

Collaborative Care

- Death Rituals
  - o Death rituals vary among cultures; facilitate such practices whenever possible.
- Pain
  - o Recognize that how clients react to and display pain varies by culture.
  - o Use an alternative to the pain scale (0 to 10), as it may not appropriately reflect pain for all cultures.
  - o Explore religious beliefs that influence the meaning of pain.
- Nutrition
  - o Provide food choices and preparation consistent with cultural beliefs.
  - o As possible, allow clients to consume foods that they view as a treatment for illness.
  - o Communicate ethnicity-related food intolerances/allergies to the dietary staff.
- Communication
  - o Improve nurse-client communication when cultural variations exist.
  - o Use facility-approved interpreters when the communication barrier is significant enough to affect the exchange of information between the nurse and the client.
  - o Use nonverbal communication with caution, as it may have a different meaning for the client than for the nurse.
  - o Apologize if cultural traditions or beliefs are violated.

- Family Patterns and Gender Roles

    o   Communicate with and include the person who has the authority to make decisions in the family.

- Culture and Life Transitions

    o   Assist families as they mark rituals (rites of passage) that symbolize cultural values. Common events expressed with cultural rituals are:

        ■   Puberty.

        ■   Pregnancy.

        ■   Childbirth.

        ■   Dying and death.

- Repatterning

    o   Accommodate clients' cultural beliefs and values as much as possible.

    o   When a cultural value or behavior hinders a client's health and wellness, attempt to repattern that belief to one that is compatible with health promotion.

    o   With knowledge of cultural differences and respect for the client and family, plan and implement appropriate interventions.

- Using an Interpreter

    o   Use only a facility-approved medical interpreter. Do not use the client's family or friends to interpret.

    o   Inform the interpreter about the reason for and the type of questions that will be asked, the expected response (brief or detailed), and with whom to converse.

    o   Allow time for the interpreter and the family to be introduced and become acquainted before starting the interview.

    o   Refrain from making comments about the family to the interpreter, as the family may understand some of the discussion.

    o   Ask one question at a time.

    o   Direct the questions to the family, not to the interpreter.

    o   Use lay terminology if possible, knowing that some words may not have an equivalent word in the client's language.

    o   Do not interrupt the interpreter, the client, or the family as they talk.

    o   Do not try to interpret answers.

    o   Following the interview, ask the interpreter for any additional thoughts about the interview and the client's and family's responses, both verbal and nonverbal.

- Addressing Spirituality

    o   Identify the client's perception of the existence of a higher power.

o   Facilitate growth in the client's abilities to connect with a higher power.

o   Assist the client to feel connected or reconnected to a higher power by:

- Allowing time and/or resources for the practice of religious rituals.

- Providing privacy for prayer, meditation, or the reading of religious materials.

o   Facilitate development of a positive outcome in a particular situation.

o   Provide stability for the person experiencing a dysfunctional spiritual mood.

o   Establish a caring presence in "being with" the client and family rather than merely performing tasks for them.

o   Support all healing relationships:

- Using a holistic approach to care – Seeing the large picture for the client

- Using client-identified spiritual resources and needs

o   Be aware of diet therapies included in spiritual beliefs.

o   Support religious rituals:

- Icons

- Statues

- Prayer rugs

- Devotional readings

- Music

o   Support restorative care:

- Prayer

- Meditation

- Grief work

o   Evaluation of care is ongoing and continuous, with a need for flexibility as the client and family process the current crisis through their spiritual identity.

CHAPTER 35: CULTURAL AND SPIRITUAL NURSING CARE

 Application Exercises

1. Nurses who are knowledgeable about the cultures prevalent in their area of practice are

    A. culturally competent.

    B. culturally congruent.

    C. culturally sensitive.

    D. culturally appropriate.

2. The belief that one's culture is superior to others is called

    A. ethnocentrism.

    B. socialization.

    C. repatterning.

    D. acculturation.

3. Which of the following is appropriate when using an interpreter to communicate with a client and his family? (Select all that apply.)

    _____ Talk to the interpreter about the family while the family is in the room.

    _____ Ask the family one question at a time.

    _____ Look at the interpreter when asking the family questions.

    _____ Use lay terms if possible.

    _____ Do not interrupt the interpreter and the family as they talk.

4. If a nurse and a client share the same religious background, the nurse should recognize that

    A. members of the same religion share similar feelings about their religion.

    B. a shared religious background generates mutual regard for one another.

    C. the same religious beliefs may influence individuals differently.

    D. they should discuss the differences and commonalities in their beliefs.

5. A client is observed crying as he reads from his devotional book. What intervention is appropriate?

    A. Contact the hospital's spiritual services.

    B. Ask him what is making him cry.

    C. Provide quiet times for these moments.

    D. Turn on the television for a distraction.

6. Match the following terms with the descriptions.

_____	Hope	A. Connectedness with a higher power, oneself, others, and the environment
_____	Spiritual distress	B. Multidimensional concept that provides comfort during a crisis
_____	Spirituality	C. A challenge to well-being due to catastrophic events
_____	Religion	D. System of beliefs practiced outwardly to express one's spirituality.

CHAPTER 35: CULTURAL AND SPIRITUAL NURSING CARE

 Application Exercises Answer Key

1. Nurses who are knowledgeable about the cultures prevalent in their area of practice are

   A. culturally competent.

   B. culturally congruent.

   C. culturally sensitive.

   D. culturally appropriate.

   Culturally sensitive means being knowledgeable about cultures prevalent in one's area of practice. Culturally competent means understanding and addressing the entire cultural context of each client within the realm of care delivery. Culturally congruent refers to care that is in synch with the client's values, lifestyle, and meanings. Culturally appropriate applying knowledge of a client's culture to care delivery.

    NCLEX® Connection: Psychosocial Integrity: Cultural Diversity

2. The belief that one's culture is superior to others is called

   A. ethnocentrism.

   B. socialization.

   C. repatterning.

   D. acculturation.

   Ethnocentrism is the belief that one's own culture is superior to others. Socialization refers to a person's upbringing within a culture that results in becoming a practicing member of the culture. Repatterning refers to helping clients shift their beliefs to make them compatible with health promotion. Acculturation refers to the degree to which a client adopts the behaviors of a new dominant culture.

    NCLEX® Connection: Psychosocial Integrity: Cultural Diversity

3. Which of the following is appropriate when using an interpreter to communicate with a client and his family? (Select all that apply.)

   _____ Talk to the interpreter about the family while the family is in the room.

   __X__ **Ask the family one question at a time.**

   _____ Look at the interpreter when asking the family questions.

   __X__ **Use lay terms if possible.**

   __X__ **Do not interrupt the interpreter and the family as they talk.**

   Asking the family one question at a time, using lay terms, and not interrupting will promote communication between the family and the nurse/interpreter. Talking to the interpreter about the family while the family is in the room and looking at the interpreter instead of the family would hinder communication between the family and the nurse/interpreter.

    NCLEX® Connection: Psychosocial Integrity: Cultural Diversity

4. If a nurse and a client share the same religious background, the nurse should recognize that

    A. members of the same religion share similar feelings about their religion.

    B. a shared religious background generates mutual regard for one another.

    C. the same religious beliefs may influence individuals differently.

    D. they should discuss the differences and commonalities in their beliefs.

It would be stereotyping to assume that all members of a specific religion had the same beliefs. Feelings and ideas about religion and spiritual matters may be quite diverse, even within a specific culture. Thus, members of any particular religion should be assessed for individual feelings and ideas. Mutual regard does not necessarily follow a shared religious background. Due to boundary issues, the nurse's beliefs are not part of a therapeutic client relationship; it is the client's beliefs that are important.

(N) NCLEX® Connection: Psychosocial Integrity: Cultural Diversity

5. A client is observed crying as he reads from his devotional book. What intervention is appropriate?

    A. Contact the hospital's spiritual services.

    B. Ask him what is making him cry.

    C. Provide quiet times for these moments.

    D. Turn on the television for a distraction.

Providing privacy and time for the reading of religious materials supports the client's spiritual health. Contacting the hospital's spiritual services presumes there is a problem. Asking the client about the crying or providing a distraction could be interpreted as discounting or being disrespectful of the client's beliefs.

(N) NCLEX® Connection: Psychosocial Integrity: Cultural Diversity

6. Match the following terms with the descriptions.

B	Hope	A.	Connectedness with a higher power, oneself, others, and the environment
C	Spiritual distress	B.	Multidimensional concept that provides comfort during a crisis
A	Spirituality	C.	A challenge to well-being due to catastrophic events
D	Religion	D.	System of beliefs practiced outwardly to express one's spirituality.

(N) NCLEX® Connection: Psychosocial Integrity: Cultural Diversity

UNIT 3	PSYCHOSOCIAL INTEGRITY
Chapter 36	Grief, Loss, and Palliative Care

Overview

- Clients experience loss in many aspects of their lives.

- Grief is the inner emotional response to loss and is exhibited in as many ways as there are individuals.

- Bereavement includes both grief and mourning (the outward display of loss) as the individual deals with the death of a significant individual in his life.

- Palliative or end-of-life care is an important aspect of nursing care and attempts to meet the client's physical and psychosocial needs.

- End-of-life issues include decision making in a highly stressful time during which the nurse must consider the desires of the client and the family. Any decisions must be shared with other health care personnel for a smooth transition during this time of stress, grief, and bereavement.

- Advance directives – Legal documents that direct end-of-life issues

   ○ Living wills – Directive documents for medical treatment per client's wishes.

   ○ Durable power of attorney for health care – A document that appoints someone to make medical decisions when the client is no longer able to do so on his own behalf.

Types of Loss

TYPE OF LOSS	DEFINITION
Necessary loss	This is part of the cycle of life that is anticipated but still may be intensely felt. This type of loss can be replaced by something different or better.
Actual loss	This is any loss of a valued person or item.
Perceived loss	This is any loss defined by the client that is not obvious to others.
Maturational loss	This is any loss normally expected due to the developmental processing of life. These are associated with normal life transitions and help to develop coping skills.
Situational loss	This is any unanticipated loss caused by an external event.

Theories of Grief

- Kübler-Ross: Five Stages of Grief

  o Denial – The client has difficulty believing a terminal diagnosis or loss.

  o Anger – The client lashes out at other people or things.

  o Bargaining – The client negotiates for more time or a cure.

  o Depression – The client is saddened over the inability to change the situation.

  o Acceptance – The client recognizes what is happening and plans for the future.

  o Stages may not be experienced in order, and the length of each stage varies from person to person.

- Worden: Four Tasks of Mourning

  o Task I: Accepting the inevitability of the loss

  o Task II: Using coping mechanisms to experience the emotional pain of the loss

  o Task III: Changing the environment to accommodate the absence of the deceased

  o Task IV: Readjusting emotional ties to new individuals and moving thoughts about the deceased to a less prominent place in everyday thoughts

  o To complete all four tasks, it should take about a year, but may vary.

Factors Influencing Loss, Grief, and Coping Ability

- The individual's current stage of development

- Interpersonal relationships and social support networks

- Type and significance of the loss

- Culture and ethnicity

- Spiritual and religious beliefs and practices

- Prior experience with loss

- Socioeconomic status

- Factors that may increase an individual's risk for dysfunctional grieving include:

  o Having a great deal of dependence on the deceased

  o The deceased dying unexpectedly at a young age, through violence, or by a socially unacceptable manner

  o Inadequate coping skills or lack of social supports

  o Lack of hope or pre-existing mental health issues, such as depression or substance abuse

Assessment

TYPES OF GRIEF	MANIFESTATIONS
Normal grief	• This grief is considered uncomplicated. • Emotions may be negative, such as anger, resentment, withdrawal, hopelessness, and guilt but should change to acceptance with time. • Some acceptance should be evident by 6 months after the loss. • Somatic complaints may include chest pain, palpitations, headaches, nausea, changes in sleep patterns, and fatigue.
Anticipatory grief	• This grief implies the "letting go" of an object or person before the loss, as in a terminal illness. • Individuals have the opportunity to grieve before the actual loss.
Dysfunctional grief (unresolved or chronic grief is a type of complicated grief)	• This grief involves difficult progression through the expected stages of grief. • Usually, the work of grief is prolonged, the symptoms of grief are more severe, and they may result in depression or exacerbate a pre-existing disorder. • The client may develop suicidal ideation, intense feelings of guilt, and lowered self-esteem. • Somatic complaints persist for an extended period of time.
Disenfranchised grief	• This grief entails an experienced loss that cannot be publicly shared or is not socially acceptable, such as suicide.

Nursing Interventions

- Facilitate Mourning

  o Grant time for the grieving process.

  o Identify expected grieving behaviors, such as crying, somatic symptoms, and anxiety.

  o Use therapeutic communication. Name the emotion the client is feeling. For example, say, "You sound as though you are angry. Anger is a normal feeling for someone who has lost a loved one. Tell me about how you are feeling."

  o Avoid communication that inhibits the open expression of feelings, such as offering false reassurance, giving advice, changing the subject, and taking the focus away from the grieving individual.

  o Assist the grieving individual to accept the reality of the loss.

  o Support efforts to "move on" in the face of the loss.

  o Encourage the building of new relationships.

  o Provide continuing support; encourage the support of family and friends.

  o Assess for signs of ineffective coping, such as refusing to leave the home months after the client's spouse has died.

- o   Share information about mourning and grieving with the client, who may not realize that her feelings, such as anger toward the deceased, are expected.

- o   Encourage attendance at bereavement or grief support groups. Provide information about available community resources.

- o   Initiate referrals for individual psychotherapy for clients who are having difficulty resolving grief.

- o   Ask the client if contacting a spiritual advisor would be acceptable or encourage the client to do so.

- o   Participate in debriefing provided by professional grief/mental health counselors.

Client Outcomes

- The client verbalizes needs to health care provider.

- The client progresses through the stages of grief in a timely manner.

PALLIATIVE CARE

- The nurse serves as an advocate for the client's sense of dignity and self-esteem by providing palliative care at the end of life.

- Palliative care improves the quality of life of clients and their families facing end-of-life issues.

- Palliative care interventions are primarily used when caring for clients who are dying and family members who are grieving.

- Palliative care may be provided by an interdisciplinary team of:

  - o   Physicians

  - o   Nurses

  - o   Social workers

  - o   Massage therapists

  - o   Occupational therapists

  - o   Music/art therapists

  - o   Touch/energy therapists

- Hospice care is a comprehensive care delivery system implemented when a client is not expected to live longer than 6 months. Further medical care aimed towards cure is stopped, and the focus becomes symptom relief and enhances quality of life.

Assessment/Data Collection

CHARACTERISTICS OF DISCOMFORT	SIGNS AND SYMPTOMS OF APPROACHING DEATH
<ul><li>Pain</li><li>Anxiety</li><li>Dyspnea</li><li>Nausea or vomiting</li><li>Dehydration</li><li>Diarrhea or constipation</li><li>Urinary incontinence</li><li>Inability to perform ADLs</li></ul>	<ul><li>Decreased level of consciousness</li><li>Muscle relaxation</li><li>Labored breathing (dyspnea, apnea, Cheyne-Stokes respirations)</li><li>Mucus collecting in large airways</li><li>Incontinence of bowel and/or bladder</li><li>Mottling occurring with poor circulation</li><li>Pupils no longer reactive to light</li><li>Pulse weakening and blood pressure dropping</li><li>Cool extremities</li><li>Perspiration</li><li>Decreased urine output</li><li>Inability to swallow</li></ul>

- Determine the client's sources of strength and hope.

- Identify the desires and expectations of the family and the client for end-of-life care.

Nursing Interventions

- Promote continuity of care and communication by limiting assigned staff changes.

- Assist the client and family to set priorities for end-of-life care.

- Physical Care

  o Give priority to controlling symptoms.

  o Administer medications that manage pain, air hunger, and anxiety.

  o Perform ongoing assessment to determine the effectiveness of treatment and the need for modifications of the treatment plan, such as lower or higher doses of medications.

  o Manage adverse/side effects of medications.

  o Reposition the client to maintain airway patency and comfort.

  o Maintain the integrity of skin and mucous membranes.

  o Provide an environment that promotes dignity and self-esteem.

    ▪ Remove products of elimination as soon as possible to maintain a clean and odor-free environment

    ▪ Offer comfortable clothing

- Provide careful grooming for hair, nails, and skin
- Encourage family members to bring in comforting possessions to make the client feel at home.

o Encourage the use of relaxation techniques, such as guided imagery and music.

o Promote decision making in food selection, activities, and health care to give the client as much control as possible.

o Encourage the client to perform ADLs as able and willing to do so.

- Psychosocial Care

  o Use an interdisciplinary approach.

  o Provide care to the client and family.

  o Use volunteers when appropriate to provide nonmedical care.

  o Use therapeutic communication to develop and maintain a nurse-client relationship.

  o Facilitate the understanding of information regarding disease progression and treatment choices.

  o Facilitate communication between the client, the family, and the provider.

  o Encourage the client to participate in religious practices that bring comfort and strength, if appropriate.

  o Assist the client in clarifying personal values in order to facilitate effective decision making.

  o Encourage the client to use coping mechanisms that have worked in the past.

  o Be sensitive to comments made in the presence of clients who are unconscious, as hearing is the last sensation lost.

- Prevention of Abandonment and Isolation

  o Prevent the fear of dying alone.

    - Make your presence known by answering call lights in a timely manner, making frequent contact.

    - Keep the client informed of procedure and assessment times.

    - Allow family members to stay overnight.

    - Determine where the client is most comfortable, such as in a room close to the nurses' station.

- Support for the Grieving Family

  o Suggest that family members plan visits to promote the client's rest.

  o Ensure that the family receives appropriate information as the treatment plan changes.

  o Provide privacy so family members have the opportunity to communicate and express feelings among themselves without including the client.

o   Determine family members' desire to provide physical care. Provide instruction as necessary.

o   Educate the family about physical changes to expect as the client moves closer to death.

Client Outcomes

- The client verbalizes pain and discomfort, and they are controlled.

- Client rests comfortably and shows minimal signs of distress.

- Client participates in care to his greatest ability.

POSTMORTEM CARE

- Nurses are responsible for following federal and state laws regarding requests for organ or tissues donation, obtaining permission for autopsy, ensuring the certification and appropriate documentation of the death, and providing postmortem (after-death) care.

 View Media Supplement: Postmortem Care (Video)

- The client's family now becomes the nurse's primary focus.

Nursing Interventions

- Care of the Body

    o   Provide care with respect and compassion while attending to the desires of the client and family per their cultural, religious, and social practices.

    o   Recognize that the provider certifies death by pronouncing the time and documenting therapies used, and actions taken prior to the death.

    o   Preparing the body for viewing includes:

        ▪   Maintaining privacy.

        ▪   Shaving facial hair if applicable and/or desired by the family.

        ▪   Removing all tubes and soiled linens (unless organs are to be donated or this is a medical examiner's case).

        ▪   Removing all personal belongings to be given to the family.

        ▪   Cleansing and aligning the body with a pillow under the head, arms outside the sheet and blanket, dentures in place, and eyes closed.

        ▪   Applying fresh linens and a gown.

        ▪   Brushing/combing the client's hair, replacing any hair pieces.

- Removing excess equipment and linens from the room.
- Dimming the lights and minimizing noise to provide a calm environment.
  - Viewing considerations include:
    - Asking the family if they would like to visit with the body, honoring any decision.
    - Clarifying where the client's personal belongings should go – With the body or to a designated person.
    - Adhering to the same procedures when the client is an infant, with the exception of:
      - Swaddling the infant's body in a clean blanket.
      - Transporting the infant in the nurse's arms or in an infant carrier.
      - Offering mementos of the infant (identification bracelets, footprints, the cord clamp, a lock of hair, photos).
  - Post Viewing
    - Apply identification tags according to facility policy.
    - Complete documentation.
    - Remain aware of visitor and staff sensibilities during transport.

- Organ Donation
  - Recognize that requests for tissue and organ donations must be made by specially trained personnel.
  - Provide support and education to family members as decisions are being made. Use private areas for any family discussions concerning donation.
  - Be sensitive to cultural and religious influences.
  - Maintain ventilatory and cardiovascular support for vital organ retrieval.

- Autopsy Considerations
  - The provider typically approaches the family about performing an autopsy.
  - The nurse's role is to answer the family's questions and support its choices.
  - Autopsies can be conducted to advance scientific knowledge regarding disease processes, which can lead to the development of new therapies.
  - The law may require an autopsy to be performed if the death is due to homicide, suicide, or accidental death, or if death occurs within 24 hr of hospital admission.
  - Most facilities require that all tubes remain in place for an autopsy.

- Cultural/Religious Beliefs
  - Identify cultural/religious beliefs of family members.
  - Be sensitive to these practices when providing postmortem care.

- Documentation and completion of forms following federal and state laws typically includes:
  - Who pronounced the death and at what time
  - Consideration of and preparation for organ donation
  - Disposition of personal articles
  - Who was notified and any decisions made
  - The location of identification tags
  - The time the body left the facility and the destination
- Care of Nurses who are Grieving
  - Caring long-term for clients can create personal attachments for nurses.
  - Nurses can use coping strategies such as:
    - Going to the client's funeral.
    - Communicating in writing to the family.
    - Attending debriefing sessions with colleagues.
    - Using stress management techniques.
    - Talking with a professional counselor.

CHAPTER 36: GRIEF, LOSS, AND PALLIATIVE CARE

 Application Exercises

1. In which stage of grief, per Kübler-Ross, is a client who is terminally ill displaying when she states that she is going to a clinic for acupuncture?

    A. Anger

    B. Depression

    C. Bargaining

    D. Acceptance

2. A client is diagnosed with terminal cancer. The nurse observes the client's family assisting with all ADLs. Which of the following rationales for self-care should the nurse communicate to the family?

    A. Allowing the client to function independently will strengthen her muscles and promote healing.

    B. The client needs to be given privacy at times for self-reflecting and organizing her life.

    C. Her sense of loss can be lessened through retaining control of certain areas of her life.

    D. Performing ADLs is required prior to discharge from an acute care facility.

3. Which of the following is a sign of impending death?

    A. Elevated blood pressure

    B. Warm extremities

    C. Tense muscles

    D. Labored breathing

Scenario: A nurse is present when a long-term resident at an assisted living facility dies at the age of 95. The client's partner also lives in the facility. The nurse has provided care for both clients for the past 5 years.

---

4. How should the nurse proceed with the client's remains?

5. What considerations should be made for the partner and other family members of the deceased?

CHAPTER 36: GRIEF, LOSS, AND PALLIATIVE CARE

 Application Exercises Answer Key

1. In which stage of grief, per Kübler-Ross, is a client who is terminally ill displaying when she states that she is going to a clinic for acupuncture?

    A. Anger

    B. Depression

    C. Bargaining

    D. Acceptance

A client who tries alternative treatments is attempting to negotiate a way to lengthen life or find cures. Lashing out at people or things occurs during the anger stage. Being withdrawn and sad occurs during the depression stage. Recognizing the end is near with thoughts for the future occurs during the acceptance stage.

 NCLEX® Connection: Psychosocial Integrity: Grief and Loss

2. A client is diagnosed with terminal cancer. The nurse observes the client's family assisting with all ADLs. Which of the following rationales for self-care should the nurse communicate to the family?

    A. Allowing the client to function independently will strengthen her muscles and promote healing.

    B. The client needs to be given privacy at times for self-reflecting and organizing her life.

    C. Her sense of loss can be lessened through retaining control of certain areas of her life.

    D. Performing ADLs is required prior to discharge from an acute care facility.

Allowing the client as much control as possible maintains dignity and self-esteem. The strengthening of muscles is not a priority of palliative care. Privacy for times of self-reflection can be achieved at times apart from performance of ADLs. Performance of ADLs is not a criterion for discharge from an acute care facility.

 NCLEX® Connection: Psychosocial Integrity: End-of-Life Care

3. Which of the following is a sign of impending death?

    A. Elevated blood pressure

    B. Warm extremities

    C. Tense muscles

    D. Labored breathing

Labored breathing, such as dyspnea, apnea, and Cheyne-Stokes respirations, are common when a client approaches death.

 NCLEX® Connection: Psychosocial Integrity: End-of-Life Care

Scenario: A nurse is present when a long-term resident at an assisted living facility dies at the age of 95. The client's partner also lives in the facility. The nurse has provided care for both clients for the past 5 years.

4. How should the nurse proceed with the client's remains?

> **Have a provider certify death. Assess and implement any cultural considerations for postmortem care. The nurse can delegate the cleansing of the body and immediate environment to assistive personnel (AP). The body is made ready for viewing after giving the partner the option of private time with the deceased client. Wash the body, keeping parts not being washed covered to respect personal dignity. If desired by the partner, shave the face. Replace linens with fresh sheets. Position the body per the facility's protocol. Pull the top sheet and blanket up to the client's chin, placing the arms outside the sheet or per the facility's protocol. Remove soiled linens, trash, and any medical equipment from the room.**

 NCLEX® Connection: Psychosocial Integrity: End-of-Life Care

5. What considerations should be made for the partner and other family members of the deceased?

> **Assess their desires for viewing and at what times. Allow family members to have as much time with the deceased as they need. Determine their wishes for processing the remains (funeral arrangements, cremation). Grant the family access to telephones and paperwork to make final arrangements.**

 NCLEX® Connection: Psychosocial Integrity: Grief and Loss

UNIT 4: PHYSIOLOGICAL INTEGRITY
Section: Basic Care and Comfort

- Hygiene
- Rest and Sleep
- Nutrition and Oral Hydration
- Mobility and Immobility
- Pain Management
- Complementary and Alternative Therapies
- Bowel Elimination
- Urinary Elimination
- Sensory Perception

NCLEX® CONNECTIONS

When reviewing the chapters in this section, keep in mind the relevant sections of the NCLEX® outline, in particular:

CLIENT NEEDS: BASIC CARE AND COMFORT

Relevant topics/tasks include:
- Assistive Devices
  - Assess the client's use of assistive devices.
- Elimination
  - Provide skin care to clients who are incontinent.
- Mobility/Immobility
  - Apply knowledge of nursing procedures and psychomotor skills when providing care to clients with immobility.
- Nutrition and Oral Hydration
  - Calculate the client's intake and output.
- Personal Hygiene
  - Assess the client for personal hygiene habits/routine.
- Rest and Sleep
  - Schedule client care activities to promote adequate rest.

UNIT 4	PHYSIOLOGICAL INTEGRITY
Section	Basic Care and Comfort
Chapter 37	Hygiene

Overview

- Personal hygiene needs vary with clients' health status, social and cultural practices, and the daily routines they follow at home. For most clients, personal hygiene includes:

  o Bathing

  o Oral care

  o Nail and foot care

  o Perineal care

  o Hair care

  o Shaving (for men)

- Because personal hygiene has a profound impact on overall health, comfort, and well-being, it is an integral component of individualized nursing care plans.

- When clients become ill, have surgery, or are injured and are unable to manage their own personal hygiene needs, it becomes the nurse's responsibility to meet those needs.

- Before beginning any personal care delivery, it is important to assess each client's ability to participate in personal hygiene. Encourage clients to participate in any way they can.

Hygiene Care

- Bathing

  o Bathe clients to cleanse the body, relax it, and enhance healing.

  o Perform a skin assessment and wound care at this time.

  o Bathe clients whose diseases and/or disabilities have exhausted them or limited their mobility.

    ▪ Complete baths are given when the client is able to tolerate it, and the client's hygiene needs warrant it.

    ▪ Partial baths are useful when the client needs cleansing of odorous or uncomfortable areas, or he can perform part of the bath independently.

- Proper oral hygiene helps decrease the risk of infection for clients living in long-term care facilities, especially form the transmission of pathogens that can cause pneumonia.

- Foot care is given to prevent skin breakdown, pain, and infection. Foot care is extremely important for clients who have diabetes mellitus and must be done by a qualified professional.

- Perineal care helps maintain skin integrity, relieve discomfort, and prevent transmission of micro-organisms (catheter care).

- Cultural and Social Practices

  o Clients vary in their hygiene preferences and practices. These include bathing routines, oral care, grooming preferences, and health beliefs. Culture also plays an important role, because some cultures have unique hygiene practices. Be sure to be respectful and observant of each client's specific cultural needs.

  o Socioeconomic status may affect clients' hygiene status. If a client is homeless, discharge instructions and follow-up care must be altered accordingly.

  o Respect each client's dignity. Many clients are dealing with a loss of control when others must provide their hygiene care. Reassuring clients and allowing them to have as much control as possible may help.

- Safety

  o Before starting any care, understand how to complete each task to avoid injuring the client. This includes knowing the equipment and what the proper techniques are for each hygiene procedure.

  o Never leave the client in a position where injury could occur during routine hygiene care. For example, avoid leaving a client who is at risk for aspiration alone with oral hygiene supplies.

- Special Considerations for Older Adult Clients

  o Older adults' skin is drier and thinner and may not tolerate as much bathing as younger adults' skin.

  o Older adults have higher incidences of infection and periodontal disease because of the weakening of the periodontal membrane.

  o Dentures must be fitted correctly, or they can cause digestive issues, pain, and discomfort. Dentures are a client's personal property. Never leave them on a meal tray or in a place where they could be damaged or lost.

  o Dry mouth is common in older adults due to decreased saliva production and medications this population commonly uses (antihypertensives, diuretics, anti-inflammatory agents, antidepressants).

  o Poor nutritional status is often due to dental problems, socioeconomic status, or a limited ability to prepare healthful foods.

Assessment/Data Collection

- Assess the client's skin for color, hydration, texture, turgor, and the presence of any lesions or other impaired integrity.

- Check the condition of the client's gums and teeth for dryness or inflammation of the oral mucosa. Does the client report any pain?

- Assess the client's skin surfaces including the feet and nails, and note the shape and size of each foot, any lesions, and areas of dryness or inflammation. Significant alterations may indicate neuropathy and/or vascular insufficiency. Are all pulses palpable and equal bilaterally?

- Identify the client's hygiene preferences to understand how the client performs hygiene at home and what additional education and care to provide.

- Assess the client for safety issues (altered positioning, decreased mobility) and the ability to participate in self-care.

Nursing Interventions

- To give a client a bed bath:

  o Collect equipment, provide for privacy, and explain the procedure to the client.

  o Apply gloves.

  o Lock the wheels on the bed.

  o Place a bath blanket over the client and remove the client's gown.

  o Obtain bath water.

  o Wash the client's face first. Allow the client to perform this task if able.

  o Perform the bath systematically by starting with the client's upper body and continuing on to the lower extremities. Keep cleaned areas covered with a blanket or towel. Change water as indicated, using fresh water to perform perineal care.

    ■ Perineal Care

      □ It is important to maintain skin integrity to relieve discomfort and prevent transmission of infection (catheter care).

      □ Principles of perineal care include:

        ▸ Providing privacy.

        ▸ Maintaining a professional demeanor.

        ▸ Removing any fecal material from the skin.

        ▸ Cleansing the client from front to back.

        ▸ Drying thoroughly.

        ▸ Retracting the foreskin of male clients to wash the tip of the penis then replacing the foreskin.

- Foot Care

  - It is important to prevent any infection or pain that may interfere with the client's gait. This care is extremely important for clients who have diabetes mellitus, and it must be done by a qualified professional.

  - Instruct the client at risk for injury to:

    - Inspect the feet daily, paying special attention to the area between the toes.

    - Use lukewarm water and dry the feet thoroughly.

    - Apply moisturizer to the feet but avoid applying it between the toes.

    - Avoid over-the-counter products that contain alcohol or other strong chemicals.

    - Wear clean cotton socks daily.

    - Check shoes for any objects, rough seams, or edges that may cause injury.

    - Cut the nails straight across and use an emery board to file nail edges.

    - Avoid self-treating corns or calluses.

    - Buy and wear comfortable shoes that do not restrict circulation.

    - Do not apply heat unless prescribed.

    - Contact the provider if any signs of infection or inflammation appear.

  - Apply lotion and powder (if neither is contraindicated), and a clean gown.

  - Document skin assessment, type of bath, and the client's response.

  - To change linens on an occupied bed:

    - Roll the bottom linens up in the bottom sheet or mattress pad under the client who is turned on his side, facing the opposite direction.

    - Apply clean bottom linens to the bed, and extend them to the middle of the bed with the remainder of the linen fan folded underneath the client.

    - Have the client roll over the linens and face the opposite direction, then remove the used linens and apply the clean linens.

    - Apply the upper sheet and blanket.

    - To remove the pillowcase, insert one hand into the opening, grab the pillow, and turn the pillowcase inside out.

    - Apply the clean pillowcase by grasping the center of the closed end, turning the case inside out, fitting the pillow into the corner of the case, and pulling the case until it is right side out over the pillow.

- Oral Hygiene

  - Clients who have fragile oral mucosa require gentle brushing and flossing.

  - Perform denture care for clients who are unable to do so themselves.

- Remove the dentures with a gloved hand, pulling down and out at the front of the upper denture, and lifting up and out at the front of the lower denture.

- Place the dentures in a denture cup or emesis basin.

- Brush them with a soft brush and denture cleaner.

- Rinse them in water.

- Store the dentures, or help the client reinsert the dentures.

- Nail Care

  o Assess the size, shape, and condition of the client's nails and nail beds.

  o Assess for cracking, clubbing, and fungus.

  o Before cutting any client's nails, check the facility's/agency's policy; some require an order from the client's provider while others allow only a podiatrist or other qualified professional to cut some or all clients' nails.

  o Foot and nail care will vary from the standard when you care for a client who has diabetes mellitus. Do not soak the feet due to the risk of infection and do not cut the nails. Instead, file them using a nail file. Do not apply lotion between the fingers or toes since the moisture can cause skin irritation and breakdown.

- Hair Care

  o Caring for the hair and scalp is important for the client's appearance and sense of well-being, and is an essential component of personal hygiene.

  o Brush or comb the client's hair daily to remove tangles, massage the scalp, stimulate circulation to the scalp, and distribute natural oils along the shaft of the hair. Use a soft-bristled brush to prevent injury or trauma to the scalp and a wide-toothed comb or hair pick to comb through tightly curled hair.

  o If the client cannot shower but can sit in a chair and lean back, shampoo the hair at the sink. For clients on bed rest, use a plastic shampoo trough. Dry or no-rinse shampoos and shampoo caps are also options for clients on bed rest.

  o Start shampooing the client's hair at the hairline and work toward the neck. To wash the hair on the back of the client's head, gently lift the head with one hand and shampoo with the other.

  o Place a folded or rolled towel behind the client's neck to pad the edge of the sink. Then rinse, comb, and dry the client's hair.

- Shaving

  o Safety is important. Clients prone to bleeding or receiving anticoagulants should use an electric razor.

  o Apply soap or shaving cream to warm, moist skin.

  o Move the razor over the skin in the direction of hair growth using long strokes on large areas of the face and short strokes around the chin and lips.

  o Be sure to communicate with the client about personal shaving preferences.

CHAPTER 37: HYGIENE

 Application Exercises

1. A nurse is caring for a client who has been transferred from a long-term care facility to an acute care setting. An indwelling urinary catheter was inserted just prior to her transfer. Which of the following tasks will help prevent the development of a nosocomial infection?

    A. Assessing the client's ability to void independently

    B. Placing an absorbent pad under the client to protect the bed in case of incontinence

    C. Frequently cleaning the client's perineal area and properly caring for her catheter

    D. Giving the client a diet high in fiber to prevent constipation

2. Which of the following are appropriate teaching measures related to care of the feet for a client who has diabetes mellitus? (Select all that apply.)

    _____ Inspect the feet daily.

    _____ Use moisturizing lotions on the feet.

    _____ Wash the feet with warm water and let them air dry.

    _____ Use over-the-counter products to treat abrasions.

    _____ Check shoes for any foreign objects.

3. A client experiences dyspnea and reports feeling tired after completing her morning care. Which of the following should the nurse include in the client's plan of care for the next day?

    A. Plan for several rest periods during morning care.

    B. Do not offer any morning care.

    C. Perform all of the client's care as quickly as possible.

    D. Ask a family member to come in to give the client a bath.

CHAPTER 37: HYGIENE

 Application Exercises Answer Key

1. A nurse is caring for a client who has been transferred from a long-term care facility to an acute care setting. An indwelling urinary catheter was inserted just prior to her transfer. Which of the following tasks will help prevent the development of a nosocomial infection?

> A. Assessing the client's ability to void independently
>
> B. Placing an absorbent pad under the client to protect the bed in case of incontinence
>
> **C. Frequently cleaning the client's perineal area and properly caring for her catheter**
>
> D. Giving the client a diet high in fiber to prevent constipation

> **Most nosocomial infections develop in the urinary tract, and regular cleaning of the perineal area along with catheter care reduces the number of micro-organisms. Assessing the client's ability to void independently, placing an absorbent pad under the client, and giving the client a diet high in fiber will not prevent a nosocomial infection.**

 NCLEX® Connection: Basic Care and Comfort: Personal Hygiene

2. Which of the following are appropriate teaching measures related to care of the feet for a client who has diabetes mellitus? (Select all that apply.)

> __X__ **Inspect the feet daily.**
>
> __X__ **Use moisturizing lotions on the feet.**
>
> _____ Wash the feet with warm water and let them air dry.
>
> _____ Use over-the-counter products to treat abrasions.
>
> __X__ **Check shoes for any foreign objects.**

> **A client who has diabetes mellitus is at increased risk for infection and should inspect the feet daily. The client should also use moisturizing lotions (but not between the toes) to help keep the skin smooth and supple. Shoes should be checked for foreign objects because decreased sensation may prevent the client from feeling an object or a rough area of the shoe that can cause an injury. The feet should be washed with warm water and dried thoroughly. Over-the-counter products often contain harmful chemicals that can cause skin impairment.**

NCLEX® Connection: Basic Care and Comfort: Personal Hygiene

3. A client experiences dyspnea and reports feeling tired after completing her morning care. Which of the following should the nurse include in the client's plan of care for the next day?

 A. Plan for several rest periods during morning care.

 B. Do not offer any morning care.

 C. Perform all of the client's care as quickly as possible.

 D. Ask a family member to come in to give the client a bath.

 Planning for several rest periods during morning care will help prevent fatigue and continue to foster independence. Fatigue and dyspnea are not reasons to eliminate morning care. Performing all of the client's care or having a family member do it will reduce the client's independence.

(N) NCLEX® Connection: Basic Care and Comfort: Personal Hygiene

UNIT 4	PHYSIOLOGICAL INTEGRITY
Section	Basic Care and Comfort
Chapter 38	**Rest and Sleep**

Overview

- Adequate amounts of sleep and rest are important for maintaining good health. People who do not get adequate sleep often experience a number of problems, including the inability to concentrate, poor judgment, moodiness, and an increased risk for accidents.

- Chronic sleep loss can increase the risk of obesity, depression, hypertension, diabetes, heart attack, and stroke.

- Nursing interventions are used to promote sleep for clients who experience sleep loss due to short term factors such as illness, pain, and hospitalization, and for clients who have chronic sleep problems.

Sleep Cycle

- The sleep cycle consists of nonrapid eye movement (NREM) sleep and rapid eye movement (REM) sleep. Typically, after a person experiences Stage 1 of NREM sleep, he cycles four to six times through the other stages of sleep during the course of a night. With each cycle, the length of time the person spends in REM sleep increases. NREM accounts for 75% to 80% of sleep time.

STAGE	CHARACTERISTICS
Stage 1 NREM	- Very light sleep - Only a few minutes long - Vital signs and metabolism beginning to diminish - Can be awakened easily - Feels relaxed and drowsy
Stage 2 NREM	- Deeper sleep - 10 to 20 min in length - Vital signs and metabolism continuing to diminish - Requires slightly more stimulation to be awakened - Increased relaxation

STAGE	CHARACTERISTICS
Stage 3 NREM	• Deep sleep • 15 to 30 min in length • Vital signs continuing to decrease • Difficult to awaken • Relaxation such that the person seldom moves
Stage 4 NREM	• Called delta sleep • Deepest sleep • 15 to 30 min in length • Vital signs very low as compared to when awake • Very difficult to awaken • Stage at which the body achieves physical rest and restoration • Stage at which enuresis and talking and walking in one's sleep occur • Repair and renewal of tissue
REM	• Occurrence of dreams • Usually begins about 90 min after falling asleep • Length increases with each sleep cycle • Average length is 20 minutes • Varying vital signs • Very difficult to awaken • Stage at which mental rest and restoration occur

Normal Developmental Sleep Patterns

AGE	SLEEP AVERAGES PER 24 HR
Birth to 3 months	16 hr a day
Infants (3 months to 1 year)	8 to 10 hr plus with two to three naps
Toddlers	12 hr with some sleep during a daytime nap
Preschoolers	12 hr with less napping during the day
School-age	11 to 12 hr for younger children with 9 to 10 hr for older ones
Adolescents	7.5 hr
Young Adults	6 to 8.5 hr
Middle Adults	6 to 8.5 hr
Older Adults	6 to 8.5 with daytime naps possibly accounting for some of the hours

- Common Sleep Disorders

  - Insomnia, the most common sleep disorder, is defined as the inability to get an adequate amount of sleep and to feel rested. The person may have difficulty falling asleep, have difficulty staying asleep, awaken too early, or not get refreshing sleep. Acute insomnia lasts for only a few days and may be due to personal stressors. Chronic insomnia lasts a month or more. Some people experience intermittent insomnia, where they are able to sleep well for a few days and then experience insomnia for a few days. Women and older adults are more likely to experience insomnia.

  - Sleep apnea is a disorder in which there are more than five apneic occurrences lasting longer than 10 seconds/hr during sleep, resulting in decreased arterial oxygen saturation levels. Sleep apnea is caused by a single disorder or a mixture of the following:

    - Central – central nervous system dysfunction that fails to trigger breathing during sleep.

    - Obstructive – occurs when the upper airway becomes occluded by relaxed structures in the mouth and throat.

  - Narcolepsy – a disorder of the sleep and wake mechanism. The person may lose the ability to stay awake. It often happens at inappropriate times and can put the person at risk for injury.

Assessment/Data Collection

- Ask the client about sleep patterns, history, and if any changes have occurred.

- Ask the client about sleep problems, which include:

  - Type of problem.

  - Symptoms.

  - Timing.

  - Seriousness.

  - Related factors.

  - How the lack of sleep has affected the client.

- Use a linear scale or visual with "best sleep" on one end and "worst sleep" on the opposite end. Also, the nurse could ask the client to rate sleep on a 0 to 10 scale.

- Assess for common factors that interfere with sleep, which include:

  - Illness – may require more sleep or disrupt sleep, such as nocturia.

  - Current life events (traveling more, change in work hours).

  - Emotional stress or mental illness (anxiety, fear).

  - Diet (caffeine consumption, heavy meals before bedtime).

  - Exercise – promotes sleep if done at least 2 hr before bedtime; otherwise, it can disrupt sleep.

o   Sleep environment that is too light, the wrong temperature, or too noisy (children, pets, loud noise, snoring partner).

o   Medications – may induce sleep but interfere with the restorative sleep cycles.

Nursing Interventions

- Assist the client in establishing and following a bedtime routine.

- Attempt to minimize the number of times the client is awakened during the night while hospitalized.

- Offer to assist the client with personal hygiene needs and/or a back rub prior to sleep to increase comfort.

- Instruct the client to:

    o   Exercise regularly at least 2 hr before bedtime.

    o   Arrange the sleep environment for comfort.

    o   Limit alcohol, caffeine, and nicotine at least 4 hr before bedtime.

    o   Limit fluids 2 to 4 hr before bedtime.

    o   Engage in muscle relaxation if anxious or stressed.

- Instruct the client with narcolepsy to:

    o   Participate in regular exercise.

    o   Eat small meals that are high in protein.

    o   Avoid activities that increase sleepiness (sitting too long, warm environments, alcohol).

    o   Avoid activities that would cause injury should the client fall asleep (driving, heights).

    o   Take naps when narcoleptic events are likely to occur.

    o   Take stimulants as prescribed by the provider.

- Apply continuous positive airway pressure (CPAP) devices as prescribed for clients with sleep apnea.

- As a last resort, suggest that the provider prescribe a pharmacological agent. Medications of choice for insomnia are benzodiazepine-like medications, which include the sedative-hypnotics zolpidem (Ambien), eszopiclone (Lunesta), and zaleplon (Sonata).

- Client Outcomes

    o   The client reports he has been successful with adapting to measure to promote sleep.

    o   The client reports he is able to fall asleep more easily and has less frequent awakenings.

    o   The client reports he is less fatigued during daytime hours.

    o   The client verbalizes feeling rested upon awakening

CHAPTER 38: REST AND SLEEP

 Application Exercises

1. A nurse is caring for a client who presents to the clinic reporting fatigue and an inability to sleep at night. Which of the following questions should the nurse ask when collecting data about the client's difficulty sleeping? (Select all that apply.)

_____ Does your lack of sleep interfere with your ability to function during the day?

_____ Do you experience confusion in the late afternoon?

_____ Do you drink coffee, tea, or other caffeinated drinks? If so, how many cups per day?

_____ Has anyone ever told you that you seem to stop breathing for a few seconds while you are asleep?

_____ Tell me about any personal stress you are experiencing.

2. Which of the following recommendations should a nurse give to a client to promote sleep and rest? (Select all that apply.)

_____ Avoid all caffeinated beverages.

_____ Participate in regular exercise each morning.

_____ Take an afternoon nap.

_____ Practice relaxation exercises before bedtime.

_____ Limit fluid intake at least 2 hr before bedtime.

3. A nurse is caring for an older adult client who has been bathing in the morning following the facility's routine. However, at home, she always takes a warm bath just before bedtime. Now she is having difficulty sleeping at night. Which of the following interventions should the nurse take first?

A. Rub her back for 15 min before bedtime.

B. Offer her warm milk and crackers at 2100.

C. Allow her to take a bath in the evening.

D. Ask her provider for a sleeping medication.

CHAPTER 38: REST AND SLEEP

 Application Exercises Answer Key

1. A nurse is caring for a client who presents to the clinic reporting fatigue and an inability to sleep at night. Which of the following questions should the nurse ask when collecting data about the client's difficulty sleeping? (Select all that apply.)

| X | **Does your lack of sleep interfere with your ability to function during the day?** |

_____ Do you experience confusion in the late afternoon?

| X | **Do you drink coffee, tea, or other caffeinated drinks? If so, how many cups per day?** |

| X | **Has anyone ever told you that you seem to stop breathing for a few seconds while you are asleep?** |

| X | **Tell me about any personal stress you are experiencing.** |

People with severe nighttime sleep problems often have difficulty concentrating during the day. Caffeinated drinks act as a stimulant and may interfere with sleep. A person who has periods of apnea may need to be referred for diagnostic studies. Personal stress may be the cause of insomnia. Confusion is not an expected finding with insomnia.

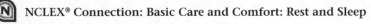 NCLEX® Connection: Basic Care and Comfort: Rest and Sleep

2. Which of the following recommendations should a nurse give to a client to promote sleep and rest? (Select all that apply.)

_____ Avoid all caffeinated beverages.

| X | **Participate in regular exercise each morning.** |

_____ Take an afternoon nap.

| X | **Practice relaxation exercises before bedtime.** |

| X | **Limit fluid intake at least 2 hr before bedtime.** |

Establishing a regular exercise routine helps promote sleep and should be completed at least 2 hr prior to sleep. Relaxation exercises can decrease stress and tension and thereby promote rest. Fluid should be limited 2 to 4 hr before bedtime to prevent nocturia. It is not necessary to avoid all caffeinated beverages but to limit consumption of these after dinner. An afternoon nap disrupts nighttime sleep.

NCLEX® Connection: Basic Care and Comfort: Rest and Sleep

3. A nurse is caring for an older adult client who has been bathing in the morning following the facility's routine. However, at home, she always takes a warm bath just before bedtime. Now she is having difficulty sleeping at night. Which of the following interventions should the nurse take first?

    A. Rub her back for 15 min before bedtime.

    B. Offer her warm milk and crackers at 2100.

    C. Allow her to take a bath in the evening.

    D. Ask her provider for a sleeping medication.

The least restrictive action is to allow the client to follow her usual bedtime routine to promote sleep. Rubbing her back, offering warm milk and crackers, and requesting a sleeping medication may be necessary if this intervention is unsuccessful.

NCLEX® Connection: Basic Care and Comfort: Rest and Sleep

UNIT 4	PHYSIOLOGICAL INTEGRITY
Section	Basic Care and Comfort
Chapter 39	Nutrition and Oral Hydration

Overview

- Nutrients provide energy for cellular metabolism and for repair, organ function, growth, and physical activity. Water, the most basic of all nutrients, is crucial for all body fluid and cellular functions.

- The proper balance of nutrients and fluid along with consideration of energy intake and requirements is essential for ensuring proper nutritional status. Malnutrition can lead to complications of health outcomes. Early recognition and treatment of malnourished or at-risk patients can have a positive influence on client outcomes.

- A nutritional assessment helps identify areas that need modification, either through adding or avoiding specific nutrients or by increasing or decreasing caloric intake. The nutritional assessment focuses on anthropometry, laboratory tests, dietary and health history, clinical observation, and client expectations.

- When planning a nutritional or hydration intervention, it is important to consider each client's beliefs and culture, the environment, and the presentation of the food, as well as any illnesses or allergies the client might have.

Basic Nutrients the Body Requires

- Carbohydrates provide most of the body's energy and fiber. Each gram produces 4 kcal. Sources include whole grain breads, baked potatoes, and brown rice.

- Fats are also used for energy and provide vitamins. No more than 30% of caloric intake should be from this source. Each gram produces 9 kcal. Sources include olive oil, salmon, and egg yolks.

- Proteins contribute to the growth and repair of body tissues. Each gram produces 4 kcal. Sources include ground beef, whole milk, and poultry.

- Vitamins must be consumed daily and are necessary for metabolism. The fat-soluble vitamins are A, D, E, and K. The water-soluble vitamins include C and B-complex (eight vitamins).

- Minerals complete essential biochemical reactions in the body (calcium, potassium, sodium, iron).

- Water replaces fluids lost through perspiration, elimination, and respiration.

Factors Affecting Nutrition and Metabolism

- Religious practices may guide a client's food preparation or choices.

- Finances may prevent clients from buying foods that are high in protein, vitamins, and minerals.

- Appetite decreases with illness, medications, pain, depression, and unpleasant environmental stimuli.

- Preferences may be determined by negative experiences with certain foods or by familiarity with foods the client has tried and liked before.

- Disease/illness can affect the client's functional ability to prepare and eat food.

- Medications can alter taste and appetite and can interfere with the absorption of certain nutrients.

- Age affects nutritional requirements.

AGE	REQUIREMENTS

Infants (Birth to 1 year)	• High energy requirements
	• Breast milk (preferred) or formula to provide:
	  ○ 108 kcal/kg of weight the first 6 months.
	  ○ 98 kcal/kg of weight the second 6 months.
	• Solid food starting at 4 to 6 months of age.
	• No cow's milk for the first year

Toddlers (12 months to 3 years) and preschoolers (3 to 6 years)	• Toddlers and preschoolers need fewer calories per kg of weight than infants. • Toddlers and preschoolers need increased protein from sources other than milk. • Calcium and phosphorus are important for bone health.
School-age (6 to 12 years)	• School-age children must be supervised to consume adequate protein and vitamins C and A. • School-age children tend to eat foods high in carbohydrates, fats, and salt.
Adolescents (13 to 20 years)	• Metabolic demands are high and require more energy. • Protein, calcium, iron, iodine, folic acid, and vitamin B needs are high. • One fourth of dietary intake comes from snacks. • Increased water consumption is important for active adolescents.
Young (20 to 40 years) and middle adults (40 to 60 years)	• There is a decreased need for most nutrients (except during pregnancy). • Calcium and iron consumption are important for women. • Good oral health is important.

AGE	REQUIREMENTS
Older adults (over 60 years)	• A slower metabolic rate requires fewer calories. • Decreased thirst sensation. • Older adults need the same amount of most vitamins and minerals as younger adults. • Calcium may be necessary and is important for both men and women.

- Eating Disorders

  - Anorexia nervosa

    - Body weight less than 85% of ideal

    - Fear of being fat

    - Feeling fat

    - With female clients, no menses for at least 3 consecutive months

  - Bulimia – a cycle of binge eating followed by purging (vomiting, using diuretics or laxatives, exercise, fasting)

  - Obesity

    - Body mass index (BMI) is determined by dividing weight (in kg) by height (in m²).

    - A BMI of 25 is the upper boundary of healthy weight. Adults who have a BMI above 30 are considered obese.

Assessment/Data Collection

- Dietary history should include:

  - Number of meals per day.

  - Fluid intake.

  - Food preferences and amounts.

  - Food preparation/purchasing practices/access to food.

  - History of indigestion, heartburn, and/or gas.

  - Allergies.

  - Taste.

  - Chewing and swallowing.

  - Appetite.

  - Elimination patterns.

  - Medication use.

  - Activity levels.

  - Religious or cultural food restrictions.

- Clinical Measures

  o Height and weight to calculate BMI and ideal body weight (IBW)

  o Laboratory values of cholesterol, triglycerides, hemoglobin, electrolytes, albumin, and nitrogen levels.

- Intake and Output (I&O)

  o Record I&O accurately.

  o Monitor I&O for any client who has fluid or electrolyte alterations.

  o Weigh clients each day at the same time, after voiding, and while wearing the same type of clothes.

  o If using bed scales, use the same amount of linen each day, and reset the scale to zero if possible.

- Subjective and objective data indicating poor nutrition:

  o Nausea, vomiting, diarrhea, and/or constipation.

  o Flaccid muscles.

  o Mental status changes.

  o Loss of appetite.

  o Change in bowel pattern.

  o Spleen or liver enlargement.

  o Dry, brittle hair.

  o Loss of subcutaneous fat.

  o Dry, scaly skin.

  o Inflammation and bleeding of gums.

  o Poor dental health.

  o Dry, dull eyes.

  o Enlarged thyroid.

  o Prominent protrusions over bony areas.

  o Weakness.

  o Change in weight.

  o Poor posture.

Nursing Interventions

- Assist the client in advancing the diet as the disease process allows.

- Teach the client about the appropriate diet regimen.

- Provide interventions to promote appetite (good oral hygiene, favorite foods, minimal environmental odors).

- Educate the client about medications that may affect nutritional intake.

- Assist the client with feeding to promote optimal independence.

- Assist with preventing aspiration.

  o Position the client in Fowler's position or in a chair.

  o Support the upper back, neck, and head.

  o Have the client tuck her chin when swallowing to help propel food down the esophagus.

  o Observe for aspiration and/or pocketing of food in the cheeks or other areas of the mouth.

  o Observe for signs of dysphagia such as coughing, choking, gagging, and drooling of food.

  o Maintain the client in semi-Fowler's position for at least 1 hr after meals.

  o Provide oral hygiene after meals/snacks.

- Provide therapeutic diets as directed by the provider/dietitian.

  o Clear liquid – liquids that leave little residue (clear fruit juices, gelatin, broth)

  o Full liquid – clear liquids plus liquid dairy products, all juice, puréed vegetables

  o Puréed – clear and full liquids plus puréed meats, fruits, and scrambled eggs

  o Mechanical soft – clear and full liquids plus diced or ground foods

  o Soft/low-residue – foods that are low in fiber and easy to digest

  o High-fiber (whole grains, raw and dried fruits)

  o Low sodium – no added salt or 1 to 2 g of sodium

  o Low cholesterol – no more than 300 mg/day of dietary cholesterol

  o Diabetic – balanced intake of protein, fats, and carbohydrates of about 1,800 calories

  o Dysphagia – puréed food and thickened liquids

  o Regular – no restrictions

- Administer and monitor enteral feedings via nasogastric, gastrostomy, or jejunostomy tubes.

- Administer and monitor parenteral nutrition to clients who are unable to use their gastrointestinal tract to acquire nutrients.

  o Types of nutrients given parenterally include:

    ■ Lipids.

    ■ Electrolytes.

- Minerals.

- Vitamins.

- Dextrose.

- Amino acids.

- Maintain fluid balance by:

  o Administering IV fluids.

  o Restricting oral fluid intake.

    - Remove the water pitcher from the bedside.

    - Tell the dietary staff the amount of fluid to be served with each meal tray.

    - Tell the staff of each shift the amount of fluid the client is allowed besides what is served with each meal.

    - Record all oral intake.

  o Encouraging oral intake of fluids.

    - Provide fresh drinking water.

    - Ask the client about beverage preferences as allowed.

CHAPTER 39: NUTRITION AND ORAL HYDRATION

 Application Exercises

1. A nurse is caring for a client who is at high risk for aspiration. Which of the following is an appropriate nursing intervention?

    A. Give the client thin liquids.

    B. Instruct the client to tuck her chin when swallowing.

    C. Have the client use a straw.

    D. Encourage the client to lie down and rest after meals.

2. Which of the following nutrients is the body's preferred energy source?

    A. Fat

    B. Protein

    C. Vitamins

    D. Carbohydrates

3. If their diets are not adequately supervised, school-age children tend to have dietary deficiencies in which of the following?

    A. Carbohydrates

    B. Fats

    C. Minerals

    D. Vitamins

4. Which of the following is appropriate for a nurse to give a client who is on a low-residue diet?

    A. Whole grains

    B. Fruits and vegetables

    C. Dairy products

    D. Nuts and legumes

5. A nurse is caring for a client who weighs 80 kg (176 lb) and is 1.6 m (5 ft 3 in) tall. Calculate her body mass index (BMI) and determine whether or not this client is obese based on her BMI.

CHAPTER 39: NUTRITION AND ORAL HYDRATION

 Application Exercises Answer Key

1. A nurse is caring for a client who is at high risk for aspiration. Which of the following is an appropriate nursing intervention?

    A. Give the client thin liquids.

    B. Instruct the client to tuck her chin when swallowing.

    C. Have the client use a straw.

    D. Encourage the client to lie down and rest after meals.

    Tucking the chin when swallowing allows food to pass down the esophagus more easily. Thin liquids and using a straw both increase the client's risk for aspiration. Sitting for an hour after meals helps prevent gastroesophageal reflux and possible aspiration of the contents after a meal.

 NCLEX® Connection: Basic Care and Comfort. Nutrition and Oral Hydration

2. Which of the following nutrients is the body's preferred energy source?

    A. Fat

    B. Protein

    C. Vitamins

    D. Carbohydrates

    Most of the body's energy comes from carbohydrates. Fat provides energy but should be less than 30% of total caloric intake. Protein is responsible for growth and repair of body tissues. Vitamins do not provide energy.

 NCLEX® Connection: Basic Care and Comfort: Nutrition and Oral Hydration

3. If their diets are not adequately supervised, school-age children tend to have dietary deficiencies in which of the following?

    A. Carbohydrates

    B. Fats

    C. Minerals

    D. Vitamins

    School-age children must have their dietary intake supervised to ensure adequate intake of protein and vitamins C and A. They tend to eat too many foods high in carbohydrates, fats, and salt.

 NCLEX® Connection: Basic Care and Comfort: Nutrition and Oral Hydration

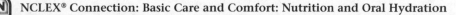

4. Which of the following is appropriate for a nurse to give a client who is on a low-residue diet?

    A. Whole grains

    B. Fruits and vegetables

    C. Dairy products

    D. Nuts and legumes

    A soft/low-residue diet consists of foods that are low in fiber and easy to digest. Dairy products are low in fiber and easy to digest. Whole grains, fruits, vegetables, nuts, and legumes all are high in fiber.

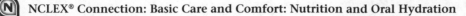 **NCLEX® Connection: Basic Care and Comfort: Nutrition and Oral Hydration**

5. A nurse is caring for a client who weighs 80 kg (176 lb) and is 1.6 m (5 ft 3 in) tall. Calculate her body mass index (BMI) and determine whether or not this client is obese based on her BMI.

    BMI = weight (kg) ÷ height (m^2). BMI = 80 ÷ 1.62^2 = 80 ÷ 2.56 = 31.25 = 31. A BMI above 30 identifies obesity, so this client is considered obese.

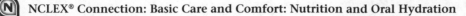 **NCLEX® Connection: Basic Care and Comfort: Nutrition and Oral Hydration**

UNIT 4	PHYSIOLOGICAL INTEGRITY
Section	Basic Care and Comfort
Chapter 40	Mobility and Immobility

Overview

- Mobility is freedom and independence in purposeful movement. Mobility refers to adapting to and having self-awareness of the environment. Functional musculoskeletal and nervous systems are essential for mobility.

- Immobility is the inability to move freely and independently at will. The risk of complications increases with the degree of immobility and the length of time of immobilization.

- Nursing interventions are designed to maintain mobility and prevent or minimize complications of immobility.

- Cutaneous stimulation in the form of cold and heat applications helps relieve pain and promote healing.

- Promoting venous return is another key component of reducing the complications of immobility.

Mobility and Immobility

- Immobility may be:
  - Temporary, such as following knee arthroplasty.
  - Permanent, such as paraplegia.
  - Sudden onset, such as a fractured arm and leg following a motor-vehicle crash.
  - Slow onset, such as multiple sclerosis.

- The principles of body mechanics are based on alignment, balance, gravity, and friction.

- Movement depends on an intact skeletal system, skeletal muscles, and nervous system.

- Assessment of the client focuses on mobility, range of motion (ROM), gait, exercise status, activity tolerance, and body alignment while standing, sitting, and lying.

- Factors affecting mobility include:
  - Alterations in muscles.
  - Injury to the musculoskeletal system.
  - Abnormal posture.

- o   Impaired central nervous system.
- o   Health status and age.
- Changes that occur in body systems include:

BODY SYSTEM	CHANGES
Integumentary	• Increased pressure on skin, which is aggravated by metabolic changes • Decreased circulation to tissue causing ischemia, which can lead to pressure ulcers
Respiratory	• Decreased respiratory movement resulting in decreased oxygenation and carbon dioxide exchange • Stasis of secretions and decreased and weakened respiratory muscles, resulting in atelectasis and hypostatic pneumonia • Decreased cough response
Cardiovascular	• Orthostatic hypotension • Less fluid volume in the circulatory system • Stasis of blood in the legs • Diminished autonomic response • Decreased cardiac output leading to poor cardiac effectiveness, which results in increased cardiac workload • Increased oxygenation requirement • Increased risk of thrombus development
Metabolic	• Altered endocrine system • Decreased basal metabolic rate • Changes in protein, carbohydrate, and fat metabolism • Decreased appetite with altered nutritional intake • Negative nitrogen balance • Decreased protein resulting in loss of muscle • Loss of weight • Alterations in calcium, fluid, and electrolytes • Resorption of calcium from bones • Decreased urinary elimination of calcium resulting in hypercalcemia

Elimination	• Genitourinary
	  o Urinary stasis
	  o Change in calcium metabolism with hypercalcemia resulting in renal calculi
	  o Decreased fluid intake, poor perineal care, and indwelling urinary catheters resulting in urinary tract infections
	• Gastrointestinal
	  o Decreased peristalsis
	• Decreased fluid intake
	• Constipation, then fecal impaction, then diarrhea

BODY SYSTEM	CHANGES
Musculoskeletal	<ul><li>Decreased muscle endurance, strength, and mass</li><li>Impaired balance</li><li>Atrophy of muscles</li><li>Decreased stability</li><li>Altered calcium metabolism</li><li>Osteoporosis</li><li>Contractures</li><li>Foot drop</li><li>Altered joint mobility</li></ul>
Neurological/ Psychosocial	<ul><li>Changes in emotional status – depression, alteration in self-concept, and anxiety</li><li>Behavioral changes – withdrawal, altered sleep/wake pattern, hostility, inappropriate laughter, and passivity</li><li>Altered sensory perception</li><li>Ineffective coping</li></ul>
Developmental	<ul><li>Infants, toddlers, and preschoolers<ul><li>Slower progression in gross motor skills and intellectual and musculoskeletal development</li><li>Body aligned with line of gravity, resulting in unbalanced posture</li></ul></li><li>Adolescents<ul><li>Imbalanced growth spurt possibly altered with immobility</li><li>Delayed development of independence</li><li>Social isolation</li></ul></li><li>Adults<ul><li>Alterations in every physiological system</li><li>Alterations in family and social systems</li><li>Alterations in job identity</li></ul></li><li>Older adults<ul><li>Alterations in balance resulting in a major risk for falls and injuries</li><li>Steady loss of bone mass resulting in weakened bones</li><li>Decreased coordination</li><li>Slower walk with smaller steps</li><li>Alterations in functional status</li><li>Increased dependence on staff and family</li></ul></li></ul>

Assessment/Data Collection and Collaborative Care

ASSESSMENT	NURSING INTERVENTIONS
Integumentary – Maintain intact skin.	
<ul><li>Observe the skin for breakdown, warmth, and change in color. Look for pallor or redness in fair-skinned clients, and purple or blue discoloration in dark-skinned clients.</li><li>Observe bony prominences.</li><li>Check skin turgor.</li><li>Use a pressure ulcer risk scale such as Norton or Braden.</li><li>Assess at least every 2 hr.</li><li>Observe for urinary or bowel incontinence.</li></ul>	<ul><li>Identify clients at risk for pressure ulcer development.</li><li>Position the client using corrective devices such as pillows, foot boots, trochanter rolls, and wedge pillows.</li><li>Turn the client every 1 to 2 hr, and use devices for support or per protocol.</li><li>Teach clients who can move independently to turn at least every 15 min.</li><li>Provide clients who are sitting in a chair with a device to decrease pressure.</li><li>Limit sitting in a chair to less than 2 hr. Instruct the client to shift his weight every 15 min.</li><li>Use a therapeutic bed or mattress for a client who is in a bed for an extended time.</li><li>Monitor nutritional intake.</li><li>Provide skin and perineal care.</li></ul>
Respiratory – Maintain airway patency, achieve optimal lung expansion and gas exchange, and mobilize airway secretions.	
<ul><li>Complete the following every 2 hr:<ul><li>Observe the client's chest wall movement for symmetry.</li><li>Auscultate breath sounds.</li><li>Observe for productive cough, and note the color, amount, and consistency of secretions.</li></ul></li></ul>	<ul><li>Reposition the client every 1 to 2 hr.</li><li>Teach the client to turn, cough, and deep breathe every 1 to 2 hr while awake.</li><li>Teach the client to yawn every hr while awake.</li><li>Teach the client to use an incentive spirometer while awake.</li><li>Remove abdominal binders every 2 hr, and ensure their correct placement.</li><li>Use chest physiotherapy.</li><li>Auscultate the lungs to determine the effectiveness of chest physiotherapy or other respiratory therapy.</li><li>Teach the client to consume at least 2,000 mL of fluid per day, unless the client's intake is restricted.</li><li>Monitor the client's ability to expectorate secretions.</li><li>Use suction if the client is unable to expectorate secretions.</li></ul>

ASSESSMENT	NURSING INTERVENTIONS
Cardiovascular – Maintain cardiovascular function, increase activity tolerance, and prevent thrombus formation.	
• Measure orthostatic blood pressure and pulse (lying to sitting to standing), and assess for vertigo. • Palpate the apical and peripheral pulses. • Auscultate the heart at the apex for S_3 (an early sign of heart failure). Older adult clients may not adapt well to immobility. • Palpate for edema in the sacrum, legs, and feet. • Palpate the skin for warmth in peripheral areas to include the nose, ear lobes, hands, and feet. • Assess for deep vein thrombosis by observing the calves for redness and palpating for warmth and tenderness. • Measure the circumference of both calves and thighs and compare in size (calf – 10 cm below the middle of the patella).	• Increase the client's activity as soon as possible. Have the client dangle his feet on side of bed or transfer to a chair. • Have the client perform isometric exercises to increase his tolerance for activity. • Change the client's position as often as possible. • Teach the client to avoid the Valsalva maneuver. • Give a stool softener as prescribed to prevent straining. • Teach range of motion (ROM) exercises such as ankle pumps or knee flexion. • Teach the client to avoid placing pillows under the knees or lower extremities, crossing the legs, wearing tight clothes around the waist or on the legs, sitting for long periods of time, and massaging the legs. • Use elastic stockings. • Use sequential compression devices (SCD) or intermittent pneumatic compression (IPC). • Increase fluid intake if not contraindicated. • Give low-dose heparin (5,000 units every 8 to 12 hr). • Contact the provider immediately if assessment data indicates venous thrombosis.

ASSESSMENT	NURSING INTERVENTIONS
Metabolic – Reduce skin injury and maintain metabolism.	
• Record anthropometric measurements of height, weight, and skin fold. • Assess I&O. • Assess food intake. • Review urinary and bowel elimination status. • Assess wound healing. • Auscultate bowel sounds. • Check skin turgor. • Review laboratory values for electrolytes, serum, total protein, and BUN.	• Provide a high-calorie and high-protein diet with vitamin B and C supplements. • Monitor and evaluate oral intake. If the client cannot eat or drink, enteral or parenteral nutritional therapy may be indicated.
Elimination – Maintain or achieve normal urinary and bowel elimination patterns.	
• Assess I&O. • Assess the bladder for distention. • Observe urine for color, amount, clarity, and frequency. • Auscultate bowel sounds. • Observe feces for color, amount, frequency, and consistency.	• Maintain hydration (at least 2,000 mL/day unless fluid is restricted.) • Teach the client to consume a diet that includes fruits and vegetables, and is high in fiber. • Give a stool softener as prescribed. Consider laxatives only as a last resort. • Provide perineal care. • Teach bladder and bowel training if needed. • Insert a straight or indwelling catheter as prescribed if the bladder is distended. • Promote urination by pouring warm water over the perineal area if the client has difficulty urinating.

ASSESSMENT	NURSING INTERVENTIONS
Musculoskeletal – Maintain or regain body alignment and stability, decrease skin and musculoskeletal system changes, achieve full or optimal ROM, and prevent contractures.	
• Assess ROM capability. • Assess muscle tone and mass. • Observe for contractures. • Monitor gait. • Monitor nutritional intake for calcium. • Monitor use of assistive devices to assist with ADLs.	• Assist/instruct the client to change position in bed at least every 2 hr and perform weight shifts in the wheelchair every 15 min. • Provide active and/or passive ROM two or three times a day. • Teach the client to perform ROM while bathing, eating, grooming, and dressing. • Monitor the client's nutritional intake of calcium. • Develop an individualized program for each client. Older adult clients may require a program that addresses the aging process. • Cluster care to promote a proper sleep-wake cycle. • Request that the provider prescribe physical therapy if the client has decreased mobility. • Advise the client to follow the physical therapy program. • Use a continuous passive motion device. Cane instructions • Maintain two points of support on the ground at all times. • Keep the cane on the stronger side of the body. • Support body weight on both legs, move the cane forward 6 to 10 inches, then move the weaker leg forward toward the cane. • Next, advance the stronger leg. Crutch instructions • Do not alter crutches after proper fit has been determined. • Follow the prescribed crutch gait. • Support body weight at the hand grips with the elbows flexed at 30°. • Position the crutches on the unaffected side when sitting or rising from a chair.

ASSESSMENT	NURSING INTERVENTIONS
Psychosocial – Maintain an acceptable sleep/wake pattern, achieve socialization, and complete self-care independently.	
<ul><li>Assess emotional status.</li><li>Assess mental status.</li><li>Assess behavior and decision-making skills.</li><li>Monitor mobility status.</li><li>Observe for unusual alterations in sleep/wake pattern.</li><li>Assess coping skills, especially for loss.</li><li>Monitor activities of daily living (ADLs).</li><li>Assess for family support and relationships.</li><li>Monitor social activities.</li></ul>	<ul><li>Assist in using usual coping skills or in developing new coping skills.</li><li>Maintain orientation to time (clock and calendar with date), person (call by name and introduce self) and place (talk about treatments, therapy, and length of stay).</li><li>Develop a schedule of therapies and place it on a calendar in the client's room.</li><li>Arrange for the client to be in a semiprivate room with an alert roommate.</li><li>Involve the client in daily care.</li><li>Provide stimuli such as books, television, newspapers, and radio.</li><li>Help the client maintain body image by performing or assisting with hygiene and grooming tasks such as shaving or applying makeup.</li><li>Have nurses and other staff interact on an informal social basis.</li><li>Recommend to the provider a referral for consultation (psychological, spiritual, or social worker), if the client is not coping well.</li></ul>

ASSESSMENT	NURSING INTERVENTIONS
Developmental – Continue expected development and achieve physical and mental stimulation.	

• Infancy through school age
  ○ Gross motor skills, and intellectual and musculoskeletal development
  ○ Body alignment and posture
  ○ Developmental tasks specific to age
• Adolescents
  ○ Growth and development specific to age
  ○ Level of independence
  ○ Social activities
• Adults
  ○ All physical systems
  ○ Family relationships
  ○ Social status
  ○ Meaning of career/job
• Older adults
  ○ Balance
  ○ Coordination
  ○ Gait
  ○ Functional status
  ○ Level of independence
  ○ Social isolation
	• Infancy through school age
	  ○ Initiate events that stimulate physical and psychosocial systems. Increase mobility, and involve play therapists in age-appropriate activities.
	  ○ Use measures to prevent falls.
	  ○ Develop strategies for maintaining or enhancing the developmental process.
	  ○ Teach the family that their perception of immobility can affect the child's progress and ability to cope.
	  ○ Encourage the parents to stay with the child.
	  ○ Incorporate the child's involvement, if it is age-appropriate, in his treatments.
	  ○ Place the child in a room with others who are age-appropriate.
	• Adolescents
	  ○ Initiate care that facilitates independence.
	  ○ Involve adolescents in decision making for ADLs.
	  ○ Provide stimuli to promote socialization (interaction with peers, use of adolescents' activity room).
	• Adults
	  ○ Provide care that promotes activity in all physical systems.
	  ○ Discuss with the family the importance of interaction with the client.
	  ○ Discuss the client's social involvement.
	  ○ Discuss the meaning of the client's career/job.
	• Older adults
	  ○ Plan care with the client and family to increase independence with ADLs and decision-making skills.
	  ○ Teach the staff to facilitate the client's independence in all activities.
	  ○ Maintain stimuli such as a clock, newspaper, calendar, and weather status.
	  ○ Encourage the family to visit to maintain socialization.
	  ○ Plan for staff to spend some time talking and listening to the client.

Application of Heat and Cold

- Therapeutic effects of heat and cold applications:

HEAT	COLD
• Increases blood flow • Increases tissue metabolism • Relaxes muscles • Eases joint stiffness and pain	• Decreases inflammation • Prevents swelling • Reduces bleeding • Reduces fever • Diminishes muscle spasms • Decreases pain by decreasing the velocity of nerve conduction

- For clients at risk for injury from heat/cold applications:

  - Use extreme caution with very young, fair-skinned, and older clients, as they have fragile skin.

  - Clients who are immobile may not be able to move away from the application if it becomes uncomfortable; they are at risk for skin injuries.

  - Clients who have impaired sensory perception may not feel pain or burning.

  - Avoid extremely long applications of either heat or cold, as they will result in a reaction opposite to the intended response.

  - Heat

    - Monitor bony prominences carefully as they are more sensitive to heat applications.

    - Avoid the use of heat applications over metal devices (pacemakers, prosthetic joints) to prevent deep tissue burns.

    - Do not apply heat to the abdomen of a pregnant woman to prevent harm to the fetus.

    - Do not place a heat application under an immobile client as this may increase the risk of burns.

  - Cold application is inappropriate for clients with cold intolerance, vascular insufficiency, and disorders aggravated by cold, such as Raynaud's phenomenon.

  - Make sure the provider has written a prescription that includes:

    - Location.

    - Duration and frequency.

    - Specific type (moist or dry).

    - Temperature to use.

Collaborative Care

- Equipment

- Heat application supplies include:

  ○ Moist

    ▪ Hot compresses – towel, bath thermometer, hot water, plastic covering, hot pack or aquathermia pad (with distilled water), and tape

    ▪ Hot soaks – water, bath thermometer, basin, and waterproof pads

    ▪ Sitz baths – sitz bath (disposable or built-in), bath thermometer, bath blanket, and towels

  ○ Dry

    ▪ Hot pack (disposable or reusable) or an aquathermia pad with distilled water, and a pillowcase

    ▪ Warming blanket

- Cold application supplies include:

  ○ Moist

    ▪ Large basin of ice

    ▪ Cold water

    ▪ Cold pack to be used in place of ice

  ○ Dry

    ▪ Ice bag, ice collar, ice glove, or a cold pack

    ▪ Cooling blanket

- Apply the application to the area.

- Make sure the client's call light is within reach, and instruct the client to report any discomfort.

- Assess the site every 5 to 10 min to check for:

  ○ Redness or pallor.

  ○ Pain or burning.

  ○ Numbness.

  ○ Shivering (with cold applications).

  ○ Blisters.

  ○ Decreased sensation.

  ○ Cyanosis (with cold applications).

- Discontinue the application if any of the above occur, or remove the application at the predetermined time (usually 15 to 20 min).

- Document:

  o Location, type, and length of the application.

  o Condition of the skin before and after the application.

  o The client's ability to tolerate the application.

PROMOTING VENOUS RETURN

- Elastic stockings or thromboembolic device (TED) hose help maintain external pressure on the muscles of the lower extremities and promote blood return to the heart.

- Sequential compression devices (SCDs) and intermittent pneumatic compression (IPC) have plastic or fabric sleeves that wrap around the leg and secure with Velcro™. The sleeves are then attached to an electric pump that alternately inflates and deflates the sleeve around the leg. These machines are set to cycle, typically a 10- to 15-second inflation and a 45- to 60-second deflation.

- Positioning techniques reduce compression of leg veins.

- ROM exercises cause skeletal muscle contractions, which promote blood return. Specific exercises that help prevent thrombophlebitis include ankle pumps, foot circles, and knee flexion.

- TED hose, SCDs, and IPC require a provider's order.

- Immobile clients should perform leg exercises, increase their fluid intake, and change positions frequently. These interventions can be implemented without a provider's order.

- When poor venous return or possible thrombus is suspected, the provider must be notified and no pressure applied to a thrombus to avoid dislodging it.

Collaborative Care

- TED hose

  o Equipment

    ▪ Tape measure

    ▪ TED hose

  o Procedure

    ▪ Perform hand hygiene.

    ▪ Assess the condition of the skin and the circulation in the client's legs.

    ▪ Measure the client's calf and/or thigh circumference and the length of the leg to select the correct size of stocking.

    ▪ Turn the stockings inside to the heel.

- Put the stocking on the foot.

- Pull the remainder of the stocking over the heel and up the leg.

- Smooth any creases or wrinkles.

- Remove the stockings and reapply them at least twice a day. Make sure the client has the necessary support to accomplish this task.

- Make sure the stockings are not too tight over the toes.

- Keep the stockings clean and dry. A postsurgical client or a client with special needs may need a second pair of hose.

- Document the application and removal of the stockings.

- SCDs and IPC

  - Equipment

    - Tape measure

    - Sequential stockings

    - Stockinette

  - Procedure

    - Perform hand hygiene.

    - Assess circulation and skin prior to application.

    - Measure around the largest part of the client's thigh to determine the stocking size.

    - Place the stockinette on first.

    - Apply the sleeves.

    - Attach the sleeves to the inflator.

    - Turn on the device.

    - Monitor circulation and skin after application.

    - Document the application and removal of the stockings.

- Positioning techniques to reduce compression of leg veins

  - Equipment – none

  - Procedure – Teach the client to avoid:

    - Crossing the legs.

    - Sitting for long periods of time.

    - Wearing restrictive clothing on the lower extremities.

    - Putting pillows behind the knees.

    - Massaging the legs.

- ROM exercises are performed hourly while the client is awake.

  o Equipment – none

  o Procedure – Teach the client to perform:

    ▪ Ankle pumps – Point the toes toward the head and then away from the head.

    ▪ Foot circles – Rotate the feet in circles at the ankles.

    ▪ Knee flexion – Flex and extend the legs at the knees.

Complications

- Thrombophlebitis/deep vein thrombosis is an inflammation of a vein (usually in the lower extremities) that results in clot formation.

  o Clinical manifestations are pain, edema, warmth, and erythema at the site.

  o Nursing actions:

    ▪ Notify the provider immediately.

    ▪ Position the client in bed with the leg elevated.

    ▪ Avoid any pressure at the site of the inflammation.

    ▪ Anticipate giving anticoagulants as prescribed.

- A pulmonary embolism is the occlusion of blood flow to one or more of the pulmonary arteries by a clot. The condition can be life-threatening. The clot or embolus often originates in the venous system of the lower extremities.

  o Clinical manifestations are shortness of breath, chest pain, hematemesis (coughing up blood), decreased blood pressure, and rapid pulse.

  o Nursing actions

    ▪ Prepare to give thrombolytics or anticoagulants as prescribed.

CHAPTER 40: MOBILITY AND IMMOBILITY

(A) Application Exercises

1. A nurse is caring for a client who has been sitting in a chair for 3 hr. Which of the following is the client at risk for developing?

    A. Stasis of secretions

    B. Muscle atrophy

    C. Pressure ulcer

    D. Fecal impaction

2. Which of the following nursing interventions should be implemented to maintain a patent airway in a client on bed rest?

    A. Perform isometric exercises.

    B. Suction every 8 hr.

    C. Give low-dose heparin as prescribed.

    D. Teach to use an incentive spirometer while awake.

3. Which of the following nursing interventions reduce the risk of thrombus development? (Select all that apply.)

    _____ Teach the client not to use the Valsalva maneuver.

    _____ Apply elastic stockings.

    _____ Review laboratory values for total protein level.

    _____ Place pillows under the client's knees and lower extremities.

    _____ Assist the client to change position often.

4. Which of the following clients would benefit from the application of cold? (Select all that apply.)

    _____ A client who has a sprained ankle

    _____ A client who has Raynaud's phenomenon

    _____ A client who just had knee arthroplasty

    _____ A client who has a toothache

    _____ A client who has a nosebleed

5. Sequential compression devices are used to

    A. prevent pressure ulcers.

    B. promote venous return.

    C. prevent muscular atrophy.

    D. increase joint mobility.

6. Identify the order in which the following steps of elastic stocking application should be completed.

_____   Perform hand hygiene.

_____   Smooth any creases or wrinkles.

_____   Pull the remainder of the stocking over the client's heel and on up his leg.

_____   Turn the stockings inside to the heel.

_____   Assess the condition of the client's skin and the circulation of his legs.

_____   Put the stocking on the client's foot.

_____   Measure the client's calf and/or thigh circumference and length of the leg, and select the correct size stocking.

CHAPTER 40: MOBILITY AND IMMOBILITY

 Application Exercises Answer Key

1. A nurse is caring for a client who has been sitting in a chair for 3 hr. Which of the following is the client at risk for developing?

    A. Stasis of secretions

    B. Muscle atrophy

    C. Pressure ulcer

    D. Fecal impaction

Unrelieved pressure over a bony prominence for too long increases the risk for skin breakdown. Sitting up in a chair will help prevent stasis of secretions. Muscle atrophy and fecal impaction would be complications for a client on prolonged bed rest.

 NCLEX® Connection: Reduction of Risk Potential, Potential for Alterations in Body Systems

2. Which of the following nursing interventions should be implemented to maintain a patent airway in a client on bed rest?

    A. Perform isometric exercises.

    B. Suction every 8 hr.

    C. Give low-dose heparin as prescribed.

    D. Teach to use an incentive spirometer while awake.

Using an incentive spirometer helps keep the airways open and prevents atelectasis. Performing isometric exercises strengthens skeletal muscles. Suctioning should not be done routinely. Low-dose heparin helps prevent thrombus formation.

NCLEX® Connection: Basic Care and Comfort, Mobility/ Immobility

3. Which of the following nursing interventions reduce the risk of thrombus development? (Select all that apply.)

    _____ Teach the client not to use the Valsalva maneuver.

    __**X**__ **Apply elastic stockings.**

    _____ Review laboratory values for total protein level.

    _____ Place pillows under the client's knees and lower extremities.

    __**X**__ **Assist the client to change position often.**

Elastic stockings promote venous return and prevent thrombus formation. Frequent position changes prevent venous stasis. The Valsalva maneuver increases the workload of the heart, but it does not affect peripheral circulation. A review of the client's total protein level is important for evaluating his ability to heal and prevent skin breakdown. Placing pillows under the knees and lower extremities further impairs circulation of the lower extremities and should be avoided.

 NCLEX® Connection: Basic Care and Comfort, Mobility/ Immobility

4. Which of the following clients would benefit from the application of cold? (Select all that apply.)

   X   **A client who has a sprained ankle**

          A client who has Raynaud's phenomenon

   X   **A client who just had knee arthroplasty**

   X   **A client who has a toothache**

   X   **A client who has a nosebleed**

A client who has a sprained ankle, a client who just had knee arthroplasty, and a client who has a toothache may benefit from the application of cold to reduce pain and decrease inflammation. A client who has a nosebleed may benefit from cold application to reduce or stop bleeding. Cold could trigger Raynaud's phenomenon.

(N) **NCLEX® Connection: Basic Care and Comfort, Nonpharmacological Comfort Interventions**

5. Sequential compression devices are used to

A. prevent pressure ulcers.

B. promote venous return.

C. prevent muscular atrophy.

D. increase joint mobility.

The purpose of sequential compression devices is to promote venous return. Sequential compression devices do not prevent bed sores or muscular atrophy, and they do not increase joint mobility.

(N) **NCLEX® Connection: Physiological Adaptation, Alterations in Body Systems**

6. Identify the order in which the following steps of elastic stocking application should be completed.

   1   Perform hand hygiene.

   7   Smooth any creases or wrinkles.

   6   Pull the remainder of the stocking over the client's heel and on up his leg.

   4   Turn the stockings inside to the heel.

   2   Assess the condition of the client's skin and the circulation of his legs.

   5   Put the stocking on the client's foot.

   3   Measure the client's calf and/or thigh circumference and length of the leg, and select the correct size stocking.

(N) **NCLEX® Connection: Physiological Adaptation, Alterations in Body Systems**

UNIT 4	PHYSIOLOGICAL INTEGRITY
Section	Basic Care and Comfort
Chapter 41	Pain Management

Overview

- Effective pain management includes the use of pharmacological and nonpharmacological pain management therapies. Invasive therapies such as nerve ablation may be appropriate for intractable cancer-related pain.

- Clients have a right to adequate assessment and management of pain. Nurses are accountable for the assessment of pain. The nurse's role is that of an advocate and educator for effective pain management.

- Nurses have a priority responsibility for the continual assessment of the client's pain level and to provide individualized interventions. They should assess the effectiveness of the interventions 30 to 60 min after implementation.

- Assessment challenges may occur with clients who are cognitively impaired or on a ventilator.

- Undertreatment of pain is a serious health care problem. Consequences of undertreatment of pain include physiological and psychological components.

  o Acute/chronic pain can cause anxiety, fear, and depression.

  o Poorly managed acute pain may lead to chronic pain syndrome.

Physiology of Pain

- Transduction is the conversion of painful stimuli to an electrical impulse through peripheral nerve fibers (nociceptors).

- Transmission occurs as the electrical impulse travels along the nerve fibers and is regulated by neurotransmitters.

- The pain threshold is the point at which a person feels pain.

- Pain tolerance is the amount of pain a person is willing to bear.

SUBSTANCES THAT INCREASE PAIN TRANSMISSION AND CAUSE AN INFLAMMATORY RESPONSE	SUBSTANCES THAT DECREASE PAIN TRANSMISSION AND PRODUCE ANALGESIA
• Substance P • Prostaglandins • Bradykinin • Histamine	• Serotonin • Endorphins

- Perception or awareness of pain occurs in various areas of the brain and is influenced by thought and emotional processes.

- Modulation occurs in the spinal cord, causing muscles to contract reflexively, moving the body away from painful stimuli.

Pain Categories

ACUTE PAIN	CHRONIC PAIN
• Acute pain is protective, temporary, usually self-limiting, and resolves with tissue healing. • Physiological responses (sympathetic nervous system) are fight-or-flight responses (tachycardia, hypertension, anxiety, diaphoresis, muscle tension). • Behavioral responses include grimacing, moaning, flinching, and guarding. • Interventions include treatment of the underlying problem.	• Chronic pain is not protective; it is ongoing or recurs frequently, lasting longer than 6 months and persisting beyond tissue healing. • Physiological responses do not usually alter vital signs, but the client may experience depression, fatigue, and a decreased level of functioning. • Psychosocial implications may lead to disability. • Chronic pain may not have a known cause, and it may not respond to interventions. • Management is aimed at symptomatic relief. • Chronic pain can be malignant or nonmalignant.
NOCICEPTIVE PAIN	NEUROPATHIC PAIN

• Nociceptive pain arises from damage to or inflammation of tissue other than that of the peripheral and central nervous systems.
• It is usually throbbing, aching, and localized.
• This pain typically responds to opioids and nonopioid medications.
• Types of nociceptive pain include:
  o Somatic – in bones, joints, muscles, skin, or connective tissues.
  o Visceral – in internal organs such as the stomach or intestines. It can cause referred pain in other body locations not associated with the stimulus.
  o Cutaneous – in the skin or subcutaneous tissue.
	• Neuropathic pain arises from abnormal or damaged pain nerves.
	• It includes phantom limb pain, pain below the level of a spinal cord injury, and diabetic neuropathy.
	• Neuropathic pain is usually intense, shooting, burning, or described as "pins and needles."
	• This pain typically responds to adjuvant medications (antidepressants, antispasmodic agents, skeletal muscle relaxants).

(S) • Risk factors for undertreatment of pain include:

  ○ Cultural and societal attitudes.

  ○ Lack of knowledge.

  ○ Fear of addiction.

  ○ Exaggerated fear of respiratory depression.

(S) • Populations at risk for undertreatment of pain include:

  ○ Infants.

  ○ Children.

(G) ○ Older adults.

  ○ Clients with substance abuse problems.

• Causes of acute and chronic pain include:

  ○ Trauma.

  ○ Surgery.

  ○ Cancer (tumor invasion, nerve compression, bone metastases, associated infections, immobility).

  ○ Arthritis.

  ○ Fibromyalgia.

  ○ Neuropathy.

  ○ Diagnostic or treatment procedures (injection, intubation, radiation).

• The pain experience is affected by:

  ○ Age.

    ▪ Infants cannot verbalize or understand their pain.

(G) ▪ Older adult clients may have multiple pathologies that cause pain and limit function.

  ○ Fatigue, which can increase sensitivity to pain.

  ○ Genetic sensitivity, which can increase or decrease the amount of pain tolerated.

  ○ Cognitive function.

    ▪ Clients who are cognitively impaired may not be able to report pain or report it accurately.

  ○ Prior experiences, which can increase or decrease sensitivity depending on whether or not adequate relief was obtained.

  ○ Anxiety and fear, which can increase sensitivity to pain.

       o   Support systems that are present and can decrease sensitivity to pain.

       o   Culture, which may influence how a client expresses pain or the meaning given to pain.

Assessment/Data Collection

- According to noted pain experts Margo McCaffery and Chris Pasero, pain is whatever the person experiencing it says it is, and it exists whenever the person says it does. The client's report of pain is the most reliable diagnostic measure of pain. Self-report using standardized pain scales is useful for clients over the age of 7 years. Specialized pain scales are available for use with younger children.

- Pain should be assessed and recorded frequently, and may be considered the fifth vital sign.

- Subjective data can be obtained using a symptom analysis.

DESCRIPTION	QUESTIONS
Location is described using anatomical terminology and landmarks.	Ask, "Where is your pain? Does it radiate anywhere else?" Ask the client to point to the location.
Quality refers to how the pain feels: sharp, dull, aching, burning, stabbing, pounding, throbbing, shooting, gnawing, tender, heavy, tight, tiring, exhausting, sickening, terrifying, torturing, nagging, annoying, intense, or unbearable.	Ask, "What does the pain feel like?" Give more than two choices ("Is the pain throbbing, burning, or stabbing?").
Intensity, strength, and severity are "measures" of the pain. Visual analog scales (description scale, number rating scale) can be used to: • Measure pain. • Monitor pain. • Evaluate the effectiveness of interventions.	Ask the following questions: • "How much pain do you have now?" • "What is the worst/best the pain has been?" • "Rate your pain on a scale of 0 to 10."
Timing – onset, duration, frequency	Ask the following questions: • "When did it start?" • "How long does it last?" • "How often does it occur?" • "Is it constant or intermittent?"
Setting – how the pain affects daily life or how activities of daily living (ADLs) affect the pain	Ask the following questions: • "Where are you when the symptoms occur?" • "What are you doing when the symptoms occur?" • "How does the pain affect your sleep?" • "How does the pain affect your ability to work and do your job?"

DESCRIPTION	QUESTIONS
Associated symptoms that should be noted include fatigue, depression, nausea, and anxiety.	Ask, "What other symptoms do you experience when you are feeling pain?"
Aggravating/relieving factors	Ask the following questions: • "What makes the pain better?" • "What makes the pain worse?" • "Are you currently taking any prescription, herbal, or over-the-counter medications?"

 View Media Supplement: Pain Assessment (Video)

- Objective Data
    - Behaviors complement self-report and assist in pain assessment of nonverbal clients.
        - Facial expressions (grimacing, wrinkled forehead), body movements (restlessness, pacing, guarding)
        - Moaning, crying
        - Decreased attention span
- Blood pressure, pulse, and respiratory rate are temporarily increased by acute pain. Eventually, increases in vital signs will stabilize despite the persistence of pain. Therefore, physiologic indicators may not be an accurate measure of pain over time.

Nonpharmacological Pain Management

- Cutaneous (skin) stimulation – transcutaneous electrical nerve stimulation (TENS), heat, cold, therapeutic touch, and massage
    - Interruption of pain pathways
    - Cold for inflammation
    - Heat to increase blood flow and to reduce stiffness
- Distraction
    - Includes ambulation, deep breathing, visitors, television, and music
- Relaxation
    - Includes meditation, yoga, and progressive muscle relaxation
- Imagery
    - Focusing on a pleasant thought to divert focus
    - Requires an ability to concentrate

- Acupuncture – vibration or electrical stimulation via tiny needles inserted into the skin and subcutaneous tissues at specific points

- Reduction of pain stimuli in the environment

- Elevation of edematous extremities to promote venous return and decrease swelling

Pharmacological Interventions

- Analgesics are the mainstay for relieving pain. The three classes of analgesics are nonopioids, opioids, and adjuvants.

- Nonopioid analgesics (acetaminophen, nonsteroidal anti-inflammatory drugs [NSAIDs], including salicylates) are appropriate for treating mild to moderate pain.

  o Be aware of the hepatotoxic effects of acetaminophen. A client with a healthy liver should take no more than 4 g/day. Therefore, the client should be aware of opioids that contain acetaminophen, such as hydrocodone bitartrate 5/acetaminophen 500 (Vicodin).

  o Monitor for salicylism (tinnitus, vertigo, decreased hearing acuity).

  o Prevent gastric upset by administering the medication with food or antacids.

  o Monitor for bleeding with long-term NSAID use.

- Opioid analgesics, such as morphine sulfate, fentanyl (Sublimaze), and codeine, are appropriate for treating moderate to severe pain (postoperative pain, myocardial infarction pain, cancer pain).

  o Managing acute severe pain with short-term (24 to 48 hr) around-the-clock administration of opioids is preferred to following a PRN schedule.

  o The parenteral route is preferred for immediate, short-term relief of acute pain. The oral route is preferred for chronic, nonfluctuating pain.

  o Consistent timing and dosing of opioid administration provide consistent pain control.

  o It is essential to monitor and intervene for adverse effects of opioid use.

    ▪ Constipation – Use a preventative approach (monitoring of bowel movements, fluids, fiber intake, exercise, stool softeners, stimulant laxatives, enemas).

    ▪ Orthostatic hypotension – Advise the client to sit or lie down if symptoms of lightheadedness or dizziness occur. Instruct the client to avoid sudden changes in position by slowly moving from a lying to a sitting or standing position. Provide assistance with ambulation as needed.

    ▪ Urinary retention – Monitor the client's I&O, assess for distention, administer bethanechol (Urecholine), and catheterize as prescribed.

    ▪ Nausea/vomiting – Administer antiemetics, advise the client to lie still and/or move slowly, and eliminate odors.

- Sedation – Monitor the client's level of consciousness and take safety precautions. Sedation usually precedes respiratory depression.

- Respiratory depression – Monitor the client's respiratory rate prior to and following administration of opioids (especially in clients who are opioid-naïve). Initial treatment of respiratory depression and sedation is generally a reduction in opioid dose. If necessary, slowly administer diluted naloxone (Narcan) as prescribed to reverse opioid effects.

- Adjuvant analgesics enhance the effects of nonopioids, help alleviate other symptoms that aggravate pain (depression, seizures, inflammation), and are useful for treating neuropathic pain.

  - Adjuvant medications include:

    - Anticonvulsants: carbamazepine (Tegretol).

    - Antianxiety agents: diazepam (Valium).

    - Tricyclic antidepressants: amitriptyline (Elavil).

    - Antihistamine: hydroxyzine (Vistaril).

    - Glucocorticoids: dexamethasone (Decadron).

    - Antiemetics: ondansetron hydrochloride (Zofran)

- Patient-controlled analgesia (PCA) is a medication delivery system that allows the client to self-administer safe doses of opioid narcotics.

  - Constant plasma levels are maintained by small, frequent doses.

  - The client experiences less lag time between identified need and delivery of medication, which increases the client's sense of control and may decrease the amount of medication needed.

  - Morphine sulfate and hydromorphone (Dilaudid) are commonly used opioids.

  - Client teaching is an important aspect of successful PCA therapy.

  - The client is the only person who should push the PCA button to prevent inadvertent overdosing.

- Other strategies for effective pain management include:

  - Taking a proactive approach by giving analgesics before pain becomes too severe. It takes less medication to prevent pain than to treat pain.

  - Instructing the client to report developing or recurrent pain and not wait until pain is severe (for PRN orders of pain medication).

  - Educating the client regarding misconceptions about pain.

  - Assisting the client to reduce fear and anxiety.

  - Creating a treatment plan that includes both nonpharmacological and pharmacological pain relief measures.

Complications and Nursing Implications

- Undertreatment of pain is a serious complication and may lead to increased anxiety with acute pain and depression with chronic pain. Assess/monitor the client for pain frequently, and intervene as appropriate.

- Sedation, respiratory depression, and coma can occur as a result of overdosing. Sedation always precedes respiratory depression.

  - o Identify high-risk clients (older adult clients, clients who are opioid-naïve).

  - o Carefully titrate doses while closely monitoring respiratory status.

  - o Stop the opioid and give the antagonist naloxone (Narcan) if the client's respirations are less than 8/min and shallow, or the client is difficult to arouse.

  - o Identify the cause of sedation.

  - o Use a sedation scale in addition to a pain rating scale to assess a client's pain, especially when administering opioids.

CHAPTER 41: PAIN MANAGEMENT

 Application Exercises

1. A nurse is assessing the pain level of a client who has come to the emergency department reporting severe abdominal pain. The nurse asks the client if he has experienced nausea and vomiting. The nurse is assessing which of the following?

    A. Presence of associated symptoms

    B. Location of the pain

    C. Pain quality

    D. Aggravating and relieving factors

2. Frequent pain assessment includes quantifying the intensity of the pain. A nurse can best assess the intensity of a client's pain by

    A. asking what precipitates the pain.

    B. questioning the client about the location of the pain.

    C. offering the client a pain scale to measure his pain.

    D. using open-ended questions to identify the sensation.

3. Which of the following statements are true regarding pain? (Select all that apply.)

    _____ All cultures have the same attitudes regarding pain.

    _____ Pain can cause feelings of anger and guilt.

    _____ It may be difficult to assess pain adequately in a client who is cognitively impaired.

    _____ A client who is sleeping could not be experiencing pain.

    _____ It is best to wait until pain is severe before administering analgesics.

4. A nurse obtaining a history from a client who has pain knows that

    A. most clients exaggerate their level of pain.

    B. pain must have an identifiable source to justify the use of opioids.

    C. objective data are essential in assessing pain.

    D. pain is whatever the client says it is.

5. Match the following types of pain with their descriptors: V = Visceral, S = Somatic, and N = Neuropathic.

    _____ Phantom limb pain

    _____ Referred pain

    _____ Fracture pain

    _____ Burning, "pins and needles" pain

    _____ Sharp, aching pain

6. A nurse is assessing a client who had surgery 3 hr ago. The client reports incisional pain of 7 on a scale of 0 to 10. His pulse, respirations, and blood pressure are elevated, and his pupils are dilated. Explain these physical findings in relation to his pain.

7. A nurse is assessing a client with pneumonia who also has a history of osteoarthritis of her knees. Although she is reporting pain of 6 on a scale of 0 to 10, her vital signs are within the expected range, and she does not show any muscle tension. Explain these physical findings in relation to her pain.

CHAPTER 41: PAIN MANAGEMENT

 Application Exercises Answer Key

1. A nurse is assessing the pain level of a client who has come to the emergency department reporting severe abdominal pain. The nurse asks the client if he has experienced nausea and vomiting. The nurse is assessing which of the following?

   A. Presence of associated symptoms

   B. Location of the pain

   C. Pain quality

   D. Aggravating and relieving factors

   Nausea and vomiting are common associated symptoms experienced with pain. The location of the pain is where the client feels the pain. Pain quality is assessed by identifying what the pain feels like, such as throbbing and aggravating. Aggravating and relieving factors are what might make the pain better or worse.

    NCLEX® Connection: Reduction of Risk Potential, System Specific Assessment

2. Frequent pain assessment includes quantifying the intensity of the pain. A nurse can best assess the intensity of a client's pain by

   A. asking what precipitates the pain.

   B. questioning the client about the location of the pain.

   C. offering the client a pain scale to measure his pain.

   D. using open-ended questions to identify the sensation.

   A pain scale can help the client measure the amount of pain he has and its intensity. Assessment of pain triggers and identification of the location of the client's pain will provide valuable information to help select pain-control interventions. But neither provides information about the intensity of pain. Asking open-ended questions is important in pain assessment, but it does not provide for consistent quantification of pain intensity.

    NCLEX® Connection: Reduction of Risk Potential, System Specific Assessment

3. Which of the following statements are true regarding pain? (Select all that apply.)

        All cultures have the same attitudes regarding pain.

** X   Pain can cause feelings of anger and guilt.**

** X   It may be difficult to assess pain adequately in a client who is cognitively impaired.**

        A client who is sleeping could not be experiencing pain.

        It is best to wait until pain is severe before administering analgesics.

Clients may experience feelings of anger and guilt with pain. Clients who are cognitively impaired may not be able to express what they are feeling. Attitudes about pain vary among different cultures. A client can still sleep even when experiencing pain; clients need less pain medication when pain is treated before it becomes severe.

Ⓝ **NCLEX® Connection: Reduction of Risk Potential, System Specific Assessment**

4. A nurse obtaining a history from a client who has pain knows that

A. most clients exaggerate their level of pain.

B. pain must have an identifiable source to justify the use of opioids.

C. objective data are essential in assessing pain.

D. pain is whatever the client says it is.

Pain is a subjective experience, and the client is the best source of information about it. A misconception about pain is that clients exaggerate their pain level. The client can experience pain without being able to identify the source. Objective data are not always present when the client is experiencing pain.

Ⓝ **NCLEX® Connection: Reduction of Risk Potential, System Specific Assessment**

5. Match the following types of pain with their descriptors: V = Visceral, S = Somatic, and N = Neuropathic.

  N   Phantom limb pain

  V   Referred pain

  S   Fracture pain

  N   Burning, "pins and needles" pain

  S   Sharp, aching pain

Ⓝ **NCLEX® Connection: Reduction of Risk Potential, System Specific Assessment**

6. A nurse is assessing a client who had surgery 3 hr ago. The client reports incisional pain of 7 on a scale of 0 to 10. His pulse, respirations, and blood pressure are elevated, and his pupils are dilated. Explain these physical findings in relation to his pain.

> **Pain elicits a physiological response from the sympathetic nervous system. The client can experience tachycardia, hypertension, anxiety, diaphoresis, muscle tension, pallor, and dilated pupils.**

 NCLEX® Connection: Reduction of Risk Potential, Changes/Abnormal Vital Signs

7. A nurse is assessing a client with pneumonia who also has a history of osteoarthritis of her knees. Although she is reporting pain of 6 on a scale of 0 to 10, her vital signs are within the expected range, and she does not show any muscle tension. Explain these physical findings in relation to her pain.

> **As the pain continues, the body is not able to sustain the level of sympathetic response, and the parasympathetic nervous system takes over. The client can still be experiencing pain without showing a physiological response to it.**

 NCLEX® Connection: Reduction of Risk Potential, Changes/Abnormal Vital Signs

UNIT 4	PHYSIOLOGICAL INTEGRITY
Section	Basic Care and Comfort
Chapter 42	Complementary and Alternative Therapies

@ Overview

- Interest in the use of complementary and alternative therapies continues to grow. These therapies are also referred to as complementary or alternative medicine (CAM).

- Alternative therapies are unconventional treatment approaches used instead of conventional medical care.

- Complementary therapies are unconventional treatment approaches used in addition to or to enhance conventional medical care.

- Many health care entities are developing programs of integrative medicine or integrative therapies to provide clients with conventional and unconventional health care choices.

- These therapies can especially be effective for chronic health problems.

- An important prerequisite for implementing complementary or alternative therapies is the client's acceptance of and involvement in the therapeutic intervention.

- Categories of CAM include:

  o Alternative medical philosophy (traditional Chinese medicine, acupuncture, homeopathy).

  o Biological and botanical therapies (diets, vitamins, minerals, herbal preparations).

  o Body manipulation (massage, touch, chiropractic therapy).

  o Mind-body therapies (biofeedback, art therapy, meditation, yoga, psychotherapy, tai chi).

  o Energy therapies (Reiki, therapeutic touch)

Nursing and CAM

- Nurses should:

  o Possess knowledge about the varieties of therapies available.

  o Be receptive to learning about a client's alternative health beliefs and practices (home remedies, cultural practices, vitamin use, modification of prescriptions).

  o Identify the client's needs for complementary or alternative therapies.

  o Incorporate complementary or alternative therapies into the client's care plan.

- Specialized licensed or certified practitioners may provide complementary or alternative therapies. These include:

THERAPY	CHARACTERISTICS
Acupuncture/pressure	Needles or pressure along meridians alters body function or produces analgesia.
Homeopathic medicine	Small doses of substances (remedies) that would produce symptoms of the disease state in a well person are given to ill clients to bring about healing.
Naturopathic medicine	Diet, exercise, environment, and herbal remedies are used to promote the natural healing of the body.
Chiropractic medicine	Clients are treated by manipulation of the spine.
Massage therapy	Relaxation and circulation are improved through stretching and loosening muscles and connective tissue.
Biofeedback	Technology is used to increase the client's awareness of various neurological body responses to minimize extremes.
Therapeutic touch	Practitioners use their hands to help bring the client's energy fields into balance.

- Nursing interventions can provide some aspects of complementary alternative therapies, including:

THERAPY	CHARACTERISTICS
Guided imagery/visualization therapy	Encourages healing and relaxation of the body by having the mind focus on images
Healing intention	Techniques that use caring, compassion, and empathy in the context of prayer to facilitate healing
Breath work	Various breathing patterns used to reduce stress and increase relaxation
Humor	A coping mechanism used to reduce tension and improve mood
Meditation	A technique used to calm the mind and body
Simple touch	Communicates presence, appreciation, and acceptance
Music therapy	Type of relaxation therapy that provides distraction from pain; earphones encourage improvement of concentration
Therapeutic communication	Allows clients to verbalize and become aware of emotions and fears in a safe, nonjudgmental environment

- Nurses evaluate the outcomes of complementary alternative therapies and revise the nursing care plan as necessary.

CHAPTER 42: COMPLEMENTARY AND ALTERNATIVE THERAPIES

 Application Exercises

1. A nurse admits a client for abdominal surgery. The client's initial vital signs are temperature 37° C (98.6° F), pulse 98/min, respirations 20/min, and blood pressure 148/88 mm Hg. The client states, "I am really worried. This is the first surgery I have ever had." Which of the following is an appropriate use of a complementary alternative intervention?

    A. Offer information and ask the client if he is interested in trying a relaxation technique.

    B. Call the provider and get permission to use relaxation techniques with the client.

    C. Provide the client with reassurance and information about the procedure.

    D. Give the client a therapeutic back massage and tell him to try to relax.

2. A nurse is caring for a client who reports back pain and tells the nurse that a friend has recommended a chiropractor. She asks the nurse what a chiropractor does to relieve back pain. Which of the following responses by the nurse is correct?

    A. "Chiropractors use their hands to manipulate the spine to treat back pain."

    B. "Chiropractors insert needles or put pressure along meridians in the back."

    C. "Chiropractors use herbal remedies to treat back pain."

    D. "Chiropractors use their hands to balance the energy fields in the back."

3. Massage therapy is an example of which category of alternative therapy?

    A. Alternative medical philosophy

    B. Biological therapy

    C. Body manipulation

    D. Mind-body therapy

4. Match the following complementary or alternative therapies with the requirements for performing the techniques.

    _____ Relaxation techniques   A. Within the scope of nursing practice

    _____ Therapeutic touch   B. Additional certification or license required

    _____ Humor

    _____ Acupuncture

    _____ Chiropractic techniques

    _____ Therapeutic communication

CHAPTER 42: COMPLEMENTARY AND ALTERNATIVE THERAPIES

 Application Exercises Answer Key

1. A nurse admits a client for abdominal surgery. The client's initial vital signs are temperature 37° C (98.6° F), pulse 98/min, respirations 20/min, and blood pressure 148/88 mm Hg. The client states, "I am really worried. This is the first surgery I have ever had." Which of the following is an appropriate use of a complementary alternative intervention?

   A. Offer information and ask the client if he is interested in trying a relaxation technique.

   B. Call the provider and get permission to use relaxation techniques with the client.

   C. Provide the client with reassurance and information about the procedure.

   D. Give the client a therapeutic back massage and tell him to try to relax.

   Providing information will help the client to make an informed decision. A provider's order is not required for relaxation therapy. Providing reassurance may negate the client's fear. Providing more information without validating this as a need may increase his anxiety. The nurse should not give any therapy without informing the client and obtaining his consent. Telling him to relax does not acknowledge the impact of his anxiety.

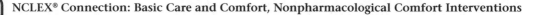 NCLEX® Connection: Basic Care and Comfort, Nonpharmacological Comfort Interventions

2. A nurse is caring for a client who reports back pain and tells the nurse that a friend has recommended a chiropractor. She asks the nurse what a chiropractor does to relieve back pain. Which of the following responses by the nurse is correct?

   A. "Chiropractors use their hands to manipulate the spine to treat back pain."

   B. "Chiropractors insert needles or put pressure along meridians in the back."

   C. "Chiropractors use herbal remedies to treat back pain."

   D. "Chiropractors use their hands to balance the energy fields in the back."

   Chiropractors use their hands to manipulate the spine. Acupuncture involves needles or pressure. Naturopathic medicine uses herbal remedies, and therapeutic touch practitioners use their hands to balance energy fields.

NCLEX® Connection: Basic Care and Comfort, Nonpharmacological Comfort Interventions

3. Massage therapy is an example of which category of alternative therapy?

    A. Alternative medical philosophy

    B. Biological therapy

    C. Body manipulation

    D. Mind-body therapy

Massage therapy is one type of body manipulation therapy. Alternative medical philosophy includes acupuncture and homeopathy. Biological therapy includes diet, vitamin and mineral supplementation, and herbal remedies. Mind-body therapy includes biofeedback, meditation, and psychotherapy.

Ⓝ NCLEX® Connection: Basic Care and Comfort, Nonpharmacological Comfort Interventions

4. Match the following complementary or alternative therapies with the requirements for performing the techniques.

__A__	Relaxation techniques	A. Within the scope of nursing practice
__B__	Therapeutic touch	B. Additional certification or license required
__A__	Humor	
__B__	Acupuncture	
__B__	Chiropractic techniques	
__A__	Therapeutic communication	

Ⓝ NCLEX® Connection: Basic Care and Comfort, Nonpharmacological Comfort Interventions

UNIT 4	PHYSIOLOGICAL INTEGRITY
Section	Basic Care and Comfort
Chapter 43	Bowel Elimination

Overview

- Interventions such as surgery, immobility, medications, and therapeutic diets may affect bowel elimination.

- Constipation is defined as bowel movements that are infrequent, hard or dry, and difficult to pass.

- Diarrhea is defined as an increased number of loose, liquid stools.

- There are objective ways to assess for the presence of constipation or diarrhea, but individual bowel patterns vary greatly.

- Various disease processes necessitate the creation of bowel diversions to allow fecal elimination to continue.

- Stool specimens are collected both for screening and for diagnostic tests, such as for the detection of occult blood, bacteria, or parasites.

Bowel Elimination Needs and Specimen Collection

- Collect stool specimens for serial fecal occult blood (guaiac) testing three times from three different defecations. Stool samples should come from fresh stools that are not contaminated with water or urine.

- Bowel diversions through ostomies are temporary or permanent openings (stomas) in the abdominal wall to allow fecal matter to pass.

- End stomas are a result of colorectal cancer or some types of bowel disease. Colostomies end in the colon, and ileostomies end in the ileum.

- Loop colostomies are performed as a medical emergency and are temporary.

- Double-barrel colostomies consist of two abdominal stomas – one proximal and one distal.

FACTORS AFFECTING NORMAL BOWEL ELIMINATION	

Age	• Infants:
	   ○ Breast milk stools – watery and yellow brown
	   ○ Formula stools – pasty and brown
	• Toddlers: bowel control at 2 to 3 years old
	• Older adults: decreased peristalsis, relaxation of sphincters

Diet	• Fiber requirement: 25 to 30 g/day • Lactose intolerance: difficulty digesting milk products
Fluids	• Fluid requirement: 2,000 to 3,000 mL/day from fluid and food sources
Physical activity	• Stimulates intestinal activity
Psychosocial factors	• Emotional distress increasing peristalsis and exacerbating chronic conditions (colitis, Crohn's disease, ulcers, irritable bowel syndrome) • Depression decreases peristalsis and can lead to constipation.
Personal habits	• Use of public toilets, false perception of the need for "one-a-day" bowel movements, lack of privacy when hospitalized
Positioning	• Normal: squatting • Immobilized client: difficulty defecating
Pain	• Normal defecation is painless. Discomfort leads to suppression of the urge to defecate. • Opioid use contributing to constipation
Pregnancy	• Growing fetus compromising intestinal space • Slower peristalsis • Straining increasing the risk of hemorrhoids
Surgery and anesthesia	• Temporary slowing of intestinal activity • Paralytic ileus – rationale for auscultating bowel sounds before advancing a client's diet
Medications	• Laxatives – to soften stool • Cathartics – to promote peristalsis • Laxative abuse leading to diarrhea and dehydration

- Diagnostic Tests

  - Visualization of the bowel

    - Colonoscopy – the large colon and sometimes a portion of the lower small bowel are visualized and may be biopsied.

    - Sigmoidoscopy – the sigmoid colon and rectum are visualized and may be biopsied.

- Preparation
  - All require the client to be NPO for 12 hr prior to the procedure and to ingest nothing but clear liquids 24 hr prior to the procedure.
  - A bowel prep using laxatives is commonly prescribed.
  - Moderate (conscious) sedation with a benzodiazepine and an opioid is commonly used, and the client is not permitted to drive home afterwards.

Collaborative Care

- Promoting healthy bowel elimination

EQUIPMENT	PROCEDURE

• Bedpans
  o Fracture pan – for supine clients and clients in body casts or leg casts
  o Regular pan – for seated clients
• Beside commode
• Toilet
• Adequate fiber in the diet
• Adequate fluid intake – minimum of 1,500 mL/day of water and/or juices
• Adequate activity – walking 15 to 20 min/day if mobile and exercises in bed or chair (pelvic tilt, single leg lifts, lower trunk rotation)
	• Encourage the client to set aside time to defecate – sometimes after a meal works best.
	• If not contraindicated or restricted, encourage the client to drink plenty of fluids and to consume a diet high in fiber to prevent constipation.
	• Wear gloves when addressing toileting needs.
	• Provide privacy.
	• Assist the client to a sitting position whether using a regular bedpan, commode, or toilet.
	• For clients using a fracture pan, raise the head of the bed to 30°.
	• If the client cannot lift his hips to get the bedpan under him, roll him onto one side, position the bedpan over his buttocks, and roll the client back onto the bedpan.
	• Encourage the client to decrease stress when sitting or rising by using an elevated toilet seat or a footstool.
	• Never leave a client lying flat on a regular bedpan.
	• After the client defecates, provide skin care to the perianal area.

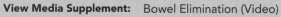

View Media Supplement: Bowel Elimination (Video)

- Specimen Collection

EQUIPMENT	PROCEDURE

• Appropriate specimen container
• Soap/cleansing solution or wipe
• Gloves
• Specimen label
• Fecal occult blood test cards
• Wooden applicator or tongue depressor
• Developer solution
• Stool collection container (bedside commode, bedpan, receptacle in toilet)
	• Fecal occult blood testing (guaiac test)
	  ○ Explain the procedure to the client.
	  ○ Ask the client to collect a specimen in the toilet receptacle, bedpan, or bedside commode.
	  ○ Apply gloves, and, with a wooden applicator, place small amounts of stool on the windows of the test card or as directed.
	  ○ Follow the facility's procedures for handling.
	    ■ Apply a label to the cards and send them to the laboratory for processing.
	    ■ Or, if for point-of-care testing, place a couple of drops of developer on the opposite side of the card as directed. A blue color is positive for blood.
	  ○ Remove the gloves and perform hand hygiene.
	• Stool for culture, parasites, and ova
	  ○ Explain the procedure to the client.
	  ○ Ask the client to collect the specimen in the toilet receptacle, bedside commode, or bedpan.
	  ○ Put on gloves.
	  ○ Use a wooden tongue depressor to transfer the stool to a specimen container.
	  ○ Label the container with the client's identifying information.
	  ○ Remove the gloves.
	  ○ Perform hand hygiene.
	  ○ Transport the specimen to the laboratory.

- Cleansing enema – The height of the bag above the rectum determines the depth of cleansing.

EQUIPMENT	PROCEDURE
<ul><li>Gloves</li><li>Lubricant</li><li>Absorbent, waterproof pads</li><li>Bedpan, beside commode, or toilet</li><li>IV pole</li><li>Enema bag with tubing or prepackaged enema</li><li>Solutions and additives – varying with the type of enema given<ul><li>Tap water or hypotonic solution<ul><li>Stimulates evacuation</li><li>Never repeated due to potential water toxicity</li></ul></li><li>Soapsuds<ul><li>Pure castile soap in tap water or normal saline</li><li>Acts as an irritant to promote bowel peristalsis</li></ul></li><li>Normal saline<ul><li>Safest due to equal osmotic pressure</li><li>Volume stimulates peristalsis</li></ul></li><li>Low-volume hypertonic<ul><li>Good for clients who cannot tolerate high-volume enemas</li><li>Fleet® – a commercially prepared hypertonic enema</li></ul></li><li>Oil retention – lubricates the rectum and colon for easier passage of stool</li><li>Medicated enemas – contains medications to be retained</li></ul></li></ul>	<ul><li>Perform hand hygiene.</li><li>Prepare the enema solution.</li><li>Pour the solution into the enema bag, allowing it to fill the tubing, and then close the clamp.</li><li>Explain the procedure to the client.</li><li>Provide privacy.</li><li>Provide quick access to a commode or bedpan.</li><li>Place absorbent pads under the client to protect the bed linens.</li><li>Position the client on the left side with the right leg flexed forward.</li><li>Put on gloves.</li><li>Lubricate the rectal tube or nozzle.</li><li>Slowly insert the rectal tube 3 to 4 in (7.5 to 10 cm). For a child, insert the tube 2 to 3 in (5 to 7.5 cm).</li><li>With the bag level with the client's hip, open the clamp.</li><li>Raise the bag 30 to 45 cm above the anus, depending on the level of cleansing desired.</li><li>Slow the flow of solution if the client reports cramping, or if fluid leaks around the tube at the anus.</li><li>If using a prepackaged solution, insert the lubricated tip into the rectum and squeeze the container until the solution is administered.</li><li>Ask the client to retain the solution for the prescribed amount of time, or until the client is no longer able to retain it.</li><li>Discard the enema bag and tubing.</li><li>Assist the client to the appropriate position to defecate.</li><li>Remove the gloves.</li><li>Perform hand hygiene.</li><li>For clients who have little or no sphincter control, administer the enema on a bedpan.</li><li>Document the results and the client's tolerance of the procedure.</li></ul>

- Ostomy Care

EQUIPMENT	PROCEDURE
• Pouch system (skin barrier and pouch) • Pouch closure clamp • Barrier pastes (optional) • Gloves • Washcloths • Towel • Warm water • Scissors • Pen	• If an enterostomal therapist (RN) is not available, educate the client about stoma care. • Perform hand hygiene. • Put on gloves. • Remove the pouch from the stoma. • Inspect the stoma. It should appear moist, shiny, and pink. The peristomal area should be intact, and the skin should appear healthy. • Use mild soap and water to cleanse the skin, then dry it gently and completely. • Apply paste if used. • Measure and draw where to cut the skin barrier, allowing only the stoma to appear through the opening. • Cut the opening in the skin barrier. • If necessary, apply barrier pastes to creases. • Apply the skin barrier and pouch. • Fold the bottom of the pouch and place the closure clamp on the pouch. • Dispose of the used pouch. Remove the gloves and perform hand hygiene.

Complications

- Constipation

  o Signs and symptoms – bowel pattern of difficult and infrequent evacuation of hard, dry feces

  o May be the result of improper diet, decreased fluid intake, lack of exercise, or side effects of certain medications.

  o Increase fiber and water consumption before treating constipation with laxatives.

  o Bulk-forming products are used before stool softeners, stimulants, or suppositories to promote bowel elimination.

  o Enemas are a last resort for stimulating defecation.

- Impaction
  - Signs and symptoms – stool that is wedged into the rectum with diarrhea fluid leaking around the impacted stool
  - Digital removal of the stool is done using a gloved and lubricated finger.
  - The stool is loosened around the edges and then removed in small pieces, allowing the client to rest as necessary.
  - When evacuating the rectum, be careful to avoid stimulating the vagus nerve.

- Diarrhea
  - Signs and symptoms – frequent, liquid stools caused by various disorders.
  - The cause must be determined and treated.
  - Medications to slow peristalsis may also be prescribed.
  - Provide good perineal care after each stool and apply a moisture barrier if indicated.
  - The client and caregivers should perform hand hygiene frequently.

- Fecal Incontinence
  - Signs and symptoms – the inability to control defecation, often caused by diarrhea
  - Assess the client for causes, such as medications, infections, or impaction.
  - Provide perineal care after each stool and apply a moisture barrier if indicated.

- Flatulence
  - Signs and symptoms – the distention of the bowel from gas accumulation (may cause cramping or a feeling of fullness)
    - Assess the client for abdominal distention and the ability to pass gas through the anus.
    - If mobile, encourage the client to ambulate to promote the passage of flatus.
    - Notify the provider if the problem continues.

- Hemorrhoids
  - Signs and symptoms – engorged, dilated blood vessels in the rectal wall caused by difficult defecation, pregnancy, liver disease, and heart failure
    - Hemorrhoids may be itchy, painful, and bloody after defecation.
    - When cleansing the perianal area, moist wipes may be more comfortable.
    - Application of prescribed ointments or creams may help.

CONSTIPATION AND DIARRHEA

(G) • For healthy clients, constipation and diarrhea are not serious. But for older adult clients and clients with pre-existing health problems, constipation and diarrhea can be serious.

- Causes of constipation include:

  o Frequent use of laxatives.

  o Advanced age.

  o Inadequate fluid intake.

  o Inadequate fiber intake.

  o Immobilization due to injury.

  o A sedentary lifestyle.

- Causes of diarrhea include:

  o Viral gastroenteritis.

  o Bacterial gastroenteritis.

  o Overuse of laxatives.

  o Use of certain antibiotics.

  o Inflammatory bowel disease.

  o Irritable bowel syndrome.

  o Food-borne pathogens.

Assessment/Data Collection

- Monitor for signs and symptoms of constipation.

  o Abdominal bloating

  o Abdominal cramping

  o Straining at defecation

- Monitor for signs and symptoms of diarrhea.

  o Signs and symptoms of dehydration (postural hypotension, dizziness when changing positions)

  o Frequent loose stools

  o Abdominal cramping

- Collect assessment data.

  o Perform a physical examination of the abdomen (bowel sounds, tenderness) daily.

  o Assess for signs and symptoms of fluid deficit.

- Assess skin integrity around the anal area.

- Collect a detailed history of the client's diet, exercise, and bowel habits.

- Perform specimen collection and diagnostic testing.

  - Fecal occult blood test – a fecal sample is obtained using medical asepsis while wearing disposable gloves. Some foods (red meat, fish, poultry, raw vegetables) and medications can cause false positive results. Bleeding can be a sign of cancer, which can be a contributing factor for constipation.

  - Digital rectal examination for impaction – the client should be positioned on the left side with the knees flexed. The examiner inserts a gloved, lubricated index finger gently into the rectum. During the procedure, the client's vital signs and response should be monitored.

  - Specimens for stool cultures – these are obtained using medical asepsis while wearing disposable gloves. The specimen should be labeled and promptly sent to the laboratory. Intestinal bacteria can be a contributing factor for diarrhea.

Collaborative Care

- Closely monitor the client's fluid status. Maintain a strict record of intake and output.

- Monitor the client for signs and symptoms of dehydration.

- Closely monitor the client's elimination pattern.

- Observe and document the character of the client's bowel movements.

- Carefully check for blood or pus. If the client is experiencing diarrhea, measure the volume of the stools.

- Administer laxatives and/or enemas as prescribed.

- Encourage the client to drink enough fluids (especially water), eat enough fiber, and exercise moderately.

- Suggest that clients who are taking antibiotics eat yogurt to help re-establish an intestinal balance of beneficial bacteria.

Complications

- Complications of constipation include:

  - Fecal impaction.

  - Development of hemorrhoids or rectal fissures.

  - Bradycardia, hypotension, and syncope associated with the Valsalva maneuver (occurs with straining/bearing down).

- o Interventions

    - ▪ Monitor constipation carefully. Instruct clients not to strain to have bowel movements. Encourage measures to treat and prevent constipation.

    - ▪ Remove fecal impactions. This is often preceded by administration of a glycerin or bisacodyl (Dulcolax) suppository.

- • Complications of diarrhea include:

    - o Signs and symptoms of dehydration and fluid and electrolyte disturbances (metabolic acidosis caused by excessive loss of bicarbonate).

    - o Skin breakdown around the anal area.

    - o Interventions

        - ▪ Replace losses as prescribed.

        - ▪ Provide appropriate care and treatment for any skin breakdown.

(G) Meeting the Needs of Older Adults

- • Older adult clients are more susceptible to developing constipation as bowel tone decreases with age, and they are more at risk for developing fecal impaction.

- • Adequate fluid and fiber intake and exercise are very important.

- • Older adult clients are less able to compensate for fluid lost due to diarrhea.

CHAPTER 43: BOWEL ELIMINATION

 Application Exercises

1. A nurse is caring for a client who will perform fecal occult blood testing at home. Which of the following should the nurse include when explaining the procedure to the client?

    A. Eating more protein is recommended prior to testing.

    B. One stool specimen is sufficient for testing.

    C. A red color change indicates a positive test.

    D. The specimen cannot be contaminated with urine.

2. A nurse is caring for a client for whom a tap water enema is prescribed, to be repeated until the return is clear. Which of the following actions should the nurse take?

    A. Clarify the order with the provider.

    B. Explain the procedure to the client.

    C. Ensure that the tap water is not too hot.

    D. Keep the amount per enema to less than 1,000 mL.

3. Which of the following foods should a nurse encourage for a client who is experiencing constipation?

    A. Macaroni and cheese

    B. Fresh fruit and whole wheat toast

    C. Beef tips and noodles

    D. Mashed potatoes and gravy

4. A nurse is caring for a client who has had diarrhea for the past 4 days. When assessing the client, the nurse should expect which of the following findings? (Select all that apply.)

    _____ Bradycardia

    _____ Hypotension

    _____ Fever

    _____ Poor skin turgor

    _____ Peripheral edema

    _____ Abdominal cramping

CHAPTER 43: BOWEL ELIMINATION

 Application Exercises Answer Key

1. A nurse is caring for a client who will perform fecal occult blood testing at home. Which of the following should the nurse include when explaining the procedure to the client?

    A. Eating more protein is recommended prior to testing.

    B. One stool specimen is sufficient for testing.

    C. A red color change indicates a positive test.

    D. The specimen cannot be contaminated with urine.

    For fecal occult blood testing at home, the stool specimens cannot be contaminated with water or urine; three specimens from three different bowel movements are required; some proteins such as red meat, fish, and poultry can alter the test results; and a blue color indicates blood in the stool.

 NCLEX® Connection: Basic Care and Comfort, Elimination

2. A nurse is caring for a client for whom a tap water enema is prescribed, to be repeated until the return is clear. Which of the following actions should the nurse take?

    A. Clarify the order with the provider.

    B. Explain the procedure to the client.

    C. Ensure that the tap water is not too hot.

    D. Keep the amount per enema to less than 1,000 mL.

    Tap water is a hypotonic solution that can cause water toxicity. It should not be repeated. The nurse should clarify the order with the provider. Explaining the procedure to the client, ensuring that the tap water is not too hot, and keeping the amount to less than 1,000 mL are not pertinent if the enema should not be repeated.

 NCLEX® Connection: Basic Care and Comfort, Elimination

3. Which of the following foods should a nurse encourage for a client who is experiencing constipation?

    A. Macaroni and cheese

    B. Fresh fruit and whole wheat toast

    C. Beef tips and noodles

    D. Mashed potatoes and gravy

    A high-fiber diet promotes normal bowel elimination. The choice of fruit and toast is the highest fiber option. Macaroni and cheese, beef tips and noodles, and mashed potatoes and gravy are lower-fiber options.

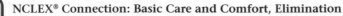 NCLEX® Connection: Basic Care and Comfort, Elimination

4. A nurse is caring for a client who has had diarrhea for the past 4 days. When assessing the client, the nurse should expect which of the following findings? (Select all that apply.)

_____ Bradycardia

__X__ **Hypotension**

__X__ **Fever**

__X__ **Poor skin turgor**

_____ Peripheral edema

__X__ **Abdominal cramping**

Prolonged diarrhea leads to dehydration, which is characterized by tachycardia, hypotension, fever, lethargy, poor skin turgor, and abdominal cramping. Peripheral edema is more likely to be caused by a fluid overload rather than a fluid deficit.

NCLEX® Connection: Basic Care and Comfort, Elimination

UNIT 4	PHYSIOLOGICAL INTEGRITY
Section	Basic Care and Comfort
Chapter 44	Urinary Elimination

Overview

- Urinary elimination is a precise system of filtration, reabsorption, and excretion. These processes help maintain fluid and electrolyte balance while filtering and excreting water-soluble wastes.

- The primary organs involved in urinary elimination are the kidneys, with the nephrons performing most of the functions of filtration and elimination. Most adults produce between 1,500 and 2,000 mL of urine per day.

- Once filtered, the urine passes through the ureters into the bladder, the storage reservoir for urine. Once an adequate amount of urine collects in the bladder (150 to 200 mL), a signal is sent to the brain to indicate the need to urinate. The person then relaxes the internal and external sphincters located at the bottom of the bladder and the urethra. Urine passes from the bladder through the urethra where it exits the body.

- Interventions such as surgery, immobility, medications, and therapeutic diets may affect a client's urinary elimination.

Urinary Diversions

- Urinary diversions – temporary or permanent, a stoma for the drainage of urine

    o Ureterostomy – one or both ureters to the abdominal surface

    o Nephrostomy – a tube from the renal pelvis to the abdominal surface

    o Pouched systems for urine diversions are similar to those for bowel diversions with similar body image concerns.

- Urinary diversions may be created for clients who have cancer of the bladder or injury to the bladder.

Factors Affecting Normal Urinary Elimination

- Age

    o Full bladder control by 4 to 5 years of age

    o Enlargement of the prostate after 40 years leading to urinary frequency, hesitancy, retention, incontinence, and urinary tract infections (UTIs).

- o Childbirth and gravity weaken the pelvic floor, putting clients at risk for prolapse of the bladder, leading to stress incontinence, which can be managed with pelvic floor (Kegel) exercises.

- o Older adult clients have:
    - Fewer nephrons
    - Loss of muscle tone of the bladder – frequency (Incontinence is not associated with normal aging, only neurological or mobility impairments.)
    - Inefficient emptying of the bladder – residual urine increasing the risk of UTIs
    - Increase in the incidence of nocturia

- Pregnancy
    - o A growing fetus compromises bladder space and compresses the bladder.
    - o There is a 30% to 50% increase in circulatory volume, which increases renal workload and output.
    - o The hormone relaxin causes relaxation of the sphincter.

- Diet
    - o An increase in sodium leads to decreased urination.
    - o Caffeine and alcohol intake lead to increased urination.

- Poor abdominal and pelvic muscle tone

- Acute and chronic disease conditions

- Spinal cord injury

- Immobility

- Psychosocial factors
    - o Emotional stress and anxiety
    - o Having to use public toilets, lack of privacy when hospitalized
    - o Not having enough time to urinate (predetermined bathroom breaks in elementary schools)

- Pain
    - o Suppression of the urge to urinate when there is pain in the urinary tract
    - o Obstruction in the ureter leading to renal colic
    - o Arthritis or painful joints causing immobility, which leads to delayed micturition

- Surgical procedures

  - Alterations in glomerular filtration rate from anesthesia/opioid analgesics, resulting in decreased urine output

  - Lower abdominal surgery creating obstructing edema and inflammation

- Medications

  - Diuretics preventing reabsorption of water

  - Antihistamines and anticholinergics causing urinary retention

  - Medications that change urine color:

    - Pyridium – orange

    - Amitriptyline – green/blue

    - Levodopa (Dopar) – brown/black

  - Chemotherapy creating a toxic environment for the kidneys

Diagnostic Tests

- Bedside sonography/bladder scanner – portable ultrasound scanner noninvasively measures bladder volume to measure residual volume after voiding

- KUB (kidneys/ureters/bladder) – x-ray to determine the size, shape, and position of the kidneys

- IVP (intravenous pyelogram) – contrast is used to view ducts, renal pelvis, ureters, bladder, and urethra. Iodine is used; therefore, it is important to determine if the client has an allergy to shellfish.

- Renal scan – view of renal blood flow and anatomy of the kidneys – no contrast

- Renal ultrasound – view of gross renal structures

- Cystoscopy – uses an endoscope to visualize the bladder and urethra

- Urodynamic testing – tests bladder muscle function by filling the bladder with CO_2 or 0.9% sodium chloride and comparing pressure readings with the client's reported sensations

Nursing Interventions

- Promoting Healthy Urinary Elimination

EQUIPMENT	PROCEDURE

• Urinal for men
• Toilet, bedpan, or commode
   ○ Fracture pan – for supine clients and clients in body or leg casts
   ○ Regular pan – for seated clients
	• Position the client in a sitting position when possible.
	• Provide for privacy needs with adequate time for urinating (generally, at least 30 min).

- I&O

EQUIPMENT	PROCEDURE
<ul><li>Hard plastic urometer on indwelling catheter sets is a reliable measuring tool on catheter bags.</li><li>Graduated cylinders, urinal, or toilet receptacle</li></ul>	<ul><li>Measure output from a bedpan, commode, or collection bag into a graduated container.</li><li>Use a receptacle to measure urine voided into the toilet.</li><li>Use markings on the side of the urinal to measure urine.</li><li>Less than 30 mL/hr for more than 2 hr is a cause for concern.</li></ul>

- Bladder retraining for the treatment of urge incontinence

EQUIPMENT	PROCEDURE
<ul><li>Clock</li></ul>	<ul><li>Use timed voidings to increase intervals between voidings/decrease voiding frequency.</li><li>Perform pelvic floor (Kegel) exercises.</li><li>Perform relaxation techniques.</li><li>Offer undergarments while the client is retraining.</li><li>Teach the client not to ignore the urge to void.</li><li>Provide positive reinforcement as the client maintains continence.</li><li>Eliminate or decrease caffeine drinks.</li><li>Take diuretics in the morning.</li></ul>

- Specimen Collection
    - Equipment
        - Appropriate specimen container
            - Nonsterile for urinalysis
            - Sterile for clean-catch midstream
        - Soap/cleansing solution or towel
        - Gloves
        - Specimen label
        - Urine collection container (catheter, urinal, receptacle in toilet, commode)

PROCEDURE	NURSING INTERVENTION
Urinalysis – random nonsterile specimen	• Explain the procedure to the client. • Ask the client to urinate. • Put on gloves. • Pour urine into the specimen container. • Label the container with the client's identifying information. • Remove gloves and perform hand hygiene. • Transport or send the specimen to the laboratory.
Clean-catch midstream (CCMS) for culture and sensitivity (C&S)	• Teach the client the technique for obtaining the specimen. • The urine sample is "caught" midstream after thorough cleansing of the urethral meatus. • The client voids some urine into a commode, bedpan, or urinal; stops; then urinates into a sterile cup. • The client needs to understand not to place his fingers in the cup and not to touch the lid.

Catheter urine specimen for C&S	• This requires a sterile specimen from a straight or indwelling catheter obtained using surgical asepsis (sterile technique).
	  o Drain the catheter's tubing of urine.
	  o Clamp the catheter's tubing below the port for 20 min.
	  o Use surgical asepsis while withdrawing the required amount from the port with a syringe.
	  o Unclamp the catheter.

Timed urine specimens	• These are usually collected for 24 hr but can be ordered for varying times. • Discard the first voiding. • Collect all other voidings in a container placed on ice. • If the client urinates and discards the urine, timing of the specimen must begin again with the next voiding.

- Straight or Indwelling Catheter Insertion

    o Equipment

        ▪ Correct size and type of catheter: usually 8 to 10 Fr for children, 14 to 16 Fr for women, and 16 to 18 Fr for men. (Use silicon or Teflon products for clients who have latex allergies.)

        ▪ Catheterization kit – with sterile drainage bag for indwelling catheter insertion

        ▪ Soap and water

        ▪ Collection container for straight catheterization

- ○ Procedure
  - Explain the procedure to the client.
  - Perform hand hygiene.
  - Establish a location in the room to set up a sterile field.
  - Provide privacy.
  - Lower the side rail, raise the bed to a comfortable height, and establish a good light source for the perineal area.
  - Position the client.
    - □ Female – supine with knees bent and apart
    - □ Male – supine with thighs abducted slightly
  - Put on gloves and wash the perineal area.
  - Remove gloves.
  - Perform hand hygiene.
  - Open the sterile package.
  - Put on sterile gloves.
  - Put antiseptic solution on the cotton balls.
  - If the manufacturer recommends it for the particular indwelling catheter, inflate the balloon with the prefilled syringe provided to check its performance and integrity, then deflate it.
  - Lubricate the lower portion of catheter.
  - Apply the sterile drape, exposing the urinary meatus.
  - Cleanse the meatus.
    - □ Female – spread the labia with the nondominant hand while wiping front-to-back with the antiseptic cotton balls held in the forceps. The hand on the labia is now contaminated and holds this position for the rest of the procedure.
    - □ Male – hold the penis with the nondominant hand and wipe in a circular motion starting at the meatus and working down the glans. Repeat three more times with clean cotton balls.
  - Insert the catheter into the meatus using the sterile hand.
  - Advance the catheter until urine returns and then continue to advance it another 2.5 to 5 cm.
  - Release the labia/penis and stabilize the catheter with the nondominant hand.
  - If using an indwelling catheter, slowly inflate the balloon, release the hand, and pull back gently.
  - Secure the catheter to the client's leg.
  - Place the drainage bag below the level of the client's bladder.

- If a straight catheterization, remove the catheter after the flow of urine has ceased.

- Dispose of drapes, equipment, and gloves.

- Replace the side rail and lower the bed.

- Perform hand hygiene.

- Closed Intermittent Irrigation

  o Prepare a sterile syringe with irrigant.

  o Clamp the catheter between the injection port and the extension tubing.

  o Cleanse the injection port with an antiseptic swab or wipe.

  o Insert the needle of the syringe with irrigant into the injection port.

  o Slowly inject the irrigant into the catheter.

  o Withdraw the syringe and remove the clamp.

  o Allow the irrigant to drain into the drainage bag.

- Routine Catheter Care

  o Equipment

    - Soap and water

    - Washcloth

    - Gloves

  o Procedure

    - Use soap and water at the insertion site.

    - Cleanse the catheter at least three times/day and after defecation.

    - Monitor the patency of the catheter.

      □ If the client reports fullness in the bladder area, check for kinks in the tubing and check for sediment in the tubing.

      □ Make sure the catheter bag/system is at a level below the client's bladder to avoid reflux.

- Condom Catheter Application

  o Equipment

    - Gloves

    - Condom catheter

    - Elastic tape

    - Leg or standard collection bag

- o   Procedure

  - ▪   Perform hand hygiene.

  - ▪   Explain the procedure to the client.

  - ▪   Adjust the height of the bed.

  - ▪   Expose the client's perineal area minimally.

  - ▪   Put on gloves.

  - ▪   Apply skin prep to the skin of the penis.

  - ▪   Hold the penis with the nondominant hand, and place the condom over the tip, allowing 2.5 cm of space between the tip of the penis and the catheter.

  - ▪   Roll down the sides of the condom over the shaft of the penis.

  - ▪   Use elastic tape in a spiral manner to secure it if needed.

  - ▪   Attach the catheter to the leg or standard collection bag.

  - ▪   Observe for the presence of urine.

  - ▪   Remove gloves and perform hand hygiene.

  - ▪   Lower the bed.

Complications and Nursing Implications

- •   Urinary tract infections (UTIs)

  - o   Most caused by *Escherichia coli*

  - o   Factors that increase the risk of UTIs:

    - ▪   Close proximity of the urethral meatus in women to the anus

    - ▪   Frequent sexual intercourse

    - ▪   Menopause decreasing estrogen levels and increasing susceptibility to UTIs

    - ▪   Uncircumcised males

    - ▪   Use of indwelling catheters

  - o   Nursing implications

    - ▪   Cleanse female clients from front to back.

    - ▪   Cleanse beneath the foreskin in males.

    - ▪   Provide regular catheter care.

CHAPTER 44: URINARY ELIMINATION

Ⓐ Application Exercises

1. A client with an indwelling catheter reports a need to urinate. Which of the following interventions should the nurse perform?

    A. Check to see if the catheter is patent.

    B. Reassure the client that it is not possible for her to urinate.

    C. Recatheterize the client with a larger-gauge catheter.

    D. Notify the provider.

2. Which of the following nursing interventions is correct when performing a 24-hr urine specimen test?

    A. Discard the first voiding.

    B. Keep all voidings in a container at room temperature for 24 hr.

    C. Ask the client to urinate and pour the urine into a specimen container.

    D. Ask the client to urinate into the toilet, stop midstream, and finish urinating into the specimen container.

3. Which of the following positions promotes a client's normal elimination?

    A. Left lateral Sims'

    B. Sitting

    C. Supine

    D. Right side-lying

4. Which of the following interventions is appropriate when a nurse performs a catheterization on a female client? (Select all that apply.)

    _____ Provide privacy.

    _____ Darken the room.

    _____ Maintain surgical asepsis throughout the procedure.

    _____ Position the client supine with knees bent and apart.

    _____ Ask the client not to talk during the procedure.

CHAPTER 44: URINARY ELIMINATION

 Application Exercises Answer Key

1. A client with an indwelling catheter reports a need to urinate. Which of the following interventions should the nurse perform?

   A. Check to see if the catheter is patent.

   B. Reassure the client that it is not possible for her to urinate.

   C. Recatheterize the client with a larger-gauge catheter.

   D. Notify the provider.

   A clogged catheter causes the bladder to fill and stimulates the need to urinate. Reassuring the client that it is not possible to urinate is a nontherapeutic response. The patency of the tube must be checked before replacing the client's catheter. It is not necessary to contact the provider. The nurse can determine whether or not the tube is patent and replace the tube if necessary without a new order.

    NCLEX® Connection: Basic Care and Comfort, Elimination

2. Which of the following nursing interventions is correct when performing a 24-hr urine specimen test?

   A. Discard the first voiding.

   B. Keep all voidings in a container at room temperature for 24 hr.

   C. Ask the client to urinate and pour the urine into a specimen container.

   D. Ask the client to urinate into the toilet, stop midstream, and finish urinating into the specimen container.

   The first voiding of the 24-hr urine specimen is discarded, and the time is noted. All voidings are collected after that and kept in a container on ice. If a urinalysis is ordered, ask the client to urinate and pour the urine into a specimen container. If a culture is ordered, ask the client to urinate first into the toilet, then stop midstream, and finish urinating in the specimen container. The specimen for a 24-hr collection is stored on ice.

    NCLEX® Connection: Basic Care and Comfort, Elimination

3. Which of the following positions promotes a client's normal elimination?

   A. Left lateral Sims'

   B. Sitting

   C. Supine

   D. Right side-lying

   The most natural and efficient way to urinate is while sitting upright. Left lateral Sims' and right lateral positions are not appropriate for urine collection. The supine position makes it difficult to empty the bladder completely.

    NCLEX® Connection: Basic Care and Comfort, Elimination

4. Which of the following interventions is appropriate when a nurse performs a catheterization on a female client? (Select all that apply.)

    X   **Provide privacy.**

            Darken the room.

    X   **Maintain surgical asepsis throughout the procedure.**

    X   **Position the client supine with knees bent and apart.**

            Ask the client not to talk during the procedure.

It is important to maintain privacy during catheterization to preserve the client's dignity. Insertion of a urinary catheter requires surgical asepsis, because the catheter is entering a sterile body cavity. Positioning the client supine with knees bent and apart facilitates insertion of the catheter. It is not necessary to darken the room. Talking will not contaminate the sterile field, so it is not necessary to ask the client not to talk.

Ⓝ NCLEX® Connection: Basic Care and Comfort, Elimination

SENSORY PERCEPTION **chapter 45**

UNIT 4	PHYSIOLOGICAL INTEGRITY
Section	Basic Care and Comfort
Chapter 45	Sensory Perception

Overview

- Sensory perception is the ability to receive and interpret sensory impressions:

    o Consciousness.

    o Arousal and awareness.

    o Memory.

    o Affect.

    o Judgment.

    o Awareness of reality.

    o Language.

- Sensory deficit is a change in reception and/or perception. Deficits can affect any of the senses. The body will often compensate for the deficit.

- Sensory deprivation is reduced sensory input either from the internal or the external environment. Sensory deprivation can be the result of illness, trauma, or isolation.

- Sensory overload is excessive, sustained, and unmanageable multisensory stimulation.

Contributing Factors

- Factors that contribute to loss of vision include presbyopia, cataracts, glaucoma, diabetic retinopathy, macular degeneration, infection, inflammation, injury, and brain tumor.

- Factors that contribute to conductive hearing loss include obstruction, tympanic membrane perforation, ear infections, and otosclerosis.

- Factors that contribute to sensorineural hearing loss include exposure to loud noises, ototoxic medications, aging, and acoustic neuroma.

Collaborative Care

- Nursing Care

    o Check for communication deficits and adjust care accordingly.

- ○ Collect equipment necessary to care for any assistive devices the client has (glasses, hearing aids).

- ○ Do not avoid communicating with clients with sensoriperceptual losses, as they tend to withdraw from interactions with others.

- ○ Equipment

  - Assistive devices

  - Orientation tools (clocks, calendars)

  - Radio, television, compact disc (CD/DVD) player, digital audio file (MP3) player

  - Large-print materials

- ○ Procedures

  - Keep the client safe and free from injury.

    - □ Make sure the call light is readily available.

    - □ Orient the client to the room.

    - □ Keep furniture clear from the path to the bathroom.

    - □ Keep personal items within reach.

    - □ Place the bed in its lowest position.

    - □ Make sure IV poles and drainage tubes/bags are easy to maneuver.

  - Learn the client's preferred alternative method of communication and make accommodations.

  - For clients who are hearing impaired:

    - □ Sit and face the client.

    - □ Avoid covering the mouth while speaking.

    - □ Have the client use hearing devices.

    - □ Speak slowly and clearly.

    - □ Do not shout.

    - □ Try lowering the pitch before increasing the volume to be heard.

    - □ Use brief sentences with simple words.

    - □ Write down what is not understood.

    - □ Minimize background noises.

    - □ Ask for a sign language interpreter if necessary.

  - For clients who are visually impaired:

    - □ Call the person by name before approaching to avoid startling him.

    - □ Identify yourself.

    - □ Stay within the client's visual field if the client has a partial loss.

- Give specific information about the location of items or areas of the building.
- Explain interventions before touching the client.
- Before leaving, inform the client of your departure.
- Carefully appraise the client's clothing and suggest changes if soiled or torn.
- Make a radio, television, compact disc (CD/DVD) player, or digital audio file (MP3) player available for the client to use.
- Describe the arrangement of the food on the tray before leaving the room.

■ For clients who have aphasia:

- Greet the client and call him by name.
- Speak clearly and slowly using short sentences.
- Do not shout.
- Pause between statements to allow the client time to understand.
- Check for comprehension.
- Ask questions that require simple answers.
- Reinforce verbal with nonverbal communication (gestures, body language).
- Allow plenty of time for the client to respond.
- Use methods implemented by speech therapists, such as a picture chart, to improve communication.
- Acknowledge any frustration in communicating that the client expresses.

■ For clients who are disoriented:

- Call the client by name and identify yourself.
- Maintain eye contact at the client's eye level.
- Use brief, simple sentences.
- Ask only one question at a time.
- Allow plenty of time for the client to respond.
- Give directions one step at a time.
- Avoid lengthy conversations.
- Provide for adequate sleep and pain management.

■ Encourage the client to verbalize feelings about sensoriperceptual loss.

■ Orient the client to time, person, place, and situation.

- Keep a clock in the room.
- Post a calendar, or write the date where it is visible.

■ Provide and/or use assistive devices as needed.

■ Provide care that the client is not able to perform (reading the menu, opening containers).

- Interdisciplinary care

  - Determine which assistive devices the client needs, and plan for their procurement while in the facility and community.

  - Consult with rehabilitation therapists, as appropriate, for restorative potential.

  - Refer the client to community-based support groups and organizations for additional resources.

Complications

- Risk for injury in the home environment

  - Teach/reinforce with the client ways to reduce hazards at home.

    - Visual – Remove throw rugs to prevent tripping hazards.

      - Keep walking pathways clear.

      - Ensure that stairways are well lit with secure handrails.

    - Auditory – Use flashing lights versus a warning sound from alarms.

    - Olfactory – Make sure smoke and carbon monoxide detectors are functioning to sense odors that are not perceived (burning food, natural gas).

    - Gustatory – Read dates on food packages to avoid contamination or spoilage that cannot be detected through taste.

    - Tactile – Protect and inspect body parts that lack sensation (burns, pressure ulcers, frostbite).

- Sensory deprivation and overload

  - Minimize overall stimuli and provide meaningful stimulation.

    - Minimize glare.

    - Manage pain effectively.

    - Allow for adequate sleep and rest periods.

    - Provide large-print materials or electronic players for audio books.

    - Amplify phones.

    - Season foods.

    - Reduce unpleasant odors.

    - Provide pleasant aromas.

    - Increase touch (if acceptable to the client) with back rubs, hand holding, range-of-motion exercises, and hair care.

    - Organize care to minimize the activity surrounding the client's bed when possible.

CHAPTER 45: SENSORY PERCEPTION

 Application Exercises

1. A nurse is caring for a client who had a recent cerebrovascular accident and has aphasia. Which of the following interventions should the nurse use to promote communication with this client? (Select all that apply.)

_____ Speak fast and loud.

_____ Minimize background noise.

_____ Write down what the client does not understand.

_____ Allow plenty of time for the client to respond.

_____ Use brief sentences with simple words.

2. A nurse is caring for a client who recently overdosed on amphetamines and is experiencing sensory overload. Which of the following interventions should the nurse implement?

A. Immediately complete a thorough assessment.

B. Put the client in a room with a client who is hearing impaired.

C. Provide a private room and limit stimulation.

D. Talk loudly to the client and encourage ambulation.

3. A form of nonverbal communication that helps to clarify verbal communication to clients is _____.

4. _____ means the client cannot speak or comprehend spoken language.

5. A client whose sensory input is reduced may experience sensory _____.

CHAPTER 45: SENSORY PERCEPTION

 Application Exercises Answer Key

1. A nurse is caring for a client who had a recent cerebrovascular accident and has aphasia. Which of the following interventions should the nurse use to promote communication with this client? (Select all that apply.)

    _____ Speak fast and loud.

    X **Minimize background noise.**

    X **Write down what the client does not understand.**

    X **Allow plenty of time for the client to respond.**

    X **Use brief sentences with simple words.**

Minimizing background noise provides a calming environment. Writing down what the client does not understand, allowing time for the client to respond, and using simple words and brief sentences help promote communication with clients who have aphasia. The client is not hearing impaired, so speaking loud will not promote communication.

 NCLEX® Connection: Psychosocial Integrity, Sensory/Perceptual Alterations

2. A nurse is caring for a client who recently overdosed on amphetamines and is experiencing sensory overload. Which of the following interventions should the nurse implement?

A. Immediately complete a thorough assessment.

B. Put the client in a room with a client who is hearing impaired.

C. Provide a private room and limit stimulation.

D. Talk loudly to the client and encourage ambulation.

Minimizing stimuli helps clients who experience sensory overload. Immediately completing a thorough assessment might overwhelm the client at this time; therefore, brief assessments done over the course of the shift are preferred. Rooming with a client who is hearing impaired and/or talking in a loud voice would increase environmental stimuli.

 NCLEX® Connection: Psychosocial Integrity, Sensory/Perceptual Alterations

3. A form of nonverbal communication that helps clarify verbal communication to clients is **gestures**.

 NCLEX® Connection: Psychosocial Integrity, Sensory/Perceptual Alterations

4. **Aphasia** means the client cannot speak or comprehend spoken language.

 NCLEX® Connection: Psychosocial Integrity, Sensory/Perceptual Alterations

5. A client whose sensory input is reduced may experience sensory **deprivation**.

NCLEX® Connection: Psychosocial Integrity, Sensory/Perceptual Alterations

UNIT 4: PHYSIOLOGICAL INTEGRITY

Section: Pharmacological and Parenteral Therapies

- Pharmacokinetics and Routes of Administration
- Safe Medication Administration and Error Reduction
- Dosage Calculation
- Intravenous Therapy
- Adverse Effects, Interactions, and Contraindications
- Individual Considerations of Medication Administration

NCLEX® CONNECTIONS

When reviewing the chapters in this section, keep in mind the relevant sections of the NCLEX® outline, in particular:

CLIENT NEEDS: MANAGEMENT OF CARE

Relevant topics/tasks include:
- Client Rights
  - Recognize the client's right to refuse treatment/procedures.
- Continuity of Care
  - Use approved abbreviations and standard terminology when documenting care.

CLIENT NEEDS: SAFETY AND INFECTION CONTROL

Relevant topics/tasks include:
- Error Prevention
  - Ensure proper identification of the client when providing care.

CLIENT NEEDS: PHARMACOLOGICAL AND PARENTERAL THERAPIES

Relevant topics/tasks include:
- Dosage Calculation
  - Perform calculations needed for medication administration.
- Expected Actions/Outcomes
  - Obtain information on prescribed medication for the client.
- Medication Administration
  - Prepare and administer medications, using the rights of medication administration.

UNIT 4	PHYSIOLOGICAL INTEGRITY
Section	Pharmacological and Parenteral Therapies
Chapter 46	Pharmacokinetics and Routes of Administration

Overview

- Pharmacokinetics refers to how medications travel through the body. Medication undergo a variety of biochemical processes that result in absorption, distribution, metabolism, and excretion.

Phases of Pharmacokinetics

- Absorption – the transmission of medications from the location of administration (gastrointestinal tract, muscle, skin, or subcutaneous tissue) to the bloodstream. The most common routes of administration are enteral (through the GI tract) and parenteral (by injection). Each of these routes will have a unique pattern of absorption.

  o The rate of medication absorption determines how soon the medication will take effect.

  o The amount of medication absorbed determines its intensity.

  o The route of administration affects the rate and amount of absorption.

ROUTES AND ABSORPTION		
ROUTE	BARRIERS TO ABSORPTION	ABSORPTION PATTERN
Oral	Medications must pass through the layer of epithelial cells that line the GI tract.	Varies greatly due to the following variables: • Stability and solubility of the medication • Gastrointestinal pH and emptying time • Presence of food in the stomach or intestines • Other medications currently being administered • Forms of medications (enteric-coated pills, liquids).

ROUTES AND ABSORPTION		
ROUTE	**BARRIERS TO ABSORPTION**	**ABSORPTION PATTERN**

Subcutaneous and intramuscular	The capillary wall has large spaces between cells; therefore, there is no significant barrier.	The rate of absorption is determined by:
		• Solubility of the medication in water:
		   ○ Highly soluble medications will be absorbed in 10 to 30 min.
		   ○ Poorly soluble medications will be absorbed slower.
		• Blood perfusion at the site of injection – sites with high blood perfusion will have rapid absorption. Sites with low blood perfusion will have slow absorption.

Intravenous	No barriers	• Immediate – administered directly into the blood. • Complete – all of it reaches the blood.

- Distribution – the transportation of medications to sites of action by bodily fluids. Distribution may be influenced by the ability to:

  ○ Travel to the site of action through the bloodstream (peripheral vascular or cardiac disease may delay medication distribution).

  ○ Leave the bloodstream by traveling between the capillaries' cells

    ■ Plasma protein binding: Medications compete for protein binding sites within the bloodstream, primarily albumin. The ability of a medication to bind to a protein can affect how much of the medication will leave and travel to target tissues. Two medications can compete for the same binding sites, resulting in toxicity.

    ■ Barriers: Medications that are lipid soluble or have a transport system can cross the blood brain barrier or the placenta.

- Metabolism – (biotransformation) changes medications into less active forms or inactive forms by the action of enzymes. This occurs primarily in the liver, but also takes place in the kidneys, lungs, bowel, and blood.

  ○ Factors influencing the rate of medication metabolism include:

    ■ Age – Infants have limited medication-metabolizing capacity. The aging process can also influence medication metabolism, but varies from individual to individual. In general, hepatic medication metabolism tends to decline with age.

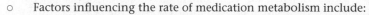

- An increase in certain medication-metabolizing enzymes – This can cause that particular medication to be metabolized sooner, requiring an increase in dosage of that medication to maintain a therapeutic level. It can also cause an increase in the metabolism of other medications that are being used concurrently.

- First-pass effect – Some medications are inactivated on their first pass through the liver and must be given by a nonenteral route because of their high first-pass effect. These medications are usually given by routes such as SL or IV.

- Similar metabolic pathways – When two medications are metabolized by the same pathway, they can interfere with the metabolism of one or both of the medications. In this way, the rate of metabolism can be decreased for one or both of the medications leading to medication accumulation.

- Nutritional status – A malnourished client may be deficient in the factors that are necessary to produce specific medication-metabolizing enzymes. Consequently, medication metabolism may be impaired.

- Outcomes of metabolism include:

    - Increased renal excretion of medication.

    - Inactivation of medications.

    - Increased therapeutic effect.

    - Activation of pro-medications into active forms.

    - Decreased toxicity when active forms of medications are converted to inactive forms.

    - Increased toxicity when inactive forms of medications are converted to active forms.

- Excretion – The elimination of medications from the body primarily through the kidneys. Elimination also takes place through the liver, lungs, bowel, and exocrine glands. Renal dysfunction may lead to an increase in duration and intensity of medication response.

- Medication responses – Plasma medication levels can be regulated to control medication responses. Medication dosing attempts to maintain plasma levels between the minimum effective concentration (MEC) and the toxic concentration. A plasma medication level is in the therapeutic range when it is effective and not toxic. Therapeutic levels are well established for many medications, and these levels can be used to monitor a client's response.

- Therapeutic index (TI) – Medications with a high TI have a wide safety margin. Therefore, there is no need for routine serum medication level monitoring. Medications with a low TI should have serum medication levels monitored closely. Monitor peak levels based on the route of administration. For example, an oral medication may have a peak of 1 to 3 hr after administration. If the medication is given intravenously, the peak time might occur within 10 min. (Refer to a drug reference or a pharmacist for specific medication peak times.) For trough levels, blood is drawn immediately before the next medication dose, regardless of the route of administration.

- Half-life (t1/2) – Refers to the period of time needed for the medication in the body to be reduced by 50%. May be affected by liver and kidney function. Usually takes four half-lives to achieve a steady state of serum concentration (medication intake = medication metabolism and excretion).

SHORT HALF-LIFE	LONG HALF-LIFE
Medications leave the body quickly – 4 to 8 hr.	Medications leave the body more slowly – 24+ hr. Greater risk for medication accumulation and toxicity.
Short-dosing interval or minimum effective concentration (MEC) will drop between doses.	Medications are given at longer intervals without a loss of therapeutic effects.
	Medications take a longer time to reach a steady state.

- Pharmacodynamics (mechanism of action) describes the interactions between medications and target cells, body systems, and organs to produce effects. These interactions result in functional changes that are considered the mechanism of action of the medication. Medications interact with cells in one of two ways.

  ○ Agonist – Medication that can mimic the receptor activity regulated by endogenous compounds. For example, morphine sulfate (Duramorph) is classified as an agonist because it activates the receptors that produce analgesia, sedation, constipation, and other effects.

  ○ Antagonist – Medication that can block normal receptor activity regulated by endogenous compounds or receptor activity caused by other medications. For example, losartan (Cozaar), an angiotensin II receptor blocker, is classified as an antagonist. Losartan works by blocking angiotensin II receptors on blood vessels, which prevents vasoconstriction.

  ○ Partial agonists – May act as an agonist/antagonist. Limited affinity to receptor site. For example, nalbuphine (Nubain) acts as an antagonist at mu receptors and an agonist at kappa receptors, causing analgesia at low doses, with minimal respiratory depression.

Routes of Administration

ROUTE OF ADMINISTRATION	NURSING IMPLICATIONS
Oral or enteral (tablets, capsules, liquids, suspensions, elixirs)	• Contraindications for oral medication administration include vomiting, absence of a gag reflex, difficulty swallowing, and a decreased level of consciousness. • Have the client sitting upright, in Fowler's or semi-Fowler's position, to facilitate swallowing. • Administer irritating medications with small amounts of food. • Do not mix with large amounts of food or beverages in case the client is unable to consume the entire quantity. • Avoid administration with contraindicated foods or beverages such as grapefruit juice. • In general, administer oral medications on an empty stomach (1 hr before meals, 2 hr after meals). • Follow the manufacturer's directions for crushing, cutting, and diluting medications. A complete list can be found at The Institute for Safe Medication Practices Web site. (http://www.ismp.org/Tools/DoNotCrush.pdf) • Enteric-coated or time-release medications must be swallowed whole. • Time-release medications must be swallowed whole to prevent faster absorption. • Use a liquid form of the medication to facilitate swallowing whenever possible.
Sublingual (under the tongue) and buccal (between the cheek and the gum)	• Instruct the client to have medication remain in place until absorbed. • The client should not eat or drink while the tablet is in place.
Liquids, suspensions, and elixirs	• Follow directions for dilution and shaking. • When administering the medication, the base of the meniscus (lowest fluid line) is at the level of the desired dose.
Transdermal – medication stored in a skin patch and absorbed through the skin producing systemic effects	Instructions to the client should include: • Apply patches as provided to ensure proper dosing. • Wash the skin with soap and water, and dry it thoroughly before applying a new patch. • Place the patch on a hairless area of the skin and rotate sites to prevent skin irritation.
Topical	• Apply with a glove, tongue blade, or cotton-tipped applicator. • Never apply with a bare hand.

ROUTE OF ADMINISTRATION	NURSING IMPLICATIONS

Instillation (drops, ointments, sprays) – generally used for eyes, ears, and nose	• Eyes
	  ○ Use medical aseptic technique when instilling medications in eyes.
	  ○ Have the client sit upright or lie supine with the head tilted slightly and looking up at the ceiling.
	  ○ Rest the dominant hand on the client's forehead, hold the dropper above the conjunctival sac about 1 to 2 cm, drop the medication into the center of the sac and have the client close her eye gently.
	  ○ Apply gentle pressure with the finger and a clean tissue on the nasolacrimal duct for 30 to 60 seconds to prevent systemic absorption of the medication.
	• Ears
	  ○ Use medical aseptic technique when administering medications into the ears.
	  ○ Have the client sit upright or maintain a side-lying position.
	  ○ Straighten the ear canal by pulling the auricle upward and outward for adults or down and back for children. Hold the dropper 1 cm above the ear canal, install medication, and then gently apply pressure with finger to tragus of ear.
	• Nose
	  ○ Use medical aseptic technique when administering medications into the nose.
	  ○ Have the client supine with the head positioned to allow the medication to enter the appropriate nasal passage.
	  ○ Use the dominant hand to instill drops, supporting the head with the nondominant hand.
	  ○ Instruct the client to breathe through the mouth, stay in a supine position, and not to blow his nose for 5 min after drop insertion.

ROUTE OF ADMINISTRATION	NURSING IMPLICATIONS
Inhalation – Administered through metered dose inhalers (MDI) or dry powder inhalers (DPI)	<ul><li>For an MDI, instruct the client to:<ul><li>Remove the cap from the inhaler.</li><li>Shake the inhaler five or six times.</li><li>Hold the inhaler with the mouthpiece at the bottom.</li><li>Hold the inhaler with the thumb near the mouthpiece and the index and middle fingers at the top.</li><li>Hold the inhaler about 2 to 4 cm (1 to 2 in) away from the front of the mouth.</li><li>Take a deep breath and then exhale.</li><li>Tilt the head back slightly, press the inhaler, and, at the same time, begin a slow, deep breath. Continue to breathe slowly and deeply for 3 to 5 seconds to facilitate delivery to the air passages.</li><li>Hold the breath for 10 seconds to allow the medication to deposit in the airways.</li><li>Take the inhaler out of the mouth and slowly exhale through pursed lips.</li><li>Resume normal breathing.</li></ul></li><li>A spacer may be used to keep the medication in the device longer thereby increasing the amount of medication delivered to the lungs and decreasing the amount of the medication in the oropharynx.</li><li>If a spacer is used:<ul><li>Remove the covers from the mouthpieces of the inhaler and of the spacer.</li><li>Insert the MDI into the end of the spacer.</li><li>Shake the inhaler five or six times.</li><li>Exhale completely, and then close the mouth around the spacer mouthpiece. Continue as with an MDI.</li></ul></li></ul>

ROUTE OF ADMINISTRATION	NURSING IMPLICATIONS

	• For a DPI:
	  ○ Do not shake the device.
	  ○ Take the cover off the mouthpiece.
	  ○ Follow the directions of the manufacturer for preparing the medication, such as turning the wheel of the inhaler.
	  ○ Exhale completely.
	  ○ Place the mouthpiece between lips and take a deep breath through the mouth.
	  ○ Hold the breath for 5 to 10 seconds
	  ○ Take the inhaler out of the mouth and slowly exhale through pursed lips.
	  ○ Resume normal breathing.
	• If more than one puff is prescribed, instruct the client to wait the length of time directed before administering the second puff.
	• Instruct the client to remove the canister and rinse the inhaler, cap, and spacer once a day with warm running water and dry it completely before using it again.

Nasogastric and gastrostomy tubes	• Check for proper tube placement.
	• Use a syringe and allow the medication to flow in by gravity or push it in with the plunger of the syringe.
	• General guidelines:
	  ○ Liquid forms of medications must be used.
	  ○ Sublingual medications should not be given.
	  ○ Do not crush specially prepared oral medications (extended/time-release, fluid-filled, enteric-coated).
	  ○ Check the compatibility of medications before mixing them.
	  ○ Do not mix medications with enteral feedings.
	• To prevent clogging, flush the tubing before and after each medication with 15 to 30 mL of water. When administration of medications is complete, flush with 30 to 60 mL of warm water.

ROUTE OF ADMINISTRATION	NURSING IMPLICATIONS

Suppositories	• Follow the manufacturer's directions for storage.
	• Wear gloves for the procedure.
	• Remove the foil wrapper, and lubricate the suppository if necessary.
	• Rectal suppositories
	  o Position the client in the left lateral position.
	  o Insert the suppository just beyond the internal sphincter.
	  o Instruct the client to retain the medication 20 to 30 min for stimulation of defecation and 60 min for systemic absorption.
	• Vaginal suppositories
	  o Position the client supine with her knees bent, her feet flat on the bed and close to her hips (modified lithotomy position).
	  o Vaginal suppositories are generally inserted with an applicator.
	  o Instruct the client to remain in the position for the prescribed amount of time.

Parenteral	General considerations for parenteral medications include: • The vastus lateralis site is usually the recommended site for infants and children < 2 years of age. • After age 2, the ventral gluteal site can be used. Both of these sites can accommodate fluid up to 2 mL. The deltoid site has a smaller muscle mass and only can accommodate up to 1 mL of fluid. • Use a needle size and length appropriate for the type of injection and the client's size. Syringe size should approximate the volume of medication. • Use a tuberculin syringe for solution volumes < 0.5 mL. • Rotate injection sites to enhance medication absorption, and document each site used. • Do not use injection sites that are edematous, inflamed or have moles, birthmarks, or scars. • If medication is given intravenously, immediately monitor the client for therapeutic, side/adverse effects. • Discard all sharps (broken ampule bottles, needle) in designated containers. Containers should be leak- and puncture-proof.

ROUTE OF ADMINISTRATION	NURSING IMPLICATIONS
Intradermal	• Usually used for tuberculin testing or checking for medication/allergy sensitivities. • May be used for some cancer immunotherapy. • Use small amounts of solution (0.01 to 0.1 mL) in a tuberculin syringe with a fine-gauge needle (26 to 27) in lightly pigmented, thin-skinned, hairless sites (inner surface of the mid-forearm or scapular area of the back) at a 10- to 15-degree angle.
Subcutaneous	• Appropriate for small doses of nonirritating, water-soluble medications. Commonly used for insulin and heparin. • Use a 3/8- to 5/8-in, 25- to 27-gauge needle or an insulin syringe of 28 to 31 gauge. Inject no more than 1.5 mL solution. For an average size client, pinch up the skin and inject at a 45- to 90-degree angle. For an obese client, use a 90-degree angle. • Sites are selected for adequate fat-pad size (abdomen, upper hips, lateral upper arms, thighs).
Intramuscular	• Appropriate for irritating medications, solutions in oils, and aqueous suspensions. • Most common sites include ventrogluteal, dorsogluteal, deltoid, and vastus lateralis (pediatric). • Use a needle size 18 to 27 (usually 22- to 25-gauge) • 1 to 1 ½ in long, and inject at a 90-degree angle. Volume injected is usually 1 to 3 mL. If a greater amount is required, it should be divided into two syringes and two different sites should be used.
Z-Track	• Type of IM injection that prevents medication from leaking back into subcutaneous tissue. • It is often used for medications that cause visible and/or permanent skin stains such as certain iron preparations.
Intravenous	• Appropriate for administration of medications, fluid, and blood products. • Vascular access devices can be for short-term use (catheters) or long-term use (infusion ports). Use 16-gauge for trauma clients, 18-gauge for surgical clients, and 22- to 24-gauge for children, older adults, medical clients, and stable postoperative clients. • Preferred sites are peripheral veins in the arm or hand. Ask the client which site he prefers. In neonates, veins of the head, lower legs, and feet may be used. After administration, immediately monitor for therapeutic, side/adverse effects.
Epidural	• Administration of intravenous opioid analgesia (morphine [Duramorph] or fentanyl [Sublimaze]). • The catheter is advanced through the needle that is inserted into the epidural space at the level of the fourth or fifth vertebrae. • Infusion pumps are necessary to administer medication.

- Advantages and Disadvantages of Different Routes

ROUTE	ADVANTAGES	DISADVANTAGES
Oral	<ul><li>Safe</li><li>Inexpensive</li><li>Easy and convenient</li></ul>	<ul><li>Oral medications have a highly variable absorption.</li><li>Inactivation can occur by the GI tract or first-pass effect.</li><li>The client must be cooperative and conscious.</li><li>Contraindications include nausea and vomiting.</li></ul>
Subcutaneous and intramuscular	<ul><li>Use for poorly soluble medications.</li><li>This route is appropriate for administering medications that are absorbed slowly for an extended period of time (depot preparations).</li></ul>	<ul><li>Intramuscular (IM) injections are associated with a higher cost.</li><li>IM injections are inconvenient.</li><li>There can be pain with the risk for local tissue damage and nerve damage.</li><li>There is a risk for infection at the injection site.</li></ul>
Intravenous	<ul><li>Onset is rapid, and absorption of the medication into the blood is immediate, which provides an immediate response.</li><li>This route allows control over the precise amount of medication given.</li><li>This route allows for administration of large volumes of fluid.</li><li>Irritating medications can be given with free-flowing IV fluid.</li></ul>	<ul><li>Intravenous (IV) injections are associated with an even higher cost.</li><li>IV injections are more inconvenient.</li><li>Absorption of the medication into the blood is immediate. This can be potentially dangerous if the wrong amount, or the wrong medication, is given.</li><li>There is an increased risk for infection or embolism with IV injections.</li></ul>

CHAPTER 46: PHARMACOKINETICS AND ROUTES OF ADMINISTRATION

 Application Exercises

1. When medications act on receptors they can do which of the following? (Select all that apply.)

_____ Mimic the action of the body's own hormones.

_____ Change the enzymes made by the target cell.

_____ Make the receptors respond in new ways.

_____ Change the receptors' molecular structure.

_____ Block the action of the body's own compounds.

2. After an oral medication has been absorbed, most of the medication is inactivated as the blood initially passes through the liver, producing little therapeutic effect. This is called

A. tolerance.

B. first-pass effect.

C. antagonism.

D. synergism.

3. Intravenous administration of a medication eliminates the need for

A. absorption.

B. distribution.

C. metabolism.

D. excretion.

4. Identify the correct client position for each of the following routes of administration.

_____ Oral   A. Lying on the left side with the right knee brought up toward the chest (Sims' position)

_____ Otic   B. Sitting, semi-Fowler's, or Fowler's position

_____ Vaginal   C. Supine with the knees bent, the feet flat on the bed and close to the hips

_____ Rectal   D. Lying on the side with the ear that is receiving the drops facing up

5. Identify the correct equipment needed for each of the following types of injections.

_____ Intradermal   A. 16- to 24-gauge catheters appropriate for most adults, smaller-gauge catheters appropriate for infants and children

_____ Subcutaneous   B. A tuberculin syringe with a fine-gauge needle (26 to 27)

_____ Intramuscular   C. A short, fine-gauge needle (3/8- to 5/8-inch, 25- to 27-gauge)

_____ Intravenous   D. Needle size 18 to 27 (1- to 1½-inch, 22- to 25-gauge)

6. Nitroglycerin (Nitrogard) tablets, which are often prescribed for clients who have cardiovascular disorders, are given sublingually. This means that the tablets are

    A. crushed and taken with a small amount of food.

    B. held under the tongue until dissolved.

    C. taken by mouth with a small amount of water.

    D. placed between the cheek and gums.

CHAPTER 46: PHARMACOKINETICS AND ROUTES OF ADMINISTRATION

(A) Application Exercises Answer Key

1. When medications act on receptors they can do which of the following? (Select all that apply.)

   X   **Mimic the action of the body's own hormones.**

          Change the enzymes made by the target cell.

          Make the receptors respond in new ways.

          Change the receptors' molecular structure.

   X   **Block the action of the body's own compounds.**

Medications can only mimic or block the action of endogenous compounds. Medications cannot alter enzymes, cause new responses by receptors, or change molecular structure.

(N) **NCLEX® Connection: Pharmacological and Parenteral Therapies, Expected Actions/Outcomes**

2. After an oral medication has been absorbed, most of the medication is inactivated as the blood initially passes through the liver, producing little therapeutic effect. This is called

    A. tolerance.

    B. first-pass effect.

    C. antagonism.

    D. synergism.

Medications that are given orally are taken directly to the liver from the GI tract via the hepatic portal circulation. Some medications will be completely inactivated as they pass through the liver, and thus no therapeutic effects will occur. These medications must be administered by a nonenteral route.

(N) **NCLEX® Connection: Pharmacological and Parenteral Therapies, Expected Actions/Outcomes**

3. Intravenous administration of a medication eliminates the need for

    A. absorption.

    B. distribution.

    C. metabolism.

    D. excretion.

Intravenous administration delivers the medication directly into the bloodstream, where it is rapidly distributed throughout the body.

(N) **NCLEX® Connection: Pharmacological and Parenteral Therapies, Expected Actions/Outcomes**

4. Identify the correct client position for each of the following routes of administration.

__B__ Oral   A. Lying on the left side with the right knee brought up toward the chest (Sims' position)

__D__ Otic   B. Sitting, semi-Fowler's, or Fowler's position

__C__ Vaginal   C. Supine with the knees bent, the feet flat on the bed and close to the hips

__A__ Rectal   D. Client lying on side with the ear that is receiving the drops facing up

NCLEX® Connection: Pharmacological and Parenteral Therapies, Medication Administration

5. Identify the correct equipment needed for each of the following types of injections.

__B__ Intradermal   A. 16- to 24-gauge catheters appropriate for most adults, smaller-gauge catheters appropriate for infants and children

__C__ Subcutaneous   B. A tuberculin syringe with a fine-gauge needle (26 to 27)

__D__ Intramuscular   C. A short, fine-gauge needle (3/8- to 5/8-inch, 25- to 27-gauge)

__A__ Intravenous   D. Needle size 18 to 27 (1- to 1 ½-inch, 22- to 25-gauge)

NCLEX® Connection: Pharmacological and Parenteral Therapies, Medication Administration

6. Nitroglycerin (Nitrogard) tablets, which are often prescribed for clients who have cardiovascular disorders, are given sublingually. This means that the tablets are

A. crushed and taken with a small amount of food.

B. held under the tongue until dissolved.

C. taken by mouth with a small amount of water.

D. placed between the cheek and gums.

Sublingual medications are correctly administered when placed under the tongue until they are dissolved. They are readily absorbed into the bloodstream for systemic effects. They should not be crushed or taken with water. Medications placed between the cheek and gums are delivered through the buccal route. The medication should dissolve and is usually used for local effects.

NCLEX® Connection: Pharmacological and Parenteral Therapies, Medication Administration

UNIT 4	PHYSIOLOGICAL INTEGRITY
Section	Pharmacological and Parenteral Therapies
Chapter 47	Safe Medication Administration and Error Reduction

Overview

- The health care providers who are legally permitted to write prescriptions in the United States include physicians, advanced practice nurses, dentists, and physician assistants. These health care providers are responsible for:

  o Obtaining the client's medical history and physical examination.

  o Diagnosing.

  o Prescribing medications.

  o Monitoring the response to therapy.

  o Modifying medication orders as necessary.

- Nurses are legally responsible for:

  o Having knowledge of federal, state (nurse practice act), and local laws, and health care facility policies that govern the prescribing, dispensing, and administration of medications.

  o Preparing, administering, and evaluating client responses to medications.

  o Developing and maintaining an up-to-date knowledge base of medications administered, including uses, mechanisms of action, routes of administration, safe dosage range, side effects, adverse responses, precautions, and contraindications.

  o Maintaining knowledge of acceptable practice and skill competency.

  o Determining accuracy of medication orders.

  o Reporting all medication errors.

  o Safeguarding and storing medications.

Medication Category and Classification

- Nomenclature

  o Chemical name – medication is named by its chemical composition

  o Generic name – official or non-proprietary name that is given by the United States Adopted Names Council. Each medication has only one generic name.

- o Trade name – brand or proprietary name that is given by the company that manufacturers the medication. One medication may have multiple trade names.

- Prescription medications are administered under the supervision of providers. These medications may be habit-forming, have potential harmful effects, and/or require supervision.

  - o Uncontrolled substances – These medications require monitoring by a provider, but do not pose a risk of abuse and/or addiction. Antibiotics are an example of uncontrolled prescription medications.

  - o Controlled substances – Medications that have a potential for abuse and dependence are categorized into schedules. Heroin is a medication in Schedule I and has no medical use in the United States. Medications categorized in Schedules II through V all have approved applications. Each level has a decreasing risk of abuse and dependence. For example, morphine (Duramorph) is a Schedule II medication that has a greater risk of abuse and dependence than phenobarbital (Luminal), which is a Schedule IV medication.

  - o The U.S. Food and Drug Administration Pregnancy Risk Category (A, B, C, D, X) classifies medications in terms of their potential harm during pregnancy, with Category A being the safest and Category X the most dangerous. Teratogenesis is most likely to occur during the first trimester. Before giving any medication to a woman who is pregnant or could be pregnant, determine whether or not it is safe for administration during pregnancy.

KNOWLEDGE REQUIRED PRIOR TO MEDICATION ADMINISTRATION	
Medication category/class	Medications are organized according to pharmacologic action, therapeutic use, body system, chemical makeup, and safe use during pregnancy. For example, lisinopril (Zestril) is classified as an angiotensin-converting enzyme inhibitor (pharmacologic action) and an antihypertensive (therapeutic use).
Mechanism of action	This is how the medication produces the desired therapeutic effect. For example, glipizide (Glucotrol) is an oral hypoglycemic agent. Glipizide lowers blood glucose levels primarily by stimulating pancreatic islet cells to release insulin.
Therapeutic effect	This is the preferred and expected effect for which the medication is administered to a specific client. One medication may have more than one therapeutic effect. For example, one client is administered acetaminophen (Tylenol) to lower fever, whereas another client may be administered this medication to relieve pain.
Side effects	Usually expected and inevitable when a medication is given at a therapeutic dose. For example, morphine (Duramorph) given for pain relief usually results in constipation. Side effects are usually identified according to body system.

KNOWLEDGE REQUIRED PRIOR TO MEDICATION ADMINISTRATION	
Adverse effects	These are undesired, inadvertent, and unexpected dangerous effects of the medication. Adverse effects are usually identified according to body system.
Toxic effects	Medications can have specific risks and manifestations of toxicity. For example, clients taking digoxin (Lanoxin) should be monitored closely for dysrhythmias, a sign of cardiotoxicity. Hypokalemia places these clients at greater risk for digoxin toxicity.
Medication interactions	Medications can interact with each other, resulting in desired or undesired effects. For example, a desired interaction would be the beta-blocker atenolol (Tenormin) used concurrently with the calcium channel blocker nifedipine (Procardia) to prevent reflex tachycardia. Take a complete medication history and be knowledgeable of clinically significant interactions.

Precautions/ Contraindications	• Medications may be contraindicated for a client with a specific disease or condition.
	   o For example, tetracyclines can stain developing teeth and should not be administered to children under 8 years of age.
	• Some medications should only be used cautiously.
	   o For example, vancomycin (Vancocin) is excreted unchanged in the kidneys and should be used cautiously for clients with renal impairment.

Preparation, dosage, administration	It is important to know any special considerations for preparation, recommended dosages, and how to administer the medication. For example, morphine (Duramorph) is available in 10 different formulations. Oral doses of morphine are generally higher than parenteral doses due to extensive first-pass effect. Clients with chronic, severe pain, as seen with cancer, are generally given oral doses of morphine.
Nursing implications	Know how to monitor therapeutic effects, prevent and treat adverse effects, provide for comfort, and instruct clients in the safe use of medications.

Medication Prescriptions

- Each facility has written policies related to medication prescriptions. Policies include which health care providers can write medication prescriptions, receive medication prescriptions, and transcribe medication prescriptions.

- Types of medication prescriptions include:

  - Routine prescription/standard prescription.

    - A routine/standard prescription identifies medications that are given on a regular schedule. It may or may not have a termination date. Without a specified termination date, the prescription will be in effect until the provider discontinues it or the client is discharged.

    - Certain medications such as opioids and antibiotics must be represcribed within a specified amount of time or will automatically be discontinued.

  - Single/one-time prescription.

    - A single/one-time prescription is to be given once at a specified time or as soon as possible. For example, a one-time prescription instructs the nurse to give warfarin (Coumadin) 5 mg PO at 1700.

  - Stat prescription.

    - A stat prescription is only given once, and it is given immediately. For example, a stat prescription instructs the nurse to give digoxin (Lanoxin) 0.125 mg IVP stat.

  - PRN prescription.

    - A PRN prescription stipulates at what dosage, what frequency, and under what conditions a medication may be given. The nurse uses clinical judgment to determine the client's need for the medication. For example, a PRN prescription instructs the nurse to give morphine (Duramorph) 2 mg IVP Q1H PRN for chest pain.

  - Standing prescriptions.

    - Standing prescriptions may be written for specific circumstances and/or for specific units. For example, the critical care unit has standing prescriptions to treat a client with asystole.

- Components of a medication prescription include:

  - The client's name.

  - The date and time of the prescription.

  - The name of the medication (may be generic or brand).

  - The dosage of the medication.

  - The route of administration.

  - The time and frequency of medication administration – exact times or number of times per day (dictated by facility policy or the specific qualities of the medication).

  - The signature of the prescribing provider.

- Communicating Medication Prescriptions

  - Origination of Medication Prescriptions

    - Medication prescriptions are written on the client's medical record by the provider or a nurse who takes a verbal or telephone prescription from a provider. If the nurse writes a medication prescription on the client's medical record, facility policy specifies how much time the provider has in which to sign the prescription (usually 24 hr). Medication prescriptions are transcribed to the medication administration record (MAR) by a nurse or other health care provider.

  - Taking a telephone prescription:

    - If possible, have a second nurse listen on an extension.

    - Ensure that the prescription is complete and correct by reading it back to the provider: the client's name, the name of the medication, the dosage, the time to be given, the frequency, and the route.

    - Remind the provider that the prescription must be signed within the specified amount of time.

    - Write the prescription in the client's medical record

- Medication Reconciliation

  - The Joint Commission requires policies and procedures for medication reconciliation. The nurse should compile a list of current medications ensuring that all medications are included, with correct dosages and frequency. This list should be compared with new medication prescriptions and reconciled to resolve any discrepancies. This list becomes the current list from which medications should be administered. This process should take place on admission, when transferring between units or facilities and at discharge.

Preassessment for Medication Therapy

- The following information should be obtained before to the initiation of medication therapy, and updated as necessary.

  - Health history

    - Age

    - Diagnosed health problems and the current reason for seeking care

    - All medications currently being taken (prescription and nonprescription): the name, dose, route, and frequency of each medication

    - Any symptoms possibly related to medication therapy

    - Use of herbal or "natural" products for medicinal purposes

    - Use of caffeine, tobacco, alcohol, and/or street drugs

    - The client's understanding of the purpose of the medications

    - All known medication and food allergies

      ○   Physical examination – a systemic physical examination provides a baseline to evaluate therapeutic effects of medication therapy and to detect possible side and adverse medication effects.

Six Rights of Safe Medication Administration

- Right client – Verify the client's identification each time a medication is given. The Joint Commission requires two client identifiers be used when administering medications. Acceptable identifiers include the client's name, an assigned identification number, telephone number, birth date, or other person-specific identifier. Bar code scanners may be used to identify clients. Check for allergies by asking the client, checking for an allergy bracelet, and checking the medication administration record.

- Right medication – Correctly interpret medication prescription (verify completeness and clarity); read labels three times: when the container is selected, when removing the dose from container, and when the container is replaced; leave unit-dose medication in its package until administration.

- Right dose – Calculate the correct medication dose; check a drug reference to ensure the dose is within the usual range.

- Right time – Give medication on time to maintain a consistent therapeutic blood level. It is generally acceptable to give the medication ½ hr before or after the scheduled time. However, refer to the drug reference or facility policy for exceptions.

- Right route – Most common routes of administration are oral, topical, subcutaneous, intramuscular (IM), and intravenous (IV). Select the correct preparation for the ordered route (otic vs ophthalmic topical ointment or drops). Know how to administer medication safely and correctly.

- Right documentation – immediately record pertinent information, including the client's response to the medication.

Additional considerations

- Assessment – Appropriate data should be collected before administering medication (apical heart rate before giving digitalis preparations). Assess the client for physical and psychosocial factors that may affect medication response.

- Education – As part of informed consent, provide accurate information about the medication therapy and its implications (therapeutic response, side/adverse effects). To individualize the teaching, determine what the client already knows about the medication, needs to know about the medication, and wants to know about the medication.

- Evaluation – determine the effectiveness of the medication based on the client's response, as well as the occurrence of side/adverse effects.

- Medication refusal – clients have the right to refuse to take a medication. Determine the reason for refusal, provide information regarding the risk of refusal, notify appropriate health care personnel, and document the refusal and actions taken.

- Resources for medication information
  - ○ Nursing drug handbooks
  - ○ Pharmacology textbooks
  - ○ Professional journals
  - ○ *The Physicians' Desk Reference (PDR)*
  - ○ Professional Web sites

Ⓢ Medication Error Prevention

- Common medication errors include:
  - ○ Wrong medication or IV fluid.
  - ○ Incorrect dose or IV rate.
  - ○ Wrong client, route, or time.
  - ○ Administration of known allergic medication.
  - ○ Omission of dose.
  - ○ Incorrect discontinuation of medication or IV fluid.
- Use the nursing process to prevent medication errors
  - ○ Assessment/Data Collection
    - ■ Ensure knowledge of medication to be administered. Use appropriate resources
      - □ Health care providers including nurses, physicians and pharmacists
      - □ Poison control centers
      - □ Sales representatives from drug companies
      - □ Nursing pharmacology textbooks and drug handbooks
      - □ *Physicians' Desk Reference*
      - □ Newsletters including *The Medical Letter on Drugs and Therapeutics* (bimonthly) and *Prescriber's Letter* (monthly)
      - □ Professional journals.
      - □ Professional Web sites.
    - ■ Obtain information about the client's medical diagnoses and conditions related to medication administration such as the ability to swallow, allergies, heart, liver, and/or kidney disorders).
      - □ Identify the client's allergies.
      - □ Obtain necessary preadministration data (heart rate, blood pressure).
      - □ Omit or delay doses as indicated by the client's condition.

- Determine if the medication prescription is complete – to include the client's name, date and time, name of medication, dosage, route of administration, time and frequency, and signature of the prescribing provider.

- Interpret the medication prescription accurately.

  □ The Institute for Safe Medication Practices is a nonprofit organization working to educate health care providers and consumers regarding safe medication practices. Tools have been developed to decrease the risk of medication errors. A complete list can be found at the organization's Web site. (http://www.ismp.org/)

    ▸ Error-Prone Abbreviation List – Certain abbreviations have been associated with a high number of medication errors.

    ▸ Confused Medication Name List – Sound-alike and look-alike medication names.

    ▸ High-Alert Medication List – Medications that, if given in error, have a high risk for resulting in significant patient harm.

- Question the provider if the prescription is unclear or seems inappropriate for the client's condition. Refuse to give a medication if it is believed to be unsafe. Notify the charge nurse or supervisor.

- Dosage changes are usually made gradually. Question the provider if abrupt and excessive changes in dosages are made.

  o Planning

  - Identify client outcomes for medication administration.

  - Set priorities.

  o Implementation

  - Avoid distractions during medication preparation (poor lighting, phones). Interruptions may increase the risk of error.

  - Check the labels for the medication name and concentration. Read labels carefully. Measure doses accurately and double-check high-alert medications such as insulin and heparin with a colleague.

 View Media Supplement: Look-alike, Sound-alike Medications (Video)

  - Doses are usually one to two tablets or one single-dose vial. Question multiple tablets or vials for a single dose.

  - Follow the six rights of medication administration consistently. Take the medication administration record (MAR) to the bedside.

  - Only give medications that have been personally prepared.

  - Encourage clients to become part of the safety net, teaching them about medications and the importance of proper identification before medications are administered. Omit or delay a dose if the client questions the size of the dose or the appearance of the medication.

- Follow correct procedures for all routes of administration.

- Communicate clearly both in writing and speaking.

- Use verbal prescriptions only for emergencies and follow facility protocol for telephone prescriptions.

- Omit or delay doses as indicated by the client's condition, and document and report appropriately.

- Follow all laws and regulations regarding controlled substances when preparing and administering medications. Keep controlled substances in a locked area. Discarding an excess of a controlled substance should be witnessed by a licensed health care provider.

- Only leave medications at a client's bedside if allowed by facility policy, such as topical medications.

    o   Evaluation

- Evaluate the client's response to a medication, and document and report appropriately.

- Recognize side/adverse effects, and document and report appropriately.

- Report all errors and implement corrective measures immediately.

        □   Complete an unusual occurrence report within the specified time frame, usually 24 hr. This report should include the client's identification, the time and place of the incident, an accurate account of the event, who was notified, what actions were taken, and the signature of the person completing the report. This report does not become a part of the client's permanent record and the report should not be referenced in another part of the record.

CHAPTER 47: MEDICATION ADMINISTRATION AND ERROR REDUCTION

 Application Exercises

1. A nurse prepares an injection of morphine (Duramorph) to give to a client who reports pain. Prior to administering the medication, the nurse is called to another room to assist another client onto a bedpan. This nurse then asks a second nurse to give the injection so that she can help the client needing the bedpan. Which of the following actions should the second nurse take?

    A. Offer to assist the client needing the bedpan.

    B. Give the injection prepared by the other nurse.

    C. Prepare another syringe and give the injection.

    D. Tell the client needing the bedpan she will have to wait for her nurse.

2. For a medication that was prescribed to be administered at 0900, which of the following are acceptable administration times? (Select all that apply.)

    _____ 0905

    _____ 0825

    _____ 1000

    _____ 0840

    _____ 0935

3. Which of the following nursing actions may prevent medication errors?

    A. Taking all medications out of the unit-dose wrappers before entering the client's room.

    B. Checking with the provider when a single dose requires administration of multiple tablets.

    C. Giving the prescribed medication and then looking up the usual dosage range.

    D. Relying on another nurse to clarify a medication prescription.

4. When implementing medication therapy, the nurse's responsibilities include which of the following? (Select all that apply.)

    _____ Observing for medication side effects

    _____ Monitoring for therapeutic effects

    _____ Prescribing the appropriate dose

    _____ Changing the dose if side effects occur

    _____ Maintaining an up-to-date knowledge base

5. A nurse should use the nursing process when administering medications to prevent errors. Match the step of the nursing action in column A with the appropriate action in column B.

    _____ Assessment/Data collection   A. Follow the six rights of medication administration consistently.

    _____ Planning   B. Recognize side/adverse effects.

    _____ Implementation   C. Identify client allergies.

    _____ Evaluation   D. Determine client outcomes.

CHAPTER 47: MEDICATION ADMINISTRATION AND ERROR REDUCTION

 Application Exercises Answer Key

1. A nurse prepares an injection of morphine (Duramorph) to give to a client who reports pain. Prior to administering the medication, the nurse is called to another room to assist another client onto a bedpan. This nurse then asks a second nurse to give the injection so that she can help the client needing the bedpan. Which of the following actions should the second nurse to take?

   A. Offer to assist the client needing the bedpan.

   B. Give the injection prepared by the other nurse.

   C. Prepare another syringe and give the injection.

   D. Tell the client needing the bedpan she will have to wait for her nurse.

   The second nurse should offer to assist the client needing the bedpan. This will allow the nurse who prepared the injection to administer it. A nurse should only administer medications that he prepared. Preparing another syringe will delay the administration of the needed pain medication. Telling the client to wait is not an acceptable option for the client needing the bedpan.

   NCLEX® Connection: Safety and Infection Control, Error Prevention

2. For a medication that was ordered at 0900, which of the following are acceptable administration times? (Select all that apply.)

__X__	**0905**
_____	0825
_____	1000
__X__	**0840**
_____	0935

   A medication may be given within 30 min of the scheduled time. 0905 and 0840 are within that window of time. 0825, 1000, and 0935 are not.

   NCLEX® Connection: Pharmacological and Parenteral Therapies, Medication Administration

3. Which of the following nursing actions may prevent medication errors?

    A. Taking all medications out of the unit-dose wrappers before entering the client's room.

    B. Checking with the provider when a single dose requires administration of multiple tablets.

    C. Giving the prescribed medication and then looking up the usual dosage range.

    D. Relying on another nurse to clarify a medication prescription.

If a single dose requires multiple tablets, it is possible that an error has occurred in the transcription of the order. Errors may be prevented by taking unit-dose medication out of the wrapper at the bedside. Looking up usual dosage range prior to giving a medication may uncover an inaccurate dosage. If the order is unclear, the nurse must contact the prescribing provider for clarification.

(N) **NCLEX® Connection: Safety and Infection Control, Error Prevention**

4. When implementing medication therapy, the nurse's responsibilities include which of the following? (Select all that apply.)

    X   **Observing for medication side effects**

    X   **Monitoring for therapeutic effects**

    _____   Prescribing the appropriate dose

    _____   Changing the dose if side effects occur

    X   **Maintaining an up-to-date knowledge base**

The nurse is responsible for observing for medication side effects, monitoring for therapeutic effects, and maintaining an up-to-date knowledge base. The prescribing provider is responsible for ordering the appropriate dose and changing the dose if side effects occur.

(N) **NCLEX® Connection: Pharmacological and Parenteral Therapies, Medication Administration**

5. A nurse should use the nursing process when administering medications to prevent errors. Match the step of the nursing action in column A with the appropriate action in column B.

    C   Assessment/Data collection   A. Follow the six rights of medication administration consistently.

    D   Planning   B. Recognize side/adverse effects.

    A   Implementation   C. Identify client allergies.

    B   Evaluation   D. Determine client outcomes.

(N) **NCLEX® Connection: Safety and Infection Control, Error Prevention**

UNIT 4	PHYSIOLOGICAL INTEGRITY
Section	Pharmacological and Parenteral Therapies
Chapter 48	Dosage Calculation

(a) Overview

- Basic medication dose conversion and calculation skills are essential for the provision of safe nursing care.

- Regardless of the dosage calculation method used, knowledge of standard conversions and recognition of availability data are used to solve a clinical problem.

- Nurses are responsible for administering the correct amount of medication by calculating the appropriate amount of medication to give. Types of calculations required include:

    o Solid oral medications

    o Liquid oral medications

    o Injectable medications

    o Correct doses based on the client's weight

    o Intravenous infusions

- Three methods for dosage calculation are presented. These include ratio and proportion, desired over have, and dimensional analysis.

- Standard conversion factors are as follows:

    o 1 mg = 1,000 mcg

    o 1 g = 1,000 mg

    o 1 kg = 1,000 g

    o 1 oz = 30 mL

    o 1 L = 1,000 mL

    o 1 tsp = 5 mL

    o 1 tbsp = 15 mL

    o 1 tbsp = 3 tsp

    o 1 kg = 2.2 lb

    o 1 gr = 60 mg

- General Rounding Guidelines

    ○ If the number to the right is equal to or greater than 5, round up by adding 1 to the number to the left.

    ○ If the number to the right is less than 5, round down by dropping the number and leaving the number to the left the same.

    ○ For dosages less than 1.0, round to the nearest hundredth.

        ■ For example: The calculated dose is 0.746 mL. Look at the number in the thousandths place (6). Six is greater than 5. To round to hundredths, add 1 to 4 and drop the 6. The rounded dose is 0.75 mL.

    ○ For dosages greater than 1.0, round to the nearest tenth.

DOSAGE CALCULATIONS USING RATIO AND PROPORTION

- Process for calculating solid, liquid and injectable dosage using ratio and proportion

    STEP 1: What is the dose needed? Dose needed = Desired

    STEP 2: What is the dose available? Dose available = Have

    STEP 3: Do the units of measurement need to be converted? Convert the unit of measurement of what is desired to the unit of measurement of what is available.

    STEP 4: Determine the quantity of the dose available. The quantity of the available dose refers to how the medication is provided, such as 2 mL or 3 tablets.

    STEP 5: Set up an equation using knowledge about basic equivalents and solve for X.

    $$\frac{\text{Have}}{\text{Quantity}} = \frac{\text{Desire}}{\text{X}}$$

    STEP 6: Reassess to determine if the amount to be given makes sense.

Solid Dosage

Ⓔ Example: The provider prescribes phenytoin (Dilantin) 0.2 g PO, TID. The amount available is 200 mg/capsule. How many capsules should the nurse give?

- Follow the steps:

    STEP 1: What is the dose needed? Dose needed = Desired

    　　0.2 g

    STEP 2: What is the dose available? Dose available = Have

    　　200 mg

    STEP 3: Do the units of measurement need to be converted?

    　　Yes (g ≠ mg)

Convert the unit of measurement of what is desired to the unit of measurement of what is available.

Desire: g

Have: mg

0.2 g = X mg

Equivalents:

1 g = 1,000 mg (1 • 1,000)

Therefore:

0.2 g = 200 mg (0.2 • 1,000)

STEP 4: What is the quantity of the dose available?

1 capsule

STEP 5: Set up an equation and solve:

$$\frac{\text{Have}}{\text{Quantity}} = \frac{\text{Desire}}{\text{X}}$$

$$\frac{200\text{ mg}}{1\text{ capsule}} = \frac{200\text{ mg}}{\text{X}}$$

Cross multiply and solve for X:

200X = 200

Isolate X by dividing both sides by 200:

$$\frac{200\text{X}}{200} = \frac{200}{200}$$

X = 1 capsule

STEP 6: Reassess to determine if the amount to be given makes sense. If there are 200 mg/capsule and the prescribed amount is 0.2 g or 200 mg, it makes sense to give 1 capsule.

The nurse should administer phenytoin 1 capsule PO 3 times per day.

Liquid Dosage

Example: The provider prescribes erythromycin estolate (Ilosone) oral suspension 0.25 g PO TID. The amount available is erythromycin oral suspension, 250 mg/mL. How many mL should the nurse administer with each dose?

- Follow the steps:

    STEP 1: What is the dose needed? Dose needed = Desired

    0.25 g

    STEP 2: What is the dose available? Dose available = Have

    250 mg

    STEP 3: Do the units of measurement need to be converted?

    Yes (g ≠ mg)

    Convert the unit of measurement of what is desired to the unit of measurement of what is available.

    Desire: g

    Have: mg

    0.25 g = X mg

    Equivalents

    1 g = 1,000 mg (1 • 1,000)

    Therefore:

    0.25 g = 250 mg (0.25 • 1,000)

    STEP 4: What is the quantity of the dose available?

    1 mL

    STEP 5: Set up an equation and solve:

    $$\frac{\text{Have}}{\text{Quantity}} = \frac{\text{Desire}}{X}$$

    $$\frac{250 \text{ mg}}{1 \text{ mL}} = \frac{250 \text{ mg}}{X}$$

Cross multiply and solve for X:

    250X = 250

    Isolate X by dividing both sides by 250:

    $$\frac{250X}{250} = \frac{250}{250}$$

    X = 1 mL

STEP 6: Reassess to determine if the amount to be given makes sense. If there are 250 mg/mL and the prescribed amount is 250 mg, it makes sense to give 1 mL.

The nurse should administer erythromycin estolate 1 mL PO 3 times a day.

Injectable Dosage

 Example: The provider prescribes heparin 8,000 units subcutaneously, Q12H. The amount available is 5,000 units/mL. How many mL should the nurse administer?

- Follow the steps:

  STEP 1: What is the dose needed? Dose needed = Desired

  8,000 units

  STEP 2: What is the dose available? Dose available = Have

  5,000 units

  STEP 3: Do the units of measurement need to be converted?

  No (units = units)

  STEP 4: What is the quantity of the dose available?

  1 mL

  STEP 5: Set up an equation and solve:

  $$\frac{\text{Have}}{\text{Quantity}} = \frac{\text{Desire}}{\text{X}}$$

  $$\frac{5,000 \text{ units}}{1 \text{ mL}} = \frac{8,000 \text{ units}}{\text{X}}$$

  Cross multiply and solve for X:

  5,000X = 8,000

  Isolate X by dividing both sides by 5,000.

  $$\frac{5,000\text{X}}{5,000} = \frac{8,000}{5,000}$$

  X = 1.6 mL

STEP 6: Reassess to determine if the amount to be given makes sense. If there are 5,000 units/mL and the prescribed amount is 8,000 units, it makes sense to give 1.6 mL.

The nurse should administer heparin 1.6 mL subcutaneously every 12 hr.

Dosages by Weight

- Process for calculating dosage by weight using ratio and proportion.

- Medications may be prescribed in daily amounts per kg of body weight such as "5 mg/kg/day," which is then divided into doses given throughout the day. The same process as for calculating oral dosages is used, but first the nurse must determine the client's weight in kg, the total daily dose, and the amount per dose.

 Example: The provider prescribes cefixime (Suprax) 8 mg/kg/day PO to be given in two divided doses. The client weighs 22 lb. The amount available is 100 mg/5 mL suspension. How many mL should the nurse administer per dose?

STEP 1: What is the client's weight in kg?

2.2 lb = 1 kg

Client weight in lb = X kg

Set up an equation:

$$\frac{2.2 \text{ lb}}{1 \text{ kg}} = \frac{\text{Client's weight in lb}}{\text{X kg}}$$

$$\frac{2.2 \text{ lb}}{1 \text{ kg}} = \frac{22 \text{ lb}}{\text{X kg}}$$

Cross multiply and solve for X:

2.2X = 22

X = 10 kg

STEP 2: What is the total daily dose?

Amount prescribed • kg weight (mg • kg) = total daily dose

8 mg • 10 kg = 80 mg

STEP 3: What is the amount per dose?

$$\frac{\text{Total daily dose}}{\text{Number of doses prescribed per day}} = \text{Amount per dose}$$

$$\frac{80 \text{ mg}}{2 \text{ doses/day}} = 40 \text{ mg/dose}$$

STEP 4: What is the dose needed? Dose needed = Desired

Desired = 40 mg

STEP 5: What is the dose available? Dose available = Have

Have = 100 mg

STEP 6: Do the units of measurement need to be converted?

No (mg = mg)

STEP 7: What is the quantity of the dose available?

Quantity = 5 mL

STEP 8: Set up an equation using knowledge about basic equivalents.

$$\frac{\text{Have}}{\text{Quantity}} = \frac{\text{Desire}}{\text{X}}$$

$$\frac{100 \text{ mg}}{5 \text{ mL}} = \frac{40 \text{ mg}}{\text{X}}$$

Cross multiply and solve for X:

100X = 200

Isolate X by dividing each side by 100.

$$\frac{100\text{X}}{100} = \frac{200}{100}$$

X = 2 mL

STEP 9: Reassess to determine if the amount to be given makes sense. If there are 100 mg/5 mL and the prescribed dose is 40 mg, it makes sense for the nurse to give 2 mL.

The nurse should administer cefixime 2 mL PO with each dose.

IV Flow Rates

- IV flow rates must be calculated for either:

  o Electronic IV pumps

    ▪ Flow rates on IV infusion pumps are set in whole mL/hr. The pump regulates the number of gtt/min based on this mL/hr setting.

    ▪ While IV infusion pumps are usually programmed for whole numbers, most pumps are able to accept decimal flow rates. This option is usually reserved for use in the critical care setting or for pediatric clients where precise dosing is essential.

- ○ Manual Infusions
  - ■ The flow rate for manual IVs is based on drops per minute.
    - □ Drops per minute is expressed as gtt/min.
  - ■ Flow rate is calculated using "drop factors" found on each manufacturer's IV tubing.
    - □ The drop factor is the number of drops per mL of liquid that an IV tubing set will drip into its drip chamber. Drops per mL is expressed as gtt/mL.
- • Rounding
  - ○ If a calculation results in a remaining decimal, round to the nearest whole number.
    - ■ If the remaining decimal is less than 0.5, round down to the nearest whole number.
      - □ For example: Round 16.3 mL/hr to 16 mL/hr.
    - ■ If the remaining decimal is 0.5 or greater, round up to the nearest whole number.
      - □ For example: Round 16.6 mL/hr to 17 mL/hr.
- • When the time in hr is known, use the following formula:

$$\frac{\text{Volume (mL)}}{\text{Time (hr)}} = \text{IV flow rate (mL/hr)}$$

Ⓔ Example: The provider prescribes dextrose 5% in water 500 mL IV to infuse over the next 4 hr. The nurse should set the IV infusion pump to deliver how many mL/hr?

STEP 1: What is the volume to be infused? Volume to be infused = Volume (mL)

500 mL

STEP 2: What is the time for the infusion? Time of infusion = Time (hr)

4 hr

STEP 3: Set up an equation and solve:

$$\frac{\text{Volume (mL)}}{\text{Time (hr)}} = \text{IV flow rate (mL/hr)}$$

$$\frac{500 \text{ mL}}{4 \text{ hr}} = 125 \text{ mL/hr}$$

STEP 4: Reassess to determine if the IV flow rate makes sense. If 500 mL is to be infused in 4 hr, it makes sense to administer 125 mL/hr.

The nurse should set the IV pump to deliver 125 mL/hr.

- When the time in minutes is known, ratio and proportion may be used to find the flow rate (mL/hr):

    STEP 1: What is the volume to be infused? Volume to be infused = Volume (mL)

    STEP 2: What is the time for the infusion? Time of infusion = Time (min)

    STEP 3: Set up an equation and solve:

$$\frac{\text{Volume (mL)}}{\text{Time (min)}} = \frac{X\ mL}{60\ min}$$

Cross multiply and solve for X:

Time (min) • X mL = Volume (mL) • 60 min

    STEP 4: Reassess to determine if the IV flow rate makes sense.

Ⓔ Example: The provider prescribes cefotaxime (Claforan) 1 g by intermittent intravenous bolus. The amount available is cefotaxime 1 g to be added to 100 mL of 0.9% sodium chloride, to infuse over 45 min. The nurse should set the IV infusion pump to deliver how many mL/hr?

- Follow these steps:

    STEP 1: What is the volume to be infused? Volume to be infused = Volume (mL)

    100 mL

    STEP 2: What is the time for the infusion? Time of infusion = Time (min)

    45 min

    STEP 3: Set up an equation and solve:

$$\frac{\text{Volume (mL)}}{\text{Time (min)}} = \frac{X\ mL}{60\ min}$$

$$\frac{100\ mL}{45\ min} = \frac{X\ mL}{60\ min}$$

Cross multiply and solve for X:

45X = 6,000

X = 133.3 or 133

    STEP 4: Reassess to determine if the IV flow rate makes sense. If 100 mL are to be infused in 45 min, it makes sense to administer 133 mL/hr.

The nurse should set the IV pump to deliver 133 mL/hr.

- Flow rates for manual IV infusions can easily be calculated using this simple formula:

$$\frac{\text{Volume to be infused}}{\text{Time (min)}} \cdot \text{Drop factor (gtt/mL)} = \text{IV flow rate (gtt/min)}$$

  STEP 1: What is the volume to be infused? Volume to be infused = Volume (mL)

  STEP 2: What is the time for the infusion? Time of infusion = Time (min)

  Convert hr to min:

$$\frac{60 \text{ min}}{1 \text{ hr}} = \frac{X \text{ min}}{\text{prescribed hr}}$$

  STEP 3: What is the drop factor on the IV tubing?

  STEP 4: Set up an equation and solve:

$$\frac{\text{Volume to be infused}}{\text{Time (min)}} \cdot \text{Drop factor (gtt/mL)} = \text{IV flow rate (gtt/min)}$$

  STEP 5: Reassess to determine if the IV flow rate makes sense.

(E) Example: The provider prescribes Lactated Ringer's 250 mL IV to infuse at 75 mL/hr. The drop factor on the manual IV tubing is 20 gtt/mL. The nurse should set the IV flow rate to deliver how many gtt/min?

- Follow these steps:

  STEP 1: What is the volume to be infused? Volume to be infused = Volume (mL)

  75 mL

  STEP 2: What is the time for the infusion? Time of infusion = Time (min)

  Convert hr to min:

$$\frac{60 \text{ min}}{1 \text{ hr}} = \frac{X \text{ min}}{\text{prescribed hr}}$$

  1 hr = 60 min

  STEP 3: What is the drop factor on the IV tubing?

  20 gtt/mL

  STEP 4: Set up an equation.

$$\frac{\text{Volume to be infused}}{\text{Time (min)}} \cdot \text{Drop factor (gtt/mL)} = \text{IV flow rate (gtt/min)}$$

$$\frac{75 \text{ mL}}{60 \text{ min}} \cdot 20 \text{ gtt/mL} = \frac{1{,}500 \text{ gtt}}{60 \text{ min}} = 25 \text{ gtt/min}$$

STEP 5: Reassess to determine if the IV flow rate makes sense.

The nurse should set the manual IV flow rate at 25 gtt/min.

Ⓔ Example: The provider prescribes ranitidine (Zantac) 150 mg by intermittent IV bolus. The amount available is dextrose 5% in water 100 mL to infuse over 30 min. The drop factor on the manual IV tubing is 10 gtt/mL. The nurse should set the IV to deliver how many gtt/min?

- Follow these steps:

    STEP 1: What is the volume to be infused? Volume to be infused = Volume (mL)

    100 mL

    STEP 2: What is the time for the infusion? Time of infusion = Time (min)

    30 min

    STEP 3: What is the drop factor on the IV tubing?

    10 gtt/mL

    STEP 4: Set up an equation.

    $$\frac{\text{Volume to be infused}}{\text{Time (min)}} \cdot \text{Drop factor (gtt/mL)} = \text{IV flow rate (gtt/min)}$$

    $$\frac{100 \text{ mL}}{30 \text{ min}} \cdot 10 \text{ gtt/mL} = \frac{1{,}000 \text{ gtt}}{30 \text{ min}} = 33.3 \text{ or } 33 \text{ gtt/min}$$

    STEP 5: Reassess to determine if the IV flow rate makes sense.

The nurse should set the manual IV flow rate at 33 gtt/min.

DOSAGE CALCULATIONS USING THE DESIRED OVER HAVE METHOD

- Process of calculating solid, liquid and injectable dosage using desire over have:

    STEP 1: What is the dose needed? Dose needed = Desired

    STEP 2: What is the dose available? Dose available = Have

    STEP 3: Do the units of measurement need to be converted? Convert the unit of measurement of what is desired to the unit of measurement of what is available.

    STEP 4: Determine the quantity of the dose available. Quantity of the available dose refers to how the medication is provided, such as 2 mL or 3 tablets.

    STEP 5: Set up an equation and solve:

    $$\frac{\text{Desired} \cdot \text{Quantity}}{\text{Have}} = \text{Amount to be given}$$

    STEP 6: Reassess to determine if the amount to be given makes sense.

Solid Dosages

(E) Example: The provider prescribes phenytoin (Dilantin) 0.2 g PO, TID. The amount available is 200 mg/capsule. How many capsules should the nurse give?

- Follow the steps:

    STEP 1: What is the dose needed? Dose needed = Desired

    0.2 g

    STEP 2: What is the dose available? Dose available = Have

    200 mg

    STEP 3: Do the units of measurement need to be converted?

    Yes (g ≠ mg)

    Convert the unit of measurement of what is desired to the unit of measurement of what is available.

    Desire: g

    Have: mg

    0.2 g = X mg

    Equivalents:

    1 g = 1,000 mg (1 • 1,000)

    Therefore:

    0.2 g = 200 mg (0.2 • 1,000)

    STEP 4: What is the quantity of the dose available?

    1 capsule

    STEP 5: Set up an equation and solve:

    Desired x Quantity = Amount to be given

    Have

    $$\frac{200 \text{ mg} \cdot 1 \text{ capsule}}{200 \text{ mg}} = X \text{ capsules}$$

    $$\frac{200 \cdot 1}{200} = \frac{200}{200} = X \text{ capsules}$$

    X = 1 capsule

STEP 6: Reassess to determine if the amount to be given makes sense. If there are 200 mg/capsule and the prescribed amount is 0.2 g or 200 mg, it makes sense to give 1 capsule.

The nurse should administer phenytoin 1 capsule PO 3 times per day.

Liquid Dosage

Example: The provider prescribes erythromycin estolate (Ilosone) oral suspension 0.25 g PO TID. The amount available is erythromycin oral suspension, 250 mg/mL. How many mL should the nurse administer with each dose?

- Follow these steps

    STEP 1: What is the dose needed? Dose needed = Desired

    0.25 g

    STEP 2: What is the dose available? Dose available = Have

    250 mg

    STEP 3: Do the units of measurement need to be converted?

    Yes (g ≠ mg)

    Convert the unit of measurement of what is desired to the unit of measurement of what is available.

    Desire: g

    Have: mg

    0.25 g = X mg

    Equivalents

    1 g = 1,000 mg (1 • 1,000)

    Therefore:

    0.25 g = 250 mg (0.25 • 1,000)

    STEP 4: What is the quantity of the dose available?

    1 mL

    STEP 5: Set up an equation and solve:

$$\frac{\text{Desired} \cdot \text{Quantity}}{\text{Have}} = \text{Amount to be given}$$

$$\frac{250 \text{ mg} \cdot 1 \text{ mL}}{250 \text{ mg}} = X \text{ mL}$$

$$\frac{250 \cdot 1}{250} = \frac{250}{250} = X \text{ mL}$$

$$X = 1 \text{ mL}$$

STEP 6: Reassess to determine if the amount to be given makes sense. If there are 250 mg/mL and the prescribed amount is 250 mg, it makes sense to give 1 mL.

The nurse should administer erythromycin estolate 1 mL PO three times a day.

Injectable Dosage

Ⓔ Example: The provider prescribes heparin 8,000 units subcutaneously Q12H. The amount available is 5,000 units/mL. How many mL should the nurse administer?

- Follow the steps:

    STEP 1: What is the dose needed? Dose needed = Desired

    8,000 units

    STEP 2: What is the dose available? Dose available = Have

    5,000 units

    STEP 3: Do the units of measurement need to be converted?

    No (units = units)

    STEP 4: What is the quantity of the dose available?

    1 mL

    STEP 5: Set up an equation and solve:

$$\frac{\text{Desired} \cdot \text{Quantity}}{\text{Have}} = \text{Amount to be given}$$

$$\frac{8,000 \text{ units} \cdot 1 \text{ mL}}{5,000 \text{ units}} = X \text{ mL}$$

$$\frac{8,000 \cdot 1}{5,000} = \frac{8,000}{5,000} = X \text{ mL}$$

$$X = 1.6 \text{ mL}$$

STEP 6: Reassess to determine if the amount to be given makes sense. If there are 5,000 units/mL and the prescribed amount is 8,000 units, it makes sense to give 1.6 mL.

The nurse should administer heparin 1.6 mL subcutaneously every 12 hr.

Dosages by Weight

- Process for calculating dosage by weight using the desired over have method:

  ○ Medications may be prescribed in daily amounts per kg of body weight such as "5 mg/kg/day," which is then divided into doses given throughout the day. The same process as for calculating oral dosages is used, but first the nurse must determine the client's weight in kg, the total daily dose, and the amount per dose.

Ⓔ Example: The provider prescribes cefixime (Suprax) 8 mg/kg/day PO to be given in two divided doses. The client weighs 22 lb. The amount available is 100 mg/5 mL suspension. How many mL should the nurse administer per dose?

STEP 1: What is the client's weight in kg?

2.2 lb = 1 kg

Client weight in lb = X kg

Set up an equation:

$$\frac{2.2\ lb}{1\ kg} = \frac{Client's\ weight\ in\ lb}{X\ kg}$$

$$\frac{2.2\ lb}{1\ kg} = \frac{22\ lb}{X}$$

Cross multiply and solve for X:

2.2X = 22

X = 10 kg

STEP 2: What is the total daily dose?

Amount prescribed • kg weight (mg • kg) = total daily dose

8 mg/kg • 10 kg = 80 mg

STEP 3: What is the amount per dose?

$$\frac{Total\ daily\ dose}{Number\ of\ doses\ prescribed\ per\ day} = Amount\ per\ dose$$

$$\frac{80\ mg}{2\ doses/day} = 40\ mg/dose$$

STEP 4: What is the dose needed? Dose needed = Desired

Desired = 40 mg

STEP 5: What is the dose available? Dose available = Have

Have = 100 mg

STEP 6: Do the units of measurement need to be converted?

No (mg = mg)

STEP 7: What is the quantity of the dose available?

Quantity = 5 mL

STEP 8: Set up an equation:

$$\frac{\text{Desired} \cdot \text{Quantity}}{\text{Have}} = \text{Amount to be given}$$

$$\frac{40 \text{ mg} \cdot 5 \text{ mL}}{100 \text{ mg}} = X \text{ mL}$$

$$\frac{40 \cdot 5}{100} = X \text{ mL}$$

$$\frac{40 \cdot 5}{100} = \frac{200}{100} = X \text{ mL}$$

$$X = 2 \text{ mL}$$

STEP 9: Reassess to determine if the amount to be given makes sense. If there are 100 mg/5 mL and the prescribed dose is 40 mg, it makes sense for the nurse to give 2 mL.

The nurse should administer cefixime 2 mL PO with each dose.

DOSAGE CALCULATIONS USING DIMENSIONAL ANALYSIS

- Dimensional analysis is a method of calculation in which a series of ratios or factors, organized in the form of fractions, are multiplied.

   o   Factors are two quantities that are related, such as 30 mg in 2 mL.

   o   In dimensional analysis, factors are expressed as fractions.

○ 30 mg in 2 mL may be expressed as:

$$\frac{30 \text{ mg}}{2 \text{ mL}} \text{ or } \frac{2 \text{ mL}}{30 \text{ mg}}$$

- One unit of measurement is converted to another unit of measurement by means of conversion factors or unit equivalence. A conversion factor is a unit equivalence such as 2.2 lb = 1 kg or 1,000 mcg = 1 mg.

  ○ Conversion factors link units of measurement of what is desired with units of measurement of what is available.

  ○ Conversion factors are arranged in the form of a fraction.

  ○ 1,000 mcg = 1 mg may be expressed as:

$$\frac{1,000 \text{ mcg}}{1 \text{ mg}} \text{ or } \frac{1 \text{ mg}}{1,000 \text{ mcg}}$$

- To create an equation using dimensional analysis:

  ○ Start with the unit of measurement that is to be calculated:

    ■ For example, to convert mcg to mg, mg are desired, so start with:

      mg =

  ○ Find the quantity with the same unit of measurement or the conversion factor with the same unit of measurement as what is desired (1 mg = 1,000 mcg) and place this (mg) in the numerator.

$$\text{mg} = \frac{1 \text{ mg}}{1,000 \text{ mcg}}$$

    ■ Remember, fractions are set up as the numerator over the denominator:

$$\frac{\text{numerator}}{\text{denominator}}$$

  ○ The fractions are arranged so that unwanted units cancel out and desired units remain.

    ■ A single quantity not associated with a related quantity is expressed as a fraction by placing it in the numerator and placing 1 in the denominator.

$$\frac{\text{X mcg}}{1}$$

  ○ If mcg are available and mg are desired, arrange the conversion factor such that mcg may be cancelled out to leave mg remaining:

$$\text{mg} = \frac{1 \text{ mg}}{1,000 \text{ mcg}} \cdot \frac{\text{X mcg}}{1}$$

Cross out the identical units that are across and diagonal:

$$mg = \frac{1 \text{ mg}}{1,000 \text{ \cancel{mcg}}} \cdot \frac{X \text{ \cancel{mcg}}}{1}$$

- o   In dimensional analysis, fractions are multiplied. To multiply fractions, first multiply across the numerator, and then multiply across the denominator. Finally, divide the numerator by the denominator.

- o   Equations involving multiple factors are arranged so that the unit of measurement in the denominator of one factor is placed in the numerator of the following factor and so on. Unwanted units are then cancelled.

    - ▪   Remember:

        - ☐   A single quantity not associated with a related quantity is expressed as a fraction by placing it in the numerator and placing 1 in the denominator.

        - ☐   Factors are two quantities that are related. Related quantities are arranged as fractions.

- ●   Process of calculating dosage using dimensional analysis:

    STEP 1: What is to be calculated?

    What is the unit of measurement that is to be calculated?

    STEP 2: What quantities are needed? Needed = desired

    The quantity needed may be the prescribed dosage.

    STEP 3: What quantities are available? Available = have

    STEP 4: Are conversion factors needed to find the units that are to be calculated?

    Conversion factors link units of measurement of what is available with units of measurement of what is to be calculated.

    STEP 5: Set up an equation of factors using needed and available quantities and the conversion factors.

    STEP 6: Multiply the numerator.

    Multiply the denominator.

    Divide the numerator by the denominator.

    STEP 7: Reassess to determine if the amount makes sense.

Solid Dosages

Ⓔ Example: The provider prescribes phenytoin (Dilantin) 0.2 g PO TID. The amount available is 200 mg/capsule. How many capsules should the nurse give?

- Follow the steps:

    STEP 1: What is to be calculated?

    What is the unit of measurement that is to be calculated?

    capsule

    STEP 2: What quantities are needed? Needed = desired

    The quantity needed may be the prescribed dosage.

    0.2 g/1

    STEP 3: What quantities are available? Available = have

    200 mg/capsule

    STEP 4: Are conversion factors needed to find what is desired?

    1,000 mg = 1 g

    STEP 5: Set up an equation of factors using needed and available quantities and the conversion factors.

    $$\text{capsule} = \frac{1 \text{ capsule}}{200 \text{ mg}} \cdot \frac{1,000 \text{ mg}}{1 \text{ g}} \cdot \frac{0.2 \text{ g}}{1}$$

    Cancel out identical units:

    $$\text{capsule} = \frac{1 \text{ capsule}}{200 \text{ \cancel{mg}}} \cdot \frac{1,000 \text{ \cancel{mg}}}{1 \text{ \cancel{g}}} \cdot \frac{0.2 \text{ \cancel{g}}}{1}$$

    STEP 6: Multiply the numerator.

    Multiply the denominator.

    Divide the numerator by the denominator.

    $$\text{capsule} = \frac{200 \text{ capsule}}{200} = 1 \text{ capsule}$$

    STEP 7: Reassess to determine if the amount to be given makes sense. If there are 200 mg/capsule and the prescribed amount is 0.2 g or 200 mg, it makes sense to give 1 capsule.

The nurse should administer phenytoin 1 capsule PO three times per day.

Liquid Dosage

(E) Example: The provider prescribes erythromycin estolate (Ilosone) oral suspension 0.25 g PO TID. The amount available is erythromycin oral suspension, 250 mg/mL. How many mL should the nurse administer with each dose?

- Follow the steps:

    STEP 1: What is to be calculated?

    What is the unit of measurement that is to be calculated?

    mL

    STEP 2: What quantities are needed? Needed = desired

    The quantity needed may be the prescribed dosage.

    0.25g/1

    STEP 3: What quantities are available? Available = have

    250 mg/mL

    STEP 4: Are conversion factors needed to find what is desired?

    1 g = 1,000 mg

    STEP 5: Set up an equation of factors using needed and available quantities and the conversion factors.

$$mL = \frac{1 \text{ mL}}{250 \text{ mg}} \cdot \frac{1,000 \text{ mg}}{1 \text{ g}} \cdot \frac{0.25 \text{ g}}{1}$$

    Cancel out identical units:

$$mL = \frac{1 \text{ mL}}{250 \text{ \cancel{mg}}} \cdot \frac{1,000 \text{ \cancel{mg}}}{1 \text{ \cancel{g}}} \cdot \frac{0.25 \text{ \cancel{g}}}{1}$$

    STEP 6: Multiply the numerator.

    Multiply the denominator.

    Divide the numerator by the denominator.

$$mL = \frac{250 \text{ mL}}{250} = 1 \text{ mL}$$

    STEP 7: Reassess to determine if the amount to be given makes sense. If there are 250 mg/mL and the prescribed amount is 250 mg, it makes sense to give 1 mL.

The nurse should administer erythromycin estolate 1 mL PO three times a day.

Injectable Dosage

(E) Example: The provider prescribes heparin 8,000 units subcutaneously Q12H. The amount available is 5,000 units/mL. How many mL should the nurse administer?

- Follow the steps:

    STEP 1: What is to be calculated?

    What is the unit of measurement that is to be calculated?

    mL

    STEP 2: What quantities are needed? Needed = desired

    The quantity needed may be the prescribed dosage.

    8,000 units/1

    STEP 3: What quantities are available? Available = have

    5,000 units /mL

    STEP 4: Are conversion factors needed to find what is desired?

    No

    STEP 5: Set up an equation of factors using needed and available quantities and the conversion factors.

    $$mL = \frac{1\ mL}{5,000\ units} \cdot \frac{8,000\ units}{1}$$

    Cancel out identical units:

    $$mL = \frac{1\ mL}{5,000\ \cancel{units}} \cdot \frac{8,000\ \cancel{units}}{1}$$

    STEP 6: Multiply the numerator.

    Multiply the denominator.

    Divide the numerator by the denominator.

    $$mL = \frac{8,000\ mL}{5,000} = 1.6\ mL$$

    STEP 7: Reassess to determine if the amount to be given makes sense. If there are 5,000 units in 1 mL and the prescribed amount 8,000 units, it makes sense to give 1.6 mL.

    The nurse should administer heparin 1.6 mL subcutaneously every 12 hr.

Dosages by Weight

- Process for calculating dosage by weight using dimensional analysis:

    ○ Medications may be prescribed in daily amounts per kg of body weight, such as "5 mg/kg/day," which is then divided into doses given throughout the day. The same process as for calculating oral dosages is used.

 Example: The provider prescribes cefixime (Suprax) 8 mg/kg/day PO to be given in two divided doses. The client weighs 22 lb. The amount available is 100 mg/5 mL suspension. How many mL should the nurse administer per dose?

- Follow these steps:

    STEP 1: What is to be calculated?

    What is the unit of measurement that is to be calculated?

    mL/dose

    STEP 2: What quantities are needed? Needed = desired

    The quantity needed may be the prescribed dosage.

    8 mg/kg/day

    STEP 3: What quantities are available? Available = have

    2 doses/day

    22 lb/1

    100 mg/5 mL

    STEP 4: Are conversion factors needed to find the units that are wanted?

    2.2 lb = 1 kg

    STEP 5: Set up an equation of factors using needed and available quantities and the conversion factors.

$$mL/dose = \frac{5\ mL}{100\ mg} \cdot \frac{8\ mg}{kg/day} \cdot \frac{1\ kg}{2.2\ lb} \cdot \frac{22\ lb}{1} \cdot \frac{1\ day}{2\ doses}$$

    Cancel out identical units:

$$mL/dose = \frac{5\ mL}{100\ \cancel{mg}} \cdot \frac{8\ \cancel{mg}}{\cancel{kg/day}} \cdot \frac{1\ \cancel{kg}}{2.2\ \cancel{lb}} \cdot \frac{22\ \cancel{lb}}{1} \cdot \frac{1\ \cancel{day}}{2\ doses}$$

STEP 6: Multiply the numerator.

Multiply the denominator.

Divide the numerator by the denominator.

$$\text{mL/dose} = \frac{5 \text{ mL} \cdot 8 \cdot 22}{100 \cdot 2.2 \cdot 2 \cdot \text{dose}} \cdot \frac{880 \text{ mL}}{440 \text{ dose}} = 2 \text{ mL/dose}$$

STEP 7: Reassess to determine if the amount to be given makes sense.

The nurse should administer cefixime 2 mL PO with each dose.

IV Flow Rates

- To determine mL/hr when administering fluid via an IV pump, the process is the same as the ratio and proportion/desired over have methods.

- When calculating gtt/min, follow these steps:

   STEP 1: What is to be calculated?

   What is the unit of measurement that is to be calculated?

   gtt/min

   STEP 2: What quantities are needed? Needed = desired

   The quantity needed may be the prescribed dosage.

   Volume (mL)/infusion time (min or hr)

   STEP 3: What quantities are available? Available = have

   Drop factor (gtt/mL)

   STEP 4: Are conversion factors needed to find what is desired?

   60 min = 1 hr

   STEP 5: Set up an equation of factors using needed and available quantities and the conversion factors.

   o   If minutes are available, the process is the same as the ratio and proportion/desired over have methods.

   o   If hours are available:

   $$\text{IV flow rate (gtt/min)} = \frac{\text{gtt}}{\text{mL}} \cdot \frac{\text{Volume (mL)}}{\text{Time (hr)}} \cdot \frac{1 \text{ hr}}{60 \text{ min}}$$

   Cancel out identical units:

   $$\text{IV flow rate (gtt/min)} = \frac{\text{gtt}}{\text{mL}} \cdot \frac{\text{Volume (mL)}}{\text{Time (hr)}} \cdot \frac{1 \text{ hr}}{60 \text{ min}}$$

STEP 6: Multiply the numerator.

Multiply the denominator.

Divide the numerator by the denominator.

STEP 7: Reassess to determine if the amount makes sense.

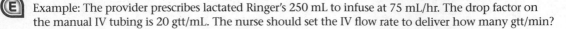 Example: The provider prescribes lactated Ringer's 250 mL to infuse at 75 mL/hr. The drop factor on the manual IV tubing is 20 gtt/mL. The nurse should set the IV flow rate to deliver how many gtt/min?

STEP 1: What is to be calculated?

What is the unit of measurement that is to be calculated?

gtt/min

STEP 2: What quantities are needed? Needed = desired

The quantity needed may be the prescribed dosage.

75 mL/hr

STEP 3: What quantities are available? Available = have

20 gtt/mL

STEP 4: Are conversion factors needed to find what is desired?

60 min = 1 hr

STEP 5: Set up an equation of factors using needed and available quantities and the conversion factors.

o   Hours are available:

$$\text{IV flow rate (gtt/min)} = \frac{20 \text{ gtt}}{1 \text{ mL}} \cdot \frac{75 \text{ mL}}{1 \text{ hr}} \cdot \frac{1 \text{ hr}}{60 \text{ min}}$$

Cancel out identical units:

$$\text{IV flow rate (gtt/min)} = \frac{20 \text{ gtt}}{1 \text{ \cancel{mL}}} \cdot \frac{75 \text{ \cancel{mL}}}{1 \text{ \cancel{hr}}} \cdot \frac{1 \text{ \cancel{hr}}}{60 \text{ min}}$$

STEP 6: Multiply the numerator.

Multiply the denominator.

Divide the numerator by the denominator.

$$\text{IV flow rate (gtt/min)} = \frac{1,500 \text{ gtt}}{60 \text{ min}} = 25 \text{ gtt/min}$$

STEP 7: Reassess to determine if the amount makes sense.

The nurse should set the manual IV flow rate at 25 gtt/min.

CHAPTER 48: DOSAGE CALCULATION

 Application Exercises

Directions: Solve each problem using ratio and proportion.

1. The provider prescribes methylprednisolone (Solu-Medrol) 5 mg by intravenous bolus Q6H. The amount available is 40 mg/2 mL. How many mL should the nurse administer for each dose?

2. The provider prescribes Lactated Ringer's 75 mL IV to be infused over 15 min. The nurse should set the IV flow rate to deliver how many mL/hr?

3. The provider prescribes 0.9% sodium chloride 250 mL IV to infuse over 30 min. The drop factor shown on the package of IV tubing is 10 gtt/mL. The nurse should set the IV flow rate to deliver how many gtt/min?

Directions: Solve each problem using the desired over have method.

4. The provider prescribes metoprolol (Lopressor) 200 mg PO every morning. The amount available is 100 mg tablets. How many tablets should the nurse administer?

5. The provider prescribes kanamycin (Kantrex) 15 mg/kg/day by mouth to be given in three divided doses. The client weights 66 lb. The amount available is 1 g/mL. How many mL should the nurse give with each dose?

6. The provider prescribes dextrose 5% in water 1,000 mL IV over 10 hr. The nurse should set the IV pump to deliver how many mL/hr?

Directions: Solve each problem using dimensional analysis.

7. The provider prescribes acetaminophen (Tylenol) 320 mg PO Q4H PRN for pain. The amount available is 160 mg/5 mL. How many mL should the nurse administer for each dose?

8. The provider prescribes Lactated Ringer's IV to infuse at 150 mL/hr. The drop factor shown on the package of IV tubing is 15 gtt/mL. The nurse should set the IV flow rate to deliver how many gtt/min?

CHAPTER 48: DOSAGE CALCULATION

 Application Exercises Answer Key

Directions: Solve each problem using ratio and proportion.

1. The provider prescribes methylprednisolone (Solu-Medrol) 5 mg by intravenous bolus administration Q6H. The amount available is 40 mg/2 mL. How many mL should the nurse administer for each dose?

> STEP 1: What is the dose needed? Dose needed = Desired
>
> 5 mg
>
> STEP 2: What is the dose available? Dose available = Have
>
> 40 mg
>
> STEP 3: Do the units of measurement need to be converted?
>
> No (mg = mg)
>
> Convert the unit of measurement of the dose desired to the unit of measurement of the dose available.
>
> STEP 4: What is the quantity of the dose available?
>
> 2 mL
>
> STEP 5: Set up an equation and solve:
>
> $$\frac{\text{Have}}{\text{Quantity}} = \frac{\text{Desire}}{X}$$
>
> $$\frac{40 \text{ mg}}{2 \text{ mL}} = \frac{5 \text{ mg}}{X}$$
>
> Cross multiply and solve for X:
>
> $40X = 10$
>
> Isolate X by dividing each side by 40.
>
> $$\frac{40X}{40} = \frac{10}{40}$$
>
> $X = 0.25 \text{ mL}$
>
> STEP 6: Reassess to determine if the amount to be given makes sense. If there is 40 mg in 2 mL and the prescribed dose is 5 mg, it makes sense to give 0.25 mL.

The nurse should administer methylprednisolone 0.25 mL IV bolus every 6 hr.

(N) NCLEX® Connection: Pharmacological and Parenteral Therapies, Dosage Calculation

2. The provider prescribes Lactated Ringer's 75 mL IV to be infused over 15 min. The nurse should set the IV flow rate to deliver how many mL/hr?

> STEP 1: What is the volume to be infused? Volume to be infused = Volume (mL)
>
> > 75 mL
>
> STEP 2: What is the time for the infusion? Time of infusion = Time (min)
>
> > 15 min
>
> STEP 3: Set up an equation and solve:
>
> > $$\frac{Volume\ (mL)}{Time\ (min)} = \frac{X\ mL}{60\ min}$$
> >
> > $$\frac{75\ mL}{15\ min} = \frac{X\ mL}{60\ min}$$
> >
> > Cross multiply and solve for X:
> >
> > 15X = 4,500
> >
> > X = 300
>
> STEP 4: Reassess to determine if the IV flow rate makes sense. If 75 mL is to be infused in 15 min, it makes sense to administer 300 mL/hr.

The nurse should set the IV pump to deliver 300 mL/hr.]

(N) **NCLEX® Connection: Pharmacological and Parenteral Therapies, Parenteral/Intravenous Therapy**

3. The provider prescribes 0.9% sodium chloride 250 mL IV to infuse over 30 min. The drop factor shown on the package of IV tubing is 10 gtt/mL. The nurse should set the IV flow rate to deliver how many gtt/min?

> STEP 1: What is the volume to be infused? Volume to be infused = Volume (mL)
>
> > 250 mL
>
> STEP 2: What is the time for the infusion? Time of infusion = Time (min)
>
> > 30 min
>
> STEP 3: What is the drop factor on the IV tubing?
>
> > 10 gtt/mL
>
> STEP 4: Set up an equation.
>
> > $$\frac{Volume\ to\ be\ infused}{Time\ (min)} \cdot Drop\ factor\ (gtt/mL) = IV\ flow\ rate\ (gtt/min)$$
> >
> > $$\frac{250\ mL}{30\ min} \cdot 10\ gtt/mL = \frac{2,500\ gtt}{30\ min} = 83.3\ or\ 83\ gtt/min$$

STEP 5: Reassess to determine if the IV flow rate makes sense.

The nurse should set the manual IV flow rate to 83 gtt/min.

Ⓝ NCLEX® Connection: Pharmacological and Parenteral Therapies, Parenteral/Intravenous Therapy

Directions: Solve each problem using the desired over have method.

4. The provider prescribes metoprolol (Lopressor) 200 mg PO every morning. The amount available is 100 mg tablets. How many tablets should the nurse administer?

STEP 1: What is the dose needed? Dose needed = Desired

200 mg

STEP 2: What is the dose available? Dose available = Have

100 mg

STEP 3: Do the units of measurement need to be converted?

No (mg = mg)

STEP 4: What is the quantity of the dose available?

1 tablet

STEP 5: Set up an equation and solve:

$$\frac{\text{Desired} \cdot \text{Quantity}}{\text{Have}} = \text{Amount to be given}$$

$$\frac{200 \text{ mg} \cdot 1 \text{ tablet}}{100 \text{ mg}} = \text{X tablets}$$

$$\frac{200 \cdot 1}{100} = \frac{200}{100} = \text{X tablets}$$

X = 2 tablets

STEP 6: Reassess to determine if the amount to be given makes sense. If there are 100 mg/tablet and the amount prescribed is 200 mg, it makes sense to give 2 tablets.

The nurse should administer metoprolol 2 tablets PO every morning.

Ⓝ NCLEX® Connection: Pharmacological and Parenteral Therapies, Dosage Calculation

5. The provider prescribes kanamycin (Kantrex) 15 mg/kg/day by mouth to be given in three divided doses. The client weights 66 lb. The amount available is 1 g/mL. How many mL should the nurse give with each dose?

STEP 1: What is the client's weight in kg?

$$\frac{2.2 \text{ lb}}{1 \text{ kg}} = \frac{\text{Client's weight in kg}}{\text{X kg}}$$

$$\frac{2.2 \text{ lb}}{1 \text{ kg}} = \frac{66 \text{ lb}}{\text{X kg}}$$

Cross multiply and solve for X:

X = 30 kg

STEP 2: What is the total daily dose?

30 mg • 15 kg = 450 mg

STEP 3: What is the amount per dose?

450 mg ÷ 3 doses = 150 mg

STEP 4: What is the dose needed? Dose needed = Desired

Desired = 150 mg

STEP 5: What is the dose available? Dose available = Have

Have = 1 g

STEP 6: Do the units of measurement need to be converted?

Yes (g ≠ mg)

Convert the unit of measurement of the dose desired to the unit of measurement of the dose available.

Desire: mg

Have: g

150 mg = X g

Equivalents:

1,000 mg = 1 g

Therefore:

150 mg = 0.15 g (150 ÷ 1,000)

Dose desired: 0.15 g

STEP 7: What is the quantity of the dose available?

Quantity = 1 mL

STEP 8: Set up an equation:

$$\frac{\text{Desired} \cdot \text{Quantity}}{\text{Have}} = \text{Amount to be given}$$

$$\frac{0.15 \text{ mg} \cdot 1 \text{ mL}}{1 \text{ g}} = X \text{ mL}$$

$$\frac{0.15 \cdot 1}{1} = \frac{0.15}{1} = X \text{ mL}$$

$$X = 0.15 \text{ mL}$$

STEP 9: Reassess to determine if the amount to be given makes sense. If there are 1,000 mg/mL and the prescribed dose is 150 mg, it makes sense to give 0.15 mL.

The nurse should administer kanamycin 0.15 mL PO with each dose.

Ⓝ **NCLEX® Connection: Pharmacological and Parenteral Therapies, Dosage Calculation**

6. The provider prescribes dextrose 5% in water 1,000 mL IV over 10 hr. The nurse should set the IV pump to deliver how many mL/hr?

STEP 1: What is the volume to be infused? Volume to be infused = Volume (mL)

1,000 mL

STEP 2: What is the time for the infusion? Time of infusion = Time (hr)

10 hr

STEP 3: Set up an equation and solve:

$$\frac{\text{Volume (mL)}}{\text{Time (hr)}} = \text{IV flow rate (mL/hr)}$$

$$\frac{1,000 \text{ mL}}{10 \text{ hr}} = 100 \text{ mL/hr}$$

STEP 4: Reassess to determine if the IV flow rate makes sense. If 1,000 mL is to be infused over 10 hr it makes sense to administer 100 mL/hr.

The nurse should set the IV pump to deliver 100 mL/hr.

Ⓝ **NCLEX® Connection: Pharmacological and Parenteral Therapies, Parenteral/Intravenous Therapy**

Directions: Solve each problem using dimensional analysis.

7. The provider prescribes acetaminophen (Tylenol) 320 mg PO Q4H PRN for pain. The amount available is 160 mg/5 mL. How many mL should the nurse administer for each dose?

STEP 1: What is to be calculated?

What is the unit of measurement that is to be calculated?

mL

STEP 2: What quantities are needed? Needed = desired

The quantity needed may be the prescribed dosage.

320 mg/1

STEP 3: What quantities are available? Available = have

160 mg/5 mL

STEP 4: Are conversion factors needed to find what is desired?

Conversion factors link units of measurement of what is available with units of measurement of what is desired.

No

STEP 5: Set up an equation of factors using needed and available quantities and the conversion factors.

$$mL = \frac{5\ mL}{160\ mg} \cdot \frac{320\ mg}{1}$$

Cancel out identical units:

$$mL = \frac{5\ mL}{160\ \cancel{mg}} \cdot \frac{320\ \cancel{mg}}{1}$$

STEP 6: Multiply the numerator.

Multiply the denominator.

Divide the numerator by the denominator.

$$mL = \frac{1{,}600\ mL}{160} = 10\ mL$$

STEP 7: Reassess to determine if the amount to be given makes sense. If there are 160 mg/5 mL and the prescribed amount is 320 mg, it makes sense to give 10 mL.

The nurse should administer acetaminophen 10 mL PO every 4 hr PRN for pain.

(N) **NCLEX® Connection: Pharmacological and Parenteral Therapies, Dosage Calculation**

8. The provider prescribes Lactated Ringer's IV to infuse at 150 mL/hr. The drop factor shown on the package of IV tubing is 15 gtt/mL. The nurse should set the IV flow rate to deliver how many gtt/min?

STEP 1: What is to be calculated?

What is the unit of measurement that is to be calculated?

gtt/min

STEP 2: What quantities are needed? Needed = desired

The quantity needed may be the prescribed dosage.

150 mL/hr

STEP 3: What quantities are available? Available = have

15 gtt/mL

STEP 4: Are conversion factors needed to find what is desired?

Conversion factors link units of measurement of what is available with units of measurement of what is desired.

60 min = 1 hr

STEP 5: Set up an equation of factors using needed and available quantities and the conversion factors.

○   Hours are available:

$$\text{IV flow rate (gtt/min)} = \frac{15 \text{ gtt}}{1 \text{ mL}} \cdot \frac{150 \text{ mL}}{1 \text{ hr}} \cdot \frac{1 \text{ hr}}{60 \text{ min}}$$

Cancel out identical units:

$$\text{IV flow rate (gtt/min)} = \frac{15 \text{ gtt}}{1 \text{ \cancel{mL}}} \cdot \frac{150 \text{ \cancel{mL}}}{1 \text{ \cancel{hr}}} \cdot \frac{1 \text{ \cancel{hr}}}{60 \text{ min}}$$

STEP 6: Multiply the numerator.

Multiply the denominator.

Divide the numerator by the denominator.

$$\text{IV flow rate (gtt/min)} = \frac{22,500 \text{ gtt}}{60 \text{ min}} = 37.5 \text{ or } 38 \text{ gtt/min}$$

STEP 7: Reassess to determine if the amount makes sense.

The nurse should set the manual IV flow rate at 38 gtt/min.

Ⓝ **NCLEX® Connection: Pharmacological and Parenteral Therapies, Parenteral/Intravenous Therapy**

UNIT 4	PHYSIOLOGICAL INTEGRITY
Section	Pharmacological and Parenteral Therapies
Chapter 49	Intravenous Therapy

Overview

- Intravenous therapy involves administering fluids via an intravenous catheter for the purpose of administering medications, supplementing fluid intake, or providing fluid replacement, electrolytes, or nutrients.

- Large-volume IV infusions are administered on a continuous basis.

- An IV medication infusion may be mixed in a large volume of fluid and given as a continuous IV infusion or mixed in a small amount of solution and given intermittently. It can also be administered as an IV bolus: The medication is given in a small amount of solution, concentrated or diluted, and injected over a short time (1 to 2 min) in emergent and nonemergent situations.

Indications and Risk Factors

- Advantages and Disadvantages of IV Therapy

ADVANTAGES	DISADVANTAGES
- Fast absorption and onset of action - Less discomfort after initial insertion - Maintains constant therapeutic blood levels - Less irritation to subcutaneous and muscle tissue	- Circulatory fluid overload is possible if the infusion is large and/or too rapid. - Immediate absorption leaves no time to correct errors. - IV administration can cause irritation to the lining of the vein. - Failure to maintain surgical asepsis can lead to local infection and septicemia.

Description of Procedure

- The provider prescribes the type of IV fluid, the volume to be infused, and either the rate at which the IV fluid should be infused or the total amount of time it should take for the fluid to be infused. The nurse regulates the IV infusion to insure the appropriate amount is administered. This can be done with an IV pump or manually.

- Large volume IV infusions are administered on a continuous basis, such as 0.9% sodium chloride IV to infuse at 100 mL/hr or 0.9% sodium chloride 1,000 mL to be given IV over 3 hr.

- A fluid bolus is a large amount of IV fluid given in a short period of time, usually less than an hour. A fluid bolus is given to rapidly replace fluid loss that could be caused by dehydration, shock, hemorrhage, burns, or trauma.

  o A large-gauge angiocatheter (18 gauge or larger) is needed to maintain the rapid rate necessary to give a fluid bolus to an adult.

- IV medication infusions may be administered in the following ways:

  o The medication may be mixed in a large volume of fluid (500 to 1,000 mL) and given as a continuous IV infusion. Potassium chloride may be administered this way.

  o The medication can be found in premixed solution bags or can be added to the IV bag by the pharmacist or the nurse.

  o Volume-controlled infusions

    ■ Some medications, such as antibiotics, are given intermittently in a small amount of solution (25 to 250 mL) through a continuous IV system, or with saline or heparin lock systems.

    ■ The medications infuse for short periods of time and are given on a scheduled basis.

    ■ These infusions can be administered by a secondary ("piggyback") IV bag or bottle or tandem setup, a volume-control administration set, or by a mini-infusion pump.

  o IV bolus dose administration

    ■ The medications are typically in small amounts of solution, concentrated or diluted, that can be injected over a short time (1 to 2 min) in emergent and nonemergent situations.

    ■ Some medications are given directly into the peripheral IV or access port to achieve an immediate medication level in the bloodstream, such as with pain medication.

    ■ Make sure medications are prepared according to the recommended concentration and administered according to the safe recommended rate.

    ■ Use extreme caution and observe for signs and symptoms of complications such as redness, burning, or increasing pain.

- Types of IV Access

  o Intravenous access can be via a peripheral or central vein (central venous access device).

  o Central venous access devices can be peripherally inserted or directly inserted into the jugular or subclavian vein.

Guidelines for Safe IV Medication Administration

- Certain medications, such as potassium chloride, can cause serious adverse reactions and should be infused on an IV pump for accurate dosage control and never given by IV bolus.

- Add medication to a new IV fluid container, not to an IV container that is already hanging.

- Never administer IV medication through tubing that is infusing blood, blood products, or parenteral nutritional solutions.

- Verify the compatibility of medications before infusing a medication through tubing that is infusing another medication.

- Needlestick Prevention

  o Be familiar with IV insertion equipment.

  o Avoid using needles when needleless systems are available.

  o Use protective safety devices when available.

  o Dispose of needles immediately in designated puncture-resistant receptacles.

  o Do not break, bend, or recap needles.

View Media Supplement: Needleless Injection System (Image)

Special Considerations

- Older adult clients, clients taking anticoagulants, or clients with fragile veins:

  - Avoid tourniquets.

  - Use a blood pressure cuff instead.

  - Do not slap the extremity to visualize veins.

  o Edema in extremities:

  - Apply digital pressure over the selected vein to displace edema.

  - Apply pressure with alcohol pad.

  - Cannulation must be quick.

  o Obese clients may require the use of anatomical landmarks to find veins.

- Preventing IV Infections

  - Use standard precautions.

  - Change IV sites according to facility policy (usually 72 hr).

  - Remove catheters as soon as they are no longer clinically indicated.

  - Change the catheter if any break in surgical aseptic technique is suspected, such as emergency insertions.

  - Use a sterile needle/catheter for each insertion attempt.

  - Avoid writing on IV bags with pens or markers, because ink could contaminate the solution.

  - Change tubing immediately if contamination is known or suspected.

- Fluids should not hang more than 24 hr unless it is a closed system (pressure bags for hemodynamic monitoring).

- Wipe all ports with alcohol or an antiseptic swab before connecting IV lines or inserting a syringe to prevent the introduction of micro-organisms into the system.

- Never disconnect tubing for convenience or to position the client.

- Do not allow ports to remain exposed to air.

- Perform hand hygiene before and after handling the IV system.

Preprocedure

- Equipment

  o Correct size catheter:

    - 16-gauge for trauma clients, rapid fluid volume

    - 18-gauge for surgical clients, rapid blood administration

    - 22- to 24-gauge for all other clients (children, adults)

  o Correct tubing

  o Infusion pump, if indicated

  o Clean gloves

  o Scissors or electric shaver for hair removal

- Nursing Actions

  o Check the provider's prescription (solution, rate).

  o Assess the client for allergies to products used in initiating and maintaining IV therapy (latex, tape, iodine).

  o Follow the six rights of medication administration (including compatibilities of all IV solutions).

  o Perform hand hygiene.

  o Examine the solution to be infused for clarity, leaks, and expiration date.

  o Don clean gloves.

  o Assess extremities and veins. If hair removal is needed, clip it with scissors or shave it with an electric shaver.

- Client Education

  o Identify the client and explain the procedure.

  o Place the client in a comfortable position.

Intraprocedure

- Nursing Actions

  - Apply a clean tourniquet or blood pressure (BP) cuff (especially for older adults) 4 to 6 inches above the proposed insertion site to compress only venous blood flow.

  - Select the vein by choosing:

    - Distal veins first on the nondominant hand

    - A site that is not painful or bruised and will not interfere with activity

    - A vein that is resilient with a soft, bouncy feeling when palpated

    - Additional methods to enhance venous access include:

      - Gravity, fist clenching, friction with alcohol, and heat.

      - Percussion with gentle tapping.

    - Avoid:

      - Varicosed veins that are permanently dilated and tortuous

      - Veins in the inner wrist with bifurcations, in flexion areas, near valves (appearing as bumps), in lower extremities, and in the antecubital fossa (except for emergency access).

      - Veins that are sclerosed or hard

      - Veins in an extremity with impaired sensitivity (scar tissue, paralysis), lymph nodes removed, recent infiltration, or an arteriovenous fistula/graft.

  - Untie the tourniquet or deflate the BP cuff.

  - Cleanse the area at the site using friction in a circular motion from the middle and outwardly with alcohol, an iodine preparation, or chlorhexidine. Allow it to air dry for 1 to 2 min.

  - Remove the cover from the catheter, grasp the plastic hub, and examine the device for smooth edges.

  - Retie the tourniquet or reinflate the BP cuff.

  - Anchor the vein below the site of insertion.

  - Pull the skin taut and hold it.

  - Warn the client of a sharp, quick stick.

  - Insert the catheter into the skin with the bevel up at an angle of 10° to 30° using a steady, smooth motion.

  - Advance the catheter through the skin and into the vein maintaining a 10° to 30° angle. Flashback of blood will confirm placement in the vein.

  - Lower the hub of the catheter close to the skin to prepare for threading it into the vein approximately ¼ in.

○ Loosen the needle from the catheter and pull back slightly on the needle so that it no longer extends past the tip of the catheter.

○ Use the thumb and index finger to advance the catheter into the vein until the hub rests against the insertion site.

○ Stabilize the IV catheter with one hand and release the tourniquet with the other.

○ Apply pressure approximately 1¼ in (3 cm) above the insertion site with the middle finger and stabilize the catheter with the index finger.

○ Remove the needle and activate the safety device.

○ Maintain pressure above the IV site and connect the appropriate equipment to the hub of the IV catheter.

○ Apply a dressing per facility protocol. The dressing is usually left in place until the catheter is removed, unless it becomes damp, loose, or soiled.

○ Avoid encircling the entire extremity with tape, and taping under the sterile dressing.

○ If a continuous IV infusion is prescribed, regulate IV infusion rate according to the provider's order.

○ Dispose of used equipment properly.

○ Document in the chart:

   ▪ The date and time of insertion

   ▪ The insertion site and appearance

   ▪ The catheter size

   ▪ The type of dressing

   ▪ The IV fluid and rate (if applicable)

   ▪ The number, locations, and conditions of site-attempted catheterizations

   ▪ The client's response.

   ▪ Sample documentation: 1/1/2010, 1635, #22-gauge IV catheter inserted into left wrist cephalic vein (1 attempt) with sterile occlusive dressing applied. IV D_5LR infusing at 100 mL/hr per infusion pump without redness or edema at the site. Tolerated without complications. S. Velez, RN

Postprocedure

- Nursing Actions

  ○ Maintaining patency of IV access

    ▪ Do not stop a continuous infusion or allow blood to back up into the catheter for any length of time. Clots can form at the tip of the needle or catheter and can be lodged against the vein wall, blocking the flow of fluid.

    ▪ Instruct the client not to manipulate the flow rate device, change the settings on the IV pump, and not to lie on the tubing.

- Make sure the IV insertion site dressing is not too tight.
- Flush intermittent IV catheters with the appropriate solution after every medication administration or every 8 to 12 hr when not in use.
- Monitor the site and infusion rate at least every hour.
  - Discontinuing IV therapy
    - Check the prescription/prepare equipment.
    - Perform hand hygiene.
    - Don clean gloves.
    - Remove the tape and dressing, stabilizing the IV catheter.
    - Clamp the IV tubing.
    - Apply a sterile gauze pad over the site without putting pressure on the vein. Do not use alcohol.
    - Using the other hand, withdraw the catheter by pulling it straight back from the site.
    - Elevate the extremity and apply pressure for 2 min.
    - Assess the site.
    - Apply tape over the gauze.
    - Use a pressure dressing, if needed.
    - Assess the catheter for intactness.
    - Document.

Complications

- Complications require notification of the provider and complete documentation. All IV infusions should be restarted with new tubing and catheters.

COMPLICATIONS	FINDINGS	TREATMENT	PREVENTION
Infiltration	Pallor, local swelling at the site, decreased skin temperature around the site, a damp dressing, a slowed infusion	• Stop the infusion and remove the catheter. • Elevate the extremity. • Encourage active range of motion. • Apply warm compresses three to four times/day. • Restart the infusion proximal to the site or in another extremity.	• Carefully select the site and catheter. • Secure the catheter.
Phlebitis/ thrombophlebitis	Edema; throbbing, burning, or pain at the site; increased skin temperature; erythema; a red line up the arm with a palpable band at the vein site; a slowed infusion	• Promptly discontinue the infusion and remove the catheter. • Elevate the extremity. • Apply warm compresses three to four times/day. • Restart the infusion proximal to the site or in another extremity. • Culture the site and catheter if drainage is present.	• Rotate sites at least every 72 hr. • Avoid the lower extremities. • Use hand hygiene. • Use surgical aseptic technique.
Hematoma	Ecchymosis at site	• Do not apply alcohol. • Apply pressure after IV catheter removal. • Use warm compress and elevation after the bleeding stops.	• Minimize tourniquet time. • Remove the tourniquet before starting the IV infusion. • Maintain pressure after IV catheter removal.

COMPLICATIONS	FINDINGS	TREATMENT	PREVENTION

Cellulitis	Pain; warmth; edema; induration; red streaking; fever, chills, and malaise	• Promptly discontinue the infusion and remove the catheter.
		• Elevate the extremity.
		• Apply warm compresses three to four times/day.
		• Obtain a specimen for culture the site and prepare the catheter for culture if drainage is present.
		• Administer as prescribed:
		  ○ Antibiotics
		  ○ Analgesics
		  ○ Antipyretics
			• Rotate sites at least every 72 hr.
			• Avoid the lower extremities.
			• Use hand hygiene.
			• Use surgical aseptic technique.

Fluid overload	Distended neck veins, increased blood pressure, tachycardia, shortness of breath, crackles in the lungs, edema	• Stop infusion. • Raise the head of the bed. • Assess vital signs. • Adjust the rate as prescribed. • Administer diuretics if prescribed.	• Use an infusion pump. • Monitor I&O.
Catheter embolus	Missing catheter tip when discontinued; severe pain at the site with migration, or no symptoms if no migration	• Place the tourniquet high on the extremity to limit venous flow. • Prepare for removal under x-ray or via surgery. • Save the catheter after removal to determine the cause.	• Do not reinsert the stylet into the catheter.

CHAPTER 49: INTRAVENOUS THERAPY

 Application Exercises

1. When assessing the IV site for infiltration, the nurse should look for which of the following findings? (Select all that apply.)

　　_____　A drop in temperature around the site

　　_____　An increased rate of infusion

　　_____　Local swelling at the site

　　_____　Reddened skin

　　_____　A damp dressing

2. What information should the nurse include when documenting the insertion of an IV catheter?

3. Match the catheter gauge with the appropriate client and use for administration.

　　_____　16-gauge　　　A. surgical clients, rapid blood administration

　　_____　18-gauge　　　B. trauma clients, rapid fluid volume

　　_____　22- to 24-gauge　C. children, older adults, and stable postoperative clients

4. A nurse is caring for a client receiving dextrose 5% in water IV at 100 mL/hr. Which of the following should the nurse observe for when assessing for fluid overload?

　　_____　Decreased blood pressure

　　_____　Tachycardia

　　_____　Shortness of breath

　　_____　Crackles heard in the lungs

　　_____　Flattened neck veins

CHAPTER 49: INTRAVENOUS THERAPY

 Application Exercises Answer Key

1. When assessing the IV site for infiltration, the nurse should look for which of the following findings? (Select all that apply.)

   X   **A drop in temperature around the site**

        A increased rate of infusion

   X   **Local swelling at the site**

        Reddened skin

   X   **A damp dressing**

A drop in skin temperature around the site, local swelling at the site, a damp dressing, a slowed infusion, and pale skin are all findings consistent with infiltration.

 NCLEX® Connection: Pharmacological and Parenteral Therapies, Parenteral/Intravenous Therapy

2. What information should the nurse include when documenting the insertion of an IV catheter?

The date and time of insertion

The insertion site and appearance

The catheter size

The type of dressing

The IV fluid and rate (if applicable)

The number, locations, and conditions of site-attempted cannulations

 NCLEX® Connection: Pharmacological and Parenteral Therapies, Parenteral/Intravenous Therapy

3. Match the catheter gauge with the appropriate client and use for administration

   B   16-gauge   A. surgical clients, rapid blood administration

   A   18-gauge   B. trauma clients, rapid fluid volume

   C   22- to 24-gauge   C. children, older adults, and stable postoperative clients

 NCLEX® Connection: Pharmacological and Parenteral Therapies, Parenteral/Intravenous Therapy

4. A nurse is caring for a client receiving dextrose 5% in water IV at 100 mL/hr. Which of the following should the nurse observe for when assessing for fluid overload?

_____ Decreased blood pressure

__X__ **Tachycardia**

__X__ **Shortness of breath**

__X__ **Crackles heard in the lungs**

_____ Flattened neck veins

Findings of fluid overload include increased blood pressure, tachycardia, shortness of breath, crackles heard in the lungs, and distended neck veins.

NCLEX® Connection: Physiological Adaptation, Fluid and Electrolyte Imbalances

UNIT 4	PHYSIOLOGICAL INTEGRITY
Section	Pharmacological and Parenteral Therapies
Chapter 50	Adverse Effects, Interactions, and Contraindications

Overview

- To ensure safe medication administration and prevent errors, nurses must know why a medication is prescribed and the intended therapeutic effect. In addition, nurses must be aware of potential side/adverse effects, interactions, contraindications, and precautions.

- Every medication has the potential to cause side effects and/or adverse effects. Side effects are usually expected when a medication is given at a therapeutic dose. Adverse effects are undesired, inadvertent, and unexpected dangerous effects of the medication. Adverse effects can occur at both therapeutic and higher than therapeutic doses.

- Medications are chemicals that affect the body. When more than one medication is given, there is a potential for an interaction. In addition, medications can interact with foods.

- Contraindications and precautions of specific medications refer to client conditions that make it unsafe or potentially harmful to administer these medications.

Side/Adverse Medication Effects

- These effects may be classified according to body systems.

SIDE/ADVERSE MEDICATION EFFECTS	NURSING IMPLICATIONS/INTERVENTIONS
Central nervous system (CNS) effects – May result from either CNS stimulation (excitement) or CNS depression.	• If CNS stimulation is expected, clients may be at risk for seizures, and precautions should be taken. • If CNS depression is likely, clients should be advised not to drive or participate in other activities that can be dangerous.
Extrapyramidal symptoms (EPS) (abnormal body movements) – May include involuntary fine motor tremors, rigidity, uncontrollable restlessness, and acute dystonias (spastic movements and/or muscle rigidity affecting the head, neck, eyes, facial area, and limbs). These may occur within a few hr or may take months to develop.	• Extrapyramidal symptoms are more often associated with medications affecting the CNS, such as those used to treat mental health disorders.

SIDE/ADVERSE MEDICATION EFFECTS	NURSING IMPLICATIONS/INTERVENTIONS
Anticholinergic effects – Many medications have side effects that are a result of muscarinic receptor blockade. Most effects are seen in the eye, smooth muscle, exocrine glands, and the heart.	• Teach clients how to manage these effects. For example, dry mouth may be relieved by sipping on liquids; photophobia can be managed by use of sunglasses; and urinary retention may be reduced by urinating before taking the medication.
Cardiovascular effects – Cardiovascular effects may involve blood vessels and the heart.	• Antihypertensives can cause orthostatic hypotension. • Instruct clients about signs of postural hypotension (lightheadedness, dizziness). If these occur, advise the client to sit or lie down. Postural hypotension can be minimized by getting up and changing positions slowly.
Gastrointestinal (GI) effects – GI effects may result from local irritation of the GI tract. Stimulation of the vomiting center also results in adverse effects.	• NSAIDs may cause GI upset. Advise the client to take with food.
Hematologic effects – Relatively common and potentially life-threatening with some groups of medications.	• Bone marrow depression/suppression is generally associated with anticancer medications and hemorrhagic disorders with anticoagulants and thrombolytics. Educate clients taking an anticoagulant about signs and symptoms of bleeding such as bruising, discolored urine/stool, petechiae, and bleeding gums. Tell them to notify the provider of any of these.
Hepatotoxicity – Since most medications are metabolized in the liver, the liver is particularly vulnerable to drug-induced injury. Damage to liver cells can impair metabolism of many medications, causing medication accumulation in the body and producing adverse effects. Many medications can alter normal values of liver function tests with no obvious clinical signs of liver dysfunction.	• When two or more medications that are hepatotoxic are combined, the risk for liver damage is increased. • Liver function tests are indicated when a client starts a medication known to be hepatotoxic and periodically thereafter.
Nephrotoxicity – May occur with a number of medications, but is primarily the result of certain antimicrobial agents and NSAIDs. Damage to the kidneys may interfere with medication excretion, leading to medication accumulation and adverse effects.	• Aminoglycosides may cause renal damage. • Monitor serum creatinine and BUN levels of clients taking an aminoglycoside.

FUNDAMENTALS FOR NURSING

SIDE/ADVERSE MEDICATION EFFECTS	NURSING IMPLICATIONS/INTERVENTIONS
Toxicity – An adverse medication effect that is considered severe and may be life threatening. It may be caused by an excessive dose, but can also occur at therapeutic dose levels.	• Liver damage will occur with an acetaminophen (Tylenol) overdose. • There is a greater risk of liver damage with chronic alcohol use. • The antidote acetylcysteine (Mucomyst) may be used to minimize liver damage.
Allergic reaction – When an individual develops an immune response to a medication. The individual has been previously exposed to the medication and has developed antibodies.	• Allergic reactions range from minor to serious. Mild rashes and hives can be treated with diphenhydramine (Benadryl). • Before administering any medications, obtain a complete medication history.
Anaphylactic reaction – A life-threatening immediate allergic reaction that causes respiratory distress, severe bronchospasm, and cardiovascular collapse.	• Treat with epinephrine, bronchodilators, and antihistamines. • Provide respiratory support and notify the provider.
Immunosuppression – A decreased or absent immune response.	• Glucocorticoids depress the immune response and increase the risk for infection. • Monitor clients taking glucocorticoids for signs and symptoms of infection.

Drug-Drug Interactions

CONSEQUENCES OF DRUG-DRUG INTERACTIONS	
TYPE OF INTERACTION	NURSING IMPLICATIONS/INTERVENTIONS
Increase therapeutic effects	• Some medications may be given together to increase therapeutic effect. Clients who have asthma are instructed to use albuterol (Proventil), a beta$_2$-adrenergic agonist inhaler, 5 min prior to using triamcinolone acetonide (Azmacort), a glucocorticoid inhaler, in order to increase the absorption of triamcinolone acetonide.
Increase adverse effects	• Clients may take two medications that have the same side effects. Taking these two medications together increases the risk of these side effects. Diazepam (Valium) and hydrocodone bitartrate 5 mg/acetaminophen 500 mg (Vicodin) both have CNS depressant effects. When these medications are used together, the client has an increased risk for CNS depression.

CONSEQUENCES OF DRUG-DRUG INTERACTIONS	
TYPE OF INTERACTION	NURSING IMPLICATIONS/INTERVENTIONS
Decrease therapeutic effects	• One medication can increase the metabolism of a second medication and therefore decrease the serum level and effectiveness of the second medication. Phenytoin (Dilantin) increases hepatic medication-metabolizing enzymes that affect warfarin (Coumadin) and thereby decreases the serum level and the effect of warfarin.
Decrease side effects	• One medication can be given to counteract the adverse effects of another medication. Ondansetron hydrochloride (Zofran), an antiemetic, may be administered to counteract the side effects of nausea and vomiting for a client receiving chemotherapy.
Increase serum levels, leading to toxicity	• One medication can decrease the metabolism of a second medication and therefore increase the serum level of the second medication. This may lead to toxicity. Fluconazole (Diflucan) inhibits hepatic medication-metabolizing enzymes that affect aripiprazole (Abilify) and thereby increases serum levels of this medication.

OVER-THE-COUNTER (OTC) MEDICATIONS	
INTERACTIONS	NURSING IMPLICATIONS/INTERVENTIONS
Ingredients in OTC medications may interact with other OTC or prescription medications.	• Obtain a complete medication history.
Inactive ingredients such as dyes, alcohol, or preservatives may cause adverse reactions.	• Instruct clients to follow the manufacturer's recommendations for dosage.
The potential for overdose exists because of the use of several preparations (including prescription medications) with similar ingredients.	
Interactions of certain prescription and OTC medications can interfere with therapeutic effects.	• Clients are advised to use caution and to check with their provider before using any OTC preparations such as antacids, laxatives, decongestants, or cough syrups. For example, antacids can interfere with the absorption of ranitidine (Zantac) and other medications. Advise clients to take antacids 1 hr apart from other medications.

Medication-Food Interactions

- Food may alter medication absorption and/or may contain substances that react with certain medications.

- Examples include:

  ○ Consuming foods with tyramine while taking monoamine oxidase inhibitors (MAOIs) can lead to hypertensive crisis. Clients taking an MAOI should be aware of such foods and avoid them.

  ○ Vitamin K can decrease the therapeutic effects of warfarin (Coumadin) and place clients at risk for developing blood clots. Clients taking warfarin should maintain a consistent intake of dietary vitamin K to avoid sudden fluctuations that could affect the action of warfarin.

  ○ Tetracycline (Tetracyn) can interact with a chelating agent such as milk, and form an insoluble, unabsorbable compound. Instruct clients not to take tetracycline within 2 hr of consuming any dairy products.

  ○ Grapefruit juice seems to act by inhibiting presystemic medication metabolism in the small bowel, thus increasing absorption of certain oral medications, either increasing effects or intensifying adverse reactions. Clients should be instructed not to drink grapefruit juice if they are taking such a medication.

Ⓢ Contraindications and Precautions

- A specific medication may be contraindicated for a client based on the client's condition. For example, penicillins are contraindicated for a client who has an allergy to this medication.

- Precautions should be taken for a client who is more likely to have an adverse reaction than another client is. For example, morphine (Duramorph) depresses respiratory function, so it should be used with caution for clients who have asthma or impaired respiratory function.

- The US Food and Drug Administration places medications in categories based on risk to a fetus.

  ○ Category A: There is no evidence of risk to fetus during pregnancy based on adequate and well-controlled studies.

  ○ Category B: There is no evidence of risk to animal fetus based on studies but there are no adequate and well-controlled studies in pregnant women.

  ○ Category C: Adverse effects have been demonstrated on animal fetuses. There are no adequate and well-controlled studies in pregnant women but use of the medication during pregnancy may be warranted based on the potential benefits.

  ○ Category D: Adverse effects have been demonstrated on human fetuses based on data from investigational or marketing experience, but use of the medication during pregnancy may be warranted based on the potential benefits.

  ○ Category X: Adverse effects have been demonstrated on animal and human fetuses based on studies and data from investigational or marketing experience. The use of the medication is contraindicated during pregnancy because the risks outweigh the potential benefits.

CHAPTER 50: ADVERSE EFFECTS, INTERACTIONS, AND CONTRAINDICATIONS

 Application Exercises

1. A nurse has just been assigned to a newly admitted client. When the nurse checks the medication administration record, she observes that the client is taking four medications. Which of the following should concern the nurse?

    A. Two of the medications cause drowsiness.

    B. The client is allergic to dairy products.

    C. There are no generic forms of the medications available.

    D. The client has difficulty swallowing four pills at one time.

2. A nurse informs a client that a prescribed medication may have side effects. Which of the following instructions should the nurse give if anticholinergic effects are among the potential side effects? (Select all that apply.)

    _____ Keep a bottle of water available.

    _____ Wear sunglasses when exposed to sunlight.

    _____ Use a soft toothbrush when brushing the teeth.

    _____ Take the medication with an antacid.

    _____ Urinate prior to taking the medication.

3. A nurse is caring for a client who has renal damage secondary to glomerulonephritis. Which of the following should the nurse monitor when administering the client's medications?

    A. Decreased efficacy of medications

    B. Delayed clearance of medications from the blood

    C. Increased risk of anaphylaxis

    D. Increased susceptibility to infection

4. A client has been recently diagnosed with hypertension and prescribed an antihypertensive medication. Which of the following instructions should the nurse give to the client in regard to taking over-the-counter (OTC) medications?

    A. Continue to take OTC medications with the antihypertensive medication.

    B. Stop taking the antihypertensive medication while taking OTC medications.

    C. Consult the provider prior to taking OTC medications.

    D. Take only one half the recommended dose of OTC medications.

CHAPTER 50: ADVERSE EFFECTS, INTERACTIONS, AND CONTRAINDICATIONS

 Application Exercises Answer Key

1. A nurse has just been assigned to a newly admitted client. When the nurse checks the medication administration record, she observes that the client is taking four medications. Which of the following should concern the nurse?

   A. Two of the medications cause drowsiness.
   B. The client is allergic to dairy products.
   C. There are no generic forms of the medications available.
   D. The client has difficulty swallowing four pills at one time.

   A drug-drug interaction can cause an increased effect. If two of these medications cause drowsiness (CNS depression), they will have a synergistic effect and increase CNS depression. Increasing CNS depression can progress from drowsiness to stupor as well as fatal respiratory depression. An allergy to dairy products should not interfere with this client's medication regimen, trade name medications can be used, and the nurse can administer each pill separately.

 NCLEX® Connection: Pharmacological and Parenteral Therapies, Adverse Effects/Contraindications/Side Effects/Interactions

2. A nurse informs a client that a prescribed medication may have side effects. Which of the following instructions should the nurse give if anticholinergic effects are among the potential side effects? (Select all that apply.)

   __X__ **Keep a bottle of water available.**
   __X__ **Wear sunglasses when exposed to sunlight.**
   _____ Use a soft toothbrush when brushing the teeth.
   _____ Take the medication with an antacid.
   __X__ **Urinate prior to taking the medication.**

   Medications that have anticholinergic effects can cause dry mouth, photophobia, and urinary retention. Keeping a bottle of water available can help alleviate dry mouth, wearing sunglasses can minimize photophobia, and urinating prior to taking the medication will allow the client to empty the bladder before possibly experiencing urinary retention. Bleeding gums is not a side effect of anticholinergic medications, so it is not necessary to use a soft toothbrush. Stomach irritation is also not experienced with anticholinergic medications, so it is not necessary to take the medication with an antacid.

NCLEX® Connection: Pharmacological and Parenteral Therapies, Adverse Effects/Contraindications/Side Effects/Interactions

3. A nurse is caring for a client who has renal damage secondary to glomerulonephritis. Which of the following should the nurse monitor when administering the client's medications?

    A. Decreased efficacy of medications

    B. Delayed clearance of medications from the blood

    C. Increased risk of anaphylaxis

    D. Increased susceptibility to infection

Renal damage can delay the excretion or clearance of medications from the blood, increasing the risk of toxicity and adverse effects. Renal damage does not result in decreased efficacy of medications, increased risk of anaphylaxis, or increased susceptibility to infection.

 NCLEX® Connection: Pharmacological and Parenteral Therapies, Adverse Effects/ Contraindications/Side Effects/Interactions

4. A client has been recently diagnosed with hypertension and prescribed an antihypertensive medication. Which of the following instructions should the nurse give to the client in regard to taking over-the-counter (OTC) medications?

    A. Continue to take OTC medications with the antihypertensive medication.

    B. Stop taking the antihypertensive medication while taking OTC medications.

    C. Consult the provider prior to taking OTC medications.

    D. Take only one half the recommended dose of OTC medications

Due to the possibility of a medication interaction between the antihypertensive and OTC medications, none should be taken unless approved by the provider. It is not safe to take some OTC medications with prescribed medications nor is it safe to discontinue a prescribed medication while taking OTC medications. Taking only one half the recommended dose of OTC medications can still cause a dangerous drug interaction and should not be done.

 NCLEX® Connection: Pharmacological and Parenteral Therapies, Medication Administration

UNIT 4	PHYSIOLOGICAL INTEGRITY
Section	Pharmacological and Parenteral Therapies
Chapter 51	Individual Considerations of Medication Administration

Overview

- Various factors may affect how clients respond to medications. It is important for nurses to recognize these factors in order to individualize nursing care when administering medications.

Factors Affecting Medication Dosages and Responses

- Body Weight – Because medications are absorbed and distributed in body tissue, individuals with a greater body mass may require larger doses.

- Age – Young children with immature liver and kidney function, and older adults, often with reduced liver and kidney function, may require proportionately smaller medication doses.

- Gender – Females may respond differently to medications than males due to a higher proportion of body fat and the effects of female hormones.

- Genetics – Genetic factors such as missing enzymes can alter the metabolism of certain medications, thus enhancing or reducing medication action.

- Biorhythmic Cycles – Responses to certain medications vary with the biologic rhythms of the body. For example, hypnotic medications work better when given at the usual sleep time than at other times.

- Tolerance – Responsiveness to a medication is reduced, and is either congenital (genetic factors) or acquired (stimulation of liver enzymes or other physiologic variations). Cross-tolerance may occur with other chemically similar medications.

- Accumulation – An increased medication concentration occurs in the body due to the inability to metabolize or excrete a medication rapidly enough, resulting in a toxic medication effect. For older adults, decreased renal function is the major cause of medication accumulation leading to toxicity.

- Psychological Factors – Emotional state and expectations can influence the effects of a medication. A term used to describe positive medication effects influenced by psychological factors is the placebo effect.

- Medical Conditions

  o Inadequate gastric acid inhibits the absorption of medications requiring an acid medium to dissolve.

  o Diarrhea causes oral medications to pass too quickly through the gastrointestinal tract to be absorbed.

  o Vascular insufficiency prevents distribution of a medication to affected tissue.

  o Liver disease/failure impairs medication metabolism, which may cause toxicity.

  o Kidney disease/failure prevents or delays medication excretion, which may cause toxicity.

Pharmacology and Children

- While most medications administered to adults are useful for children, the dosages are different. Pediatric dosages are based on body weight or body surface area (BSA). Neonates (< 1 month old) and infants (1 month to 1 year old) have immature liver and kidney function, alkaline gastric juices, and an immature blood-brain barrier. Certain medication dosages are based on age due to a greater risk for decreased skeletal bone growth, acute cardiopulmonary failure, or hepatic toxicity.

- Additional pharmacokinetic factors specific to children include:

  o Decreased gastric acid production and slower gastric emptying time

  o Decreased first-pass medication metabolism

  o Increased absorption of topical medications (greater body surface area and thinner skin)

  o Lower blood pressure (more blood flow to the liver and brain and less to the kidneys)

  o Higher body water content (dilutes water-soluble medications)

  o Decreased serum protein-binding sites (until age 1). There may be an increase in the serum drug level of protein-binding drugs

- Be particularly alert when administering medications to children due to the risk for medication errors.

  o Dosages are usually based on weight or BSA.

  o Most medications are not tested on children.

  o Adult medication forms and concentrations may require dilution, calculation, preparation, and administration of very small doses.

  o Limited sites exist for IV medication administration.

ⓖ Pharmacology and Older Adults (65+ Years)

- Physiologic changes associated with aging that impact pharmacokinetics include:

  - Increased gastric pH (alkaline)

  - Decreased gastrointestinal motility and gastric emptying time

  - Decreased blood flow through the cardiovascular system, liver, and kidneys

  - Decreased hepatic enzyme function

  - Decreased kidney function and glomerular filtration rate

  - Decreased protein-binding sites

  - Decreased body water, increased body fat, and decreased lean body mass

- Other factors affecting medication therapy for older adults include:

  - Impaired memory or altered mental state

  - Changes in vision and hearing

  - Decreased mobility and dexterity

  - Poor adherence

  - Reduced financial resources

  - Polypharmacy – The practice of taking several medications simultaneously (prescribed and/or over the counter [OTC]) together with diminished bodily functions and some medical conditions. This can contribute to the potential for medication toxicity.

- Nursing interventions for older adults include:

  - Decreasing the risk of adverse medication effects.

    - Obtain a complete medication history and include all OTC medications.

    - Make sure the medication therapy starts at the lowest possible dose.

    - Assess/monitor for therapeutic and adverse effects.

    - Assess/monitor for drug-drug and drug-food interactions.

    - Document findings.

    - Notify the provider of adverse effects.

  - Promoting adherence.

    - Give clear and concise instructions, verbally and in writing.

    - Ensure that the dosage form is appropriate. Administer liquid forms to clients who have difficulty swallowing.

    - Provide clearly marked containers that are easy to open.

    - Assist the client to set up a daily calendar with the use of pill containers.

    - Suggest that the client obtain assistance from a friend, neighbor, or relative.

(S) Pharmacology – Pregnancy and Lactation

- Pregnancy – Any medication ingested by a woman who is pregnant will be distributed to the fetus, as well. Medications are classified according to potential harm to the fetus. In general, most medications should be considered potentially harmful to the fetus; therefore, the benefits of maternal medication administration must be weighed against possible fetal risk. Medications are most commonly used during pregnancy as nutritional supplements (iron, vitamins, minerals) and for the treatment of nausea, vomiting, gastric acidity, and mild discomforts. Chronic medical conditions such as diabetes or hypertension must be managed with careful maternal-fetal monitoring. Live virus vaccines (measles, mumps, polio, rubella, yellow fever) are contraindicated due to possible teratogenic effects.

- Lactation – Most medications taken by lactating women are secreted in breast milk. Drugs with an extended half-life or those that are known to be harmful to the infant should be avoided. For medications that are safe, give the medication immediately after breastfeeding to minimize medication concentration in the next feeding.

CHAPTER 51: INDIVIDUAL CONSIDERATIONS OF MEDICATION ADMINISTRATION

 Application Exercises

1. A nurse is providing teaching to an older adult client to promote adherence with medication administration. Which of the following instructions should be included? (Select all that apply.)

_____ Only take medications when not feeling well.

_____ Place pills in daily pill holders.

_____ Contact the provider if side effects occur.

_____ Ask a relative to assist periodically.

_____ Refill prescriptions when the current supply is completed.

2. A nurse is caring for a client who says that his pain medication is not working like it used to. The nurse should recognize that the client is experiencing

A. the placebo effect.

B. tolerance.

C. accumulation.

D. dependence.

3. A nurse is preparing medications for a preschool child. Which of the following factors should the nurse recognize as altering how a preschool child is affected by a medication? (Select all that apply.)

_____ Increased gastric acid production

_____ Lower blood pressure

_____ Higher body water content

_____ Increased absorption of topical medications

_____ Increased first-pass medication metabolism

CHAPTER 51: INDIVIDUAL CONSIDERATIONS OF MEDICATION ADMINISTRATION

 Application Exercises Answer Key

1. A nurse is providing teaching to an older adult client to promote adherence with medication administration. Which of the following instructions should be included? (Select all that apply.)

	Only take medications when not feeling well.
__X__	**Place pills in daily pill holders.**
__X__	**Contact the provider if side effects occur.**
__X__	**Ask a relative to assist periodically.**
	Refill prescriptions when the current supply is completed.

Placing pills in a daily pill holder reminds the client to take the pills as scheduled. The provider should be notified of side effects to determine if medications need to be adjusted; and assistance from a relative will provide emotional support. The client should take medications on a regular schedule. Prescriptions should be filled prior to the completion of the current supply to prevent a gap in treatment.

 NCLEX® Connection: Health Promotion and Maintenance, Aging Process

2. A nurse is caring for a client who says that his pain medication is not working like it used to. The nurse should recognize that the client is experiencing

    A. the placebo effect.

    B. tolerance.

    C. accumulation.

    D. dependence.

Tolerance occurs over time and the client will experience a decrease in responsiveness to a medication. The placebo effect occurs when the client experiences a positive effect due to psychological factors. Accumulation occurs with an increase in medication concentration in the body due to the inability to metabolize or excrete a medication rapidly enough, resulting in a toxic medication effect. Dependence is experienced as a psychological or physiological need for the medication.

 NCLEX® Connection: Pharmacological and Parenteral Therapies, Medication Administration

3. A nurse is preparing medications for a preschool child. Which of the following factors should the nurse recognize as altering how a preschool child is affected by a medication? (Select all that apply.)

_____	Increased gastric acid production
__X__	**Lower blood pressure**
__X__	**Higher body water content**
__X__	**Increased absorption of topical medications**
_____	Increased first-pass medication metabolism

Children have lower blood pressure, higher body water content, and experience an increase in absorption of topical medications. Children have decreased gastric acid production and decreased first-pass metabolism.

NCLEX® Connection: Health Promotion and Maintenance, Aging Process

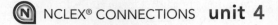

UNIT 4: PHYSIOLOGICAL INTEGRITY

Section: Reduction of Risk Potential

- Specimen Collection for Glucose Monitoring
- Respiratory Management
- Nasogastric Intubation and Enteral Feedings

NCLEX® CONNECTIONS

When reviewing the chapters in this section, keep in mind the relevant sections of the NCLEX® outline, in particular:

CLIENT NEEDS: BASIC CARE AND COMFORT	CLIENT NEEDS: REDUCTION OF RISK POTENTIAL	CLIENT NEEDS: PHYSIOLOGICAL ADAPTATION

Relevant topics/tasks include:
• Nutrition and Oral Hydration
  ○ Provide client nutrition through continuous or intermittent tube feedings.
	Relevant topics/tasks include:
	• Laboratory Values
	  ○ Obtain specimens other than blood for diagnostic testing.
	• Potential for Alterations in Body Systems
	  ○ Identify the client's potential for skin breakdown.
	• Potential for Complications of Diagnostic Tests/Treatments/Procedures
	  ○ Position the client to prevent complications following tests/treatments/procedures.
		Relevant topics/tasks include:
		• Fluid and Electrolyte Imbalances
		  ○ Manage the care of the client with a fluid and electrolyte imbalance.

UNIT 4	PHYSIOLOGICAL INTEGRITY
Section	Reduction of Risk Potential
Chapter 52	Specimen Collection for Glucose Monitoring

Overview

- Monitoring blood glucose levels is an essential component in the care of clients who have diabetes mellitus.

- Glucose monitoring can be performed through blood glucose testing or urine testing.

  o Blood glucose testing is the preferred method of monitoring blood glucose levels.

  o Urine testing is not an effective measure of glucose level as glucose levels must be greater than 180 mg/dL before glucose appears in the urine.

- Clients who are able and willing to continue monitoring independently can learn how to self-monitor blood glucose levels. Required abilities include:

  o Alertness or the ability to comprehend and give a return demonstration of the process

  o Adequate finger dexterity

  o Adequate visual acuity

Blood Glucose Testing

- For blood glucose testing of clients who have diabetes mellitus, a glucometer or a blood glucose meter is used with small test strips to "read" the blood sample. These systems require proper calibration, storage of supplies, and matching of lot numbers.

- Indications

  o Regular testing is necessary for clients who have diabetes mellitus to manage the disease by maintaining safe blood glucose levels.

- Interpretation of Findings

  o Usually, a blood glucose level greater than 250 mg/dL indicates hyperglycemia.

  o Usually, a blood glucose level less than 70 mg/dL indicates hypoglycemia.

  o Poor storage of glucose test strips can lead to falsely high and low readings. Typically, these test strips come in a vial to store at room temperature or as directed by the manufacturer.

- Preprocedure

  - Nursing Actions

    - Check the client's record and prescription for:

      - Frequency and type of test

        - Testing times vary based on the goals of management and the complexity of the client's hypoglycemic medication schedule.

      - Results from previous tests – norms and ranges

      - Actions to be taken based on results

    - Review the client's medication profile.

      - Note anticoagulant usage.

      - Note the times and dose of hypoglycemic agents.

      - Note the use of steroids or medications that can elevate blood glucose levels.

    - Gather materials and prepare the equipment.

      - Blood glucose meter

      - Meter and reagent strip compatible with the meter

      - Washcloth and soap

      - Gloves

      - Sterile lancet

      - Cotton ball

    - Review the meter and the manufacturer's instructions.

    - Check the strip solution's expiration date.

    - Calibrate the meter and run a control sample per facility/agency protocol. This is usually performed when a new bottle of test strips is opened.

    - Explain the procedure to the client.

    - Evaluate the selected puncture site for:

      - Integrity of the skin

      - Compromised circulation or other condition

    - Perform hand hygiene and put on gloves.

- Intraprocedure

  - Nursing Actions

    - Select a site from which to collect the blood sample.

      - Outer edge of a fingertip (most common site)

      - Ear lobe (alternate site)

    - Rotate sites with each testing area to avoid ongoing tenderness at the site.

- Wrap the site in a warm, moist towel to enhance circulation if indicated.

- Cleanse the site with warm water and soap and allow it to dry. Alcohol can interfere with results and should be avoided.

- Pierce the skin using a sterile lancet (or a lancet injector device).

- Place a drop of blood on the test strip.

  □ Follow the procedure outlined by the manufacturer of the blood glucose meter for applying blood to the strip.

  □ If necessary, gently milk the finger to squeeze out a drop. (Forceful milking or squeezing can cause lysis of the blood cells.) Do not touch the site directly to stimulate bleeding.

  □ Do not smear blood onto the strip, as this can cause an inaccurate reading.

- Allow the meter to process the reading. (Time varies with the meter.)

- Apply a cotton ball over the puncture site.

- Note the reading, turn off the meter, and dispose of the cotton ball, test strip, and gloves.

- Postprocedure

  ○ Nursing Actions

    - Perform hand hygiene.

    - Document the meter's reading.

    - Check prescription for medication or treatment actions and implement as indicated.

Urine Glucose Testing

- Glucose in the urine can be measured with urinalysis strips and a glucose reading scale.

- Indications

  ○ Urine glucose testing is usually performed at home by clients who have diabetes mellitus at times of acute illness or stress to identify the presence of ketones.

- Interpretation of Findings

  ○ If the test is positive for ketones, it indicates uncontrolled blood glucose.

- Preprocedure

  ○ Nursing Actions

    - If testing urine, evaluate the client's ability to urinate.

    - Verify the order for frequency and actions to be taken based on the results.

- Gather materials and prepare the equipment.
  - Sterile urine sample bottle
  - Urinalysis strips and the container with the glucose reading scale
  - Gloves
- Check the strip's expiration date.
- Explain the procedure to the client.
- Perform hand hygiene and put on gloves.

- Intraprocedure
  - Nursing Actions
    - Assist the client as needed with urine sample collection.
    - Dip the reagent strip into the urine sample.
    - Compare the strip's color change with the ranges on the container within the instructed time (usually 1 to 5 seconds).
    - Document the results.

- Postprocedure
  - Nursing Actions
    - Dispose of the remaining urine sample, test strip, and gloves.
    - Perform hand hygiene.
    - Check prescription for medication or treatment actions and implement as indicated.

CHAPTER 52: SPECIMEN COLLECTION FOR GLUCOSE MONITORING

 Application Exercises

1. Which of the following directions should the nurse give to a client who is learning self-monitoring of blood glucose (SMBG)? (Select all that apply.)

_____ Perform SMBG once daily at bedtime.

_____ Warm the hand before puncturing the finger.

_____ Calibrate the glucose monitor each time a new bottle of strips is opened.

_____ Wipe the hand with an alcohol swab.

_____ Prick the outer edge of the fingertip for a blood sample.

2. Which of the following medications can alter the results of blood glucose testing?

A. Amoxicillin (Amoxil)

B. Dexamethasone (Decadron)

C. Morphine (Duramorph)

D. Acetaminophen (Tylenol)

3. A client has an admission blood glucose reading of 350 mg/dL. The client has no history of elevated blood glucose, and there is an insulin order. Which of the following actions should the nurse take first?

A. Check the client's level of consciousness.

B. Check the client's dietary orders.

C. Review the client's recent nutritional intake.

D. Notify the provider.

CHAPTER 52: SPECIMEN COLLECTION FOR GLUCOSE MONITORING

 Application Exercises Answer Key

1. Which of the following directions should the nurse give to a client who is learning self-monitoring of blood glucose (SMBG)? (Select all that apply.)

         Perform SMBG once daily at bedtime.

   X   **Warm the hand before puncturing the finger.**

   X   **Calibrate the glucose monitor each time a new bottle of strips is opened.**

         Wipe the hand with an alcohol swab.

   X   **Prick the outer edge of the fingertip for a blood sample.**

Warming the hand prior to obtaining a blood sample increases circulation and helps ensure an adequate sample. The monitor should be calibrated each time a new bottle of strips is opened. The outer edge of the fingertip is an appropriate site for blood sampling. SMBG should be performed based on the client's medication schedule. It may be done as often as before each meal and at bedtime. Monitoring once a day at bedtime does not provide enough information to monitor blood glucose control. The hand should be washed with warm water and soap. Alcohol can interfere with the blood glucose reading.

 NCLEX® Connection: Reduction of Risk Potential, Diagnostic Tests

2. Which of the following medications can alter the results of blood glucose testing?

A. Amoxicillin (Amoxil)

B. Dexamethasone (Decadron)

C. Morphine (Duramorph)

D. Acetaminophen (Tylenol)

Dexamethasone is a steroid that may raise blood glucose. Amoxicillin, morphine, and acetaminophen should not affect blood glucose levels.

 NCLEX® Connection: Reduction of Risk Potential, Diagnostic Tests

3. A client has an admission blood glucose reading of 350 mg/dL. The client has no history of elevated blood glucose, and there is an insulin order. Which of the following actions should the nurse take first?

A. Check the client's level of consciousness.

B. Check the client's dietary orders.

C. Review the client's recent nutritional intake.

D. Notify the provider.

Using "assessment first," the nurse should further assess the client for any other manifestations of hyperglycemia. Checking the client's dietary orders, reviewing the client's nutritional intake, and notifying the provider are important interventions but are not the priority.

NCLEX® Connection: Reduction of Risk Potential, System Specific Assessment

 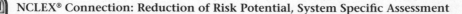

UNIT 4	PHYSIOLOGICAL INTEGRITY
Section	Reduction of Risk Potential
Chapter 53	Respiratory Management

Overview

- Managing respiratory compromise includes performing a respiratory assessment along with obtaining a complete set of vital signs, including oxygen saturation (indicated via pulse oximetry) and administration of oxygen (via a variety of delivery devices).

- Oxygen is used to maintain adequate cellular oxygenation. It is used to treat many acute and chronic respiratory problems (hypoxemia, cystic fibrosis, asthma) and for those at risk for developing hypoxia (those recovering from surgery, those who have a respiratory illness, those with circulatory impairment).

- Maintaining a patent airway is a nursing priority. It involves mobilizing secretions, suctioning the airway, and managing artificial airways (endotracheal tubes, tracheostomy tubes) to promote adequate gas exchange and lung expansion.

- Sputum specimens are collected both for screening and for diagnostic tests, such as for the detection of cancer and tuberculosis.

PULSE OXIMETRY AND OXYGEN THERAPY

Overview

- A pulse oximeter is a battery- or electric-operated device with a sensor probe that is attached securely to the client's fingertip, toe, bridge of nose, earlobe, or forehead with a clip or band.

- A pulse oximeter measures arterial oxygen saturation (SaO_2) via a wave of infrared light that measures light absorption by oxygenated and deoxygenated hemoglobin in arterial blood. SaO_2 and SpO_2 are used interchangeably.

- Oxygen is a tasteless and colorless gas that accounts for 21% of atmospheric air.

- Oxygen is administered to maintain adequate cellular oxygenation. It is used to treat many acute and chronic respiratory problems.

- Oxygen flow rates are varied in an attempt to maintain an SaO_2 of 95% to 100% using the lowest amount of oxygen to achieve the goal without putting the client at risk for complications.

- Supplemental oxygen may be delivered by a variety of methods based on the client's particular circumstances. The percentage of oxygen delivered to the client is expressed as the fraction of inspired oxygen (FiO_2).

Pulse Oximetry

- Noninvasive measurement of the oxygen saturation of the blood

- Indications

  - Potential Diagnosis

    - Pulse oximetry is indicated for conditions or situations in which a client's respiratory status should be monitored, such as during the immediate postoperative period.

  - Client Presentation

    - The following signs and symptoms indicate that oxygen saturation should be monitored:

      - Increased work of breathing

      - Wheezing

      - Coughing

      - Cyanosis

- Interpretation of Findings

  - The expected reference range for SaO_2 is 95% to 100%. Acceptable levels may range from 91% to 100%. Some illness states may even allow for an SaO_2 of 85% to 89%.

  - Values may be slightly lower for older adult clients and clients who have dark skin.

  - Additional reasons for low readings include hypothermia, poor peripheral blood flow, too much light (sun, infrared lamps), low hemoglobin levels, movement, edema, and nail polish.

  - An SaO_2 below 91% requires interventions to help the client regain acceptable SaO_2 levels. An SaO_2 below 86% is an emergency. An SaO_2 below 80% is life-threatening. The lower the SaO_2 level, the less accurate the value.

- Nursing Actions

  - Preparation of the Client

    - Perform hand hygiene and provide privacy.

    - Find an appropriate probe site. It must be dry and have adequate circulation.

    - Be sure the client is in a comfortable position, supporting the arm if a finger is used as a probe site.

  - Ongoing Care

    - Apply the sensor probe to the site.

    - Press the power switch on the oximeter.

    - Note the pulse reading and compare it with the client's radial pulse. Any discrepancy warrants further assessment.

- Allow time for the readout to stabilize, then record this value as the oxygen saturation.

- Remove the probe, turn off the oximeter, and store it appropriately.

- If continuous monitoring is required, make sure the alarms are set for a low and a high limit, they are functioning, and the sound is audible. Every 4 hr, assess the skin under the probe and move the sensor to another location.

  o Interventions

  - Document findings and report abnormal findings to the provider.

  - If a client's SaO_2 is less than 90% (indicating hypoxemia):

    □ Confirm that the sensor probe is properly placed.

    □ Confirm that the oxygen delivery system is functioning and that the client is receiving the prescribed oxygen levels.

    □ Place the client in semi-Fowler's or Fowler's position to maximize ventilation.

    □ Encourage deep breathing.

    □ Report significant findings to the provider.

    □ Remain with the client and provide emotional support to decrease anxiety.

Oxygen Therapy

- Oxygen is administered to maintain adequate cellular oxygenation. It is used to treat many acute and chronic respiratory problems.

  o Hypoxemia

  - Hypoxemia is an inadequate level of oxygen in the blood. Hypovolemia, hypoventilation, and interruption of arterial flow can lead to hypoxemia.

  - Clinical signs and symptoms of hypoxemia include:

EARLY	LATE
• Tachypnea	• Confusion and stupor
• Tachycardia	• Cyanotic skin and mucous membranes
• Restlessness	• Bradypnea
• Pale skin and mucous membranes	• Bradycardia
• Elevated blood pressure	• Hypotension
• Symptoms of respiratory distress of accessory muscles, nasal flaring, tracheal tugging, adventitious lung sounds)	• Cardiac dysrhythmias

- Indications

  o Diagnoses

    ▪ Acute and chronic respiratory conditions that make the client unable to maintain an adequate oxygen saturation.

  o Client Outcomes

    ▪ The client maintains an SaO_2 of 95% to 100%.

    ▪ The client maintains patent airway.

- Nursing Actions

  o Preparation of the Client

    ▪ Explain all procedures to the client.

    ▪ Place the client in semi-Fowler's or Fowler's or position to facilitate breathing and promote chest expansion.

    ▪ Ensure that all equipment is working properly.

    ▪ Apply oxygen as indicated.

    ▪ Monitor the client's respiratory rate and pattern, level of consciousness, and SaO_2.

  o Ongoing Care

    ▪ Provide oxygen therapy at the lowest liter flow that will correct hypoxemia.

    ▪ Assess/monitor respiratory rate, rhythm, effort, and lung sounds to determine the client's need for supplemental oxygen.

      ☐ Signs and symptoms of hypoxemia are shortness of breath, anxiety, tachypnea, tachycardia, restlessness, pallor to cyanosis of the skin and mucous membranes, adventitious breath sounds, and confusion.

      ☐ Signs and symptoms of hypercarbia (elevated levels of CO_2) are restlessness, hypertension, and headache.

    ▪ Auscultate the lungs for the presence or absence of breath sounds and adventitious sounds, such as crackles and wheezes.

    ▪ Assess/monitor oxygenation status with pulse oximetry and arterial blood gases (ABGs).

    ▪ Apply the oxygen delivery device prescribed. Assess the proper fit of the mask to ensure a secure seal over the client's nose and mouth.

    ▪ Promote good oral hygiene and provide as needed.

    ▪ Promote turning, coughing, deep breathing, and the use of incentive spirometry and suctioning.

    ▪ Promote rest and decrease environmental stimuli.

    ▪ Provide emotional support for clients who appear anxious.

    ▪ Assess nutritional status; provide supplements as prescribed.

- Assess/monitor the client's skin integrity; provide moisture and pressure-relief devices as indicated.

- Assess/monitor and document the client's response to oxygen therapy.

- Titrate oxygen to maintain the recommended oxygen saturation.

- Discontinue supplemental oxygen gradually.

- Monitor for signs and symptoms of respiratory depression such as decreased respiratory rate and decreased level of consciousness and notify the provider if present.

  ○ Interventions

- Administer the prescribed amount of oxygen using appropriate equipment.

- Low-flow oxygen delivery systems deliver varying amounts of oxygen based on the delivery method and the client's breathing pattern.

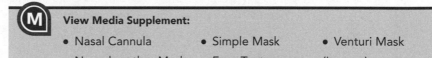

View Media Supplement:

- Nasal Cannula
- Simple Mask
- Venturi Mask
- Nonrebreather Mask
- Face Tent
- (Images)

LOW-FLOW OXYGEN DELIVERY SYSTEMS – HOW MUCH OXYGEN IS ACTUALLY DELIVERED VARIES WITH THE DELIVERY METHOD AND THE CLIENT'S BREATHING PATTERN.			
FRACTION OF INSPIRED OXYGEN (FiO_2)	ADVANTAGES	DISADVANTAGES	NURSING INTERVENTIONS
Nasal cannula (a length of tubing with two small prongs for insertion into the nares)			
• It delivers an FiO_2 of 24% to 44% at a flow rate of 1 to 6 L/min.	• It is a safe, simple, and easy-to-apply method. • It is comfortable and well-tolerated. • The client is able to eat, talk, and ambulate.	• The FiO_2 varies with the flow rate, and rate and depth of the client's breathing. • Extended use may lead to skin breakdown and dry mucous membranes. • It is easily dislodged.	• Assess the patency of the nares. • Ensure that the prongs fit in the nares properly. • Use water-soluble gel to prevent dry nares. • Provide humidification for flow rates of 4 L/min and above.

LOW-FLOW OXYGEN DELIVERY SYSTEMS – HOW MUCH OXYGEN IS ACTUALLY DELIVERED VARIES WITH THE DELIVERY METHOD AND THE CLIENT'S BREATHING PATTERN.			
FRACTION OF INSPIRED OXYGEN (FIO$_2$)	**ADVANTAGES**	**DISADVANTAGES**	**NURSING INTERVENTIONS**
Simple face mask (covers the client's nose and mouth)			
• It delivers an FiO$_2$ of 40% to 60% at flow rates of 5 to 8 L/min. • The minimum flow rate is 5 L/min to ensure flushing of CO$_2$ from the mask.	• A face mask is easy to apply and may be more comfortable than a nasal cannula. • It is a simple delivery method. • It is more comfortable than a nasal cannula.	• Flow rates of 5 L/min or lower may result in rebreathing of CO$_2$. • It is poorly tolerated by clients who have anxiety or claustrophobia. • Eating, drinking, and talking are impaired. • Use with caution for clients who have a high risk of aspiration or airway obstruction.	• Assess proper fit to ensure a secure seal over the nose and mouth. • Make sure the client wears the nasal cannula during meals.
Partial rebreather mask (covers the client's nose and mouth)			
• It delivers an FiO$_2$ of 60% to 75% at flow rates of 6 to 11 L/min.	• The mask has a reservoir bag attached with no valve, which allows the client to rebreathe up to 1/3 of exhaled air together with room air.	• Complete deflation of the reservoir bag during inspiration causes CO$_2$ buildup. • The FiO$_2$ varies with the client's breathing pattern. • Poorly tolerated by clients who have anxiety or claustrophobia. • Eating, drinking, and talking are impaired.	• Keep the bag from deflating by adjusting the oxygen flow rate to keep the reservoir bag inflated. • Assess proper fit to ensure a secure seal over nose and mouth. • Make sure the client uses a nasal cannula during meals. • Use with caution for clients who have a high risk of aspiration or airway obstruction.

FRACTION OF INSPIRED OXYGEN (FIO$_2$)	ADVANTAGES	DISADVANTAGES	NURSING INTERVENTIONS
LOW-FLOW OXYGEN DELIVERY SYSTEMS – HOW MUCH OXYGEN IS ACTUALLY DELIVERED VARIES WITH THE DELIVERY METHOD AND THE CLIENT'S BREATHING PATTERN.			
Nonrebreather mask (covers the client's nose and mouth)			
It delivers an FiO$_2$ of 80% to 95% at flow rates of 10 to 15 L/min to keep the reservoir bag 2/3 full during inspiration and expiration.	• It delivers the highest O$_2$ concentration possible (except for intubation). • A one-way valve situated between the mask and reservoir allows the client to inhale maximum O$_2$ from the reservoir bag. The two exhalation ports have flaps covering them that prevent room air from entering the mask.	• The valve and flap on the mask must be intact and functional during each breath. • It is poorly tolerated by clients who have anxiety or claustrophobia. • Eating, drinking, and talking are impaired. • Use with caution for clients who have a high risk of aspiration or airway obstruction.	• Perform an hourly assessment of the valve and flap. • Assess proper fit to ensure a secure seal over the nose and mouth. • Make sure the client uses a nasal cannula during meals.

FRACTION OF INSPIRED OXYGEN (FIO$_2$)	ADVANTAGES	DISADVANTAGES	NURSING INTERVENTIONS
HIGH-FLOW OXYGEN DELIVERY SYSTEMS – WHEN PROPERLY FITTED, THESE DEVICES DELIVER PRECISE AMOUNTS OF OXYGEN.			
Venturi mask (covers the client's nose and mouth)			
It delivers an FiO$_2$ of 24% to 55% at flow rates of 2 to 10 L/min via different size adaptors.	• It delivers the most precise oxygen concentration. • Humidification is not required. • It is best suited for clients who have chronic lung disease.	• Use is expensive.	• Assess frequently to ensure an accurate flow rate. • Make sure the tubing is free of kinks.

HIGH-FLOW OXYGEN DELIVERY SYSTEMS – WHEN PROPERLY FITTED, THESE DEVICES DELIVER PRECISE AMOUNTS OF OXYGEN.			
FRACTION OF INSPIRED OXYGEN (FIO$_2$)	ADVANTAGES	DISADVANTAGES	NURSING INTERVENTIONS
Aerosol mask, face tent (fits loosely around the face and neck), and tracheostomy collar (a small mask that covers the surgically created opening of the trachea)			
• They deliver an FiO$_2$ of 24% to 100% at flow rates of at least 10 L/min. • They provide high humidification with oxygen delivery.	• Use with clients who do not tolerate masks well. • Useful for clients who have facial trauma, burns, and thick secretions.	• High humidification requires frequent monitoring.	• Empty condensation from the tubing often. • Ensure adequate water in the humidification canister. • Make sure the tubing does not pull on the tracheostomy.

- Complications
  - Oxygen Toxicity
    - Oxygen toxicity may result from high concentrations of oxygen (typically above 50%), long durations of oxygen therapy (typically more than 24 to 48 hr), and the severity of the client's lung disease.
    - Signs and symptoms include a nonproductive cough, substernal pain, nasal stuffiness, nausea, vomiting, fatigue, headache, sore throat, and hypoventilation.
    - Nursing Actions
      - Use the lowest level of oxygen necessary to maintain an adequate SaO$_2$.
      - Monitor ABGs and notify the primary care provider if SaO$_2$ levels are outside the expected reference range.
      - Use an oxygen mask with continuous positive airway pressure (CPAP), bilevel positive airway pressure (BiPAP), or positive end-expiratory pressure (PEEP) as prescribed while the client is on a mechanical ventilator to help decrease the amount of needed oxygen.
      - FiO$_2$ should be decreased as soon as the client's condition permits.
  - Oxygen-induced hypoventilation
    - Oxygen-induced hypoventilation may develop in clients with chronic obstructive pulmonary disease (COPD) who have chronic hypoxemia and hypercarbia. Clients with COPD rely on low levels of arterial oxygen as their primary drive for breathing. Providing supplemental oxygen at high levels can decrease or eliminate their respiratory drive.

- Nursing Actions
  - Monitor the client's respiratory rate and pattern, level of consciousness, and SaO_2.
  - Provide oxygen therapy at the lowest liter flow that corrects hypoxemia.
  - If the client tolerates it, use a Venturi mask to deliver precise oxygen levels.
  - Notify the provider of impending respiratory depression such as a decreased respiratory rate and a decreased level of consciousness.

- Combustion
  - Oxygen is combustible.
  - Nursing Actions
    - Post "No Smoking" or "Oxygen in Use" signs to alert others of the fire hazard.
    - Know where the closest fire extinguisher is located.
    - Educate the client and others about the fire hazard of smoking with oxygen use.
    - Have the client wear a cotton gown because synthetic or wool fabrics can generate static electricity.
    - Ensure that all electric devices (razors, hearing aids, radios) are working well.
    - Make sure all electric machinery (monitors, suction machines) is grounded.
    - Do not use volatile, flammable materials (alcohol, acetone) near clients receiving oxygen.

SPECIMEN COLLECTION AND AIRWAY CLEARANCE

Overview

- Mucosal secretion buildup or aspiration of emesis can obstruct a client's airway.
  - Adequate hydration and coughing help the client maintain airway patency.
  - Clients at risk for developing airway compromise include: infants, clients with neuromuscular disorders, clients who are quadriplegic, and clients with cystic fibrosis.
  - Nursing interventions that mobilize secretions and maintain airway patency include assistance with coughing, hydration, positioning, humidification, nebulizer therapy, chest physiotherapy, and suctioning.
  - These interventions promote adequate gas exchange and lung expansion.
- Sputum specimens can be collected by suctioning during coughing.
- Indications that the client needs help maintaining airway clearance include signs of hypoxemia (restlessness, irritability, tachypnea, tachycardia, cyanosis, decreased level of consciousness, decreased SaO_2 levels), adventitious breath sounds, visible secretions, and absence of spontaneous cough.

- Whenever possible, the client should be encouraged to cough. Coughing is more effective than artificial suctioning at moving secretions into the upper trachea and laryngopharynx.

- Humidification of oxygen moistens the airways, which loosens and mobilizes pulmonary secretions.

- Nebulization breaks up medications (bronchodilators, mucolytic agents) into minute particles that are then dispersed throughout the respiratory tract.

- Chest physiotherapy (CPT) involves the use of chest percussion, vibration, and postural drainage to assist the client to mobilize secretions. Chest percussion and vibration facilitate movement of secretions into the central airways. For postural drainage, the client assumes one or more positions (a total of nine) to allow gravity to assist with the removal of secretions from specific areas of the lung.

- Early-morning postural drainage mobilizes secretions that have accumulated through the night.

- Suctioning can be accomplished orally, nasally, or endotracheally. Suctioning is not performed on a routine basis but only when indicated.

- Surgical asepsis must be maintained when performing any form of tracheal suctioning to avoid bacterial contamination of the airway.

Sputum specimen collection

- Collection of sputum for analysis

- Indications

  - For cytology to identify aberrant cells or cancer

  - For culture and sensitivity to grow and identify micro-organisms and the antibiotics effective against them

  - To identify acid-fast bacillus (AFB) to diagnose tuberculosis (TB) (requires three consecutive morning samples)

- Interpretation of Findings

  - Presence of bacteria indicating infection

  - Presence of cancer cells

- Nursing Actions

  - Preparation of the Client

    - Check the provider's prescription.

    - Obtain specimens early in the morning.

    - Wait 1 to 2 hr after the client eats to obtain a specimen to decrease the likelihood of emesis or aspiration.

    - Perform chest physiotherapy to help mobilize secretions.

- Use a sterile specimen container, a label, a laboratory requisition slip, a biohazard bag for delivery of the specimen to the laboratory, clean gloves, and a mask and goggles if necessary.

- Use a container with a preservative to obtain a specimen for cytology.

- Use a sterile container for routine cultures and acid-fast bacillus (AFB) testing.

  o Ongoing Care

- Perform hand hygiene, provide privacy, and explain the procedure to the client.

- Assist the client to Fowler's position.

- Have the client rinse her mouth of any oral contaminant.

- Assess the client's ability to cough and expectorate secretions. If the client is unable to cough effectively, obtain an order to collect the specimen by endotracheal suctioning. Attach a sputum trap between the suction catheter and the wall unit's tubing.

- Instruct the client to breathe deeply two to four times, then cough deeply to raise the sputum from the lungs.

- Have the client expectorate the sputum (1 to 2 tsp) into the sterile cup without contamination.

- If an inadequate amount of sputum is collected, repeat the specimen collection after the client takes several deep breaths and coughs.

- Maintaining sterility, place the lid on the specimen cup, label it, and place it in the biohazard bag.

- Specimens should be delivered to the laboratory within 30 min.

- Document interventions and the client's response.

Chest Physiotherapy

- The use of a set of techniques that include percussion, vibration, postural drainage with gravity, and positioning to loosen respiratory secretions and move them into the central airways where they can be removed by coughing or suctioning.

- Percussion – The use of cupped hands to clap rhythmically on the chest to break up secretions

- Vibration – The use of a shaking movement applied during exhalation to help remove secretions

- Postural drainage – The use of various positions to allow secretions to drain by gravity

- Indications

  o Client Presentation

    - Clients with thick secretions who are unable to clear their airways

    - Contraindicated for clients who are pregnant; have a rib, chest, head, or neck injury; have increased intracranial pressure; have had recent abdominal surgery; or have a pulmonary embolism

  o Client Outcomes

    - The client maintains a patent airway.

    - The client maintains an SaO_2 of 95% to 100%.

- Preprocedure

  o Nursing Actions

    - Schedule treatments 1 hr before meals or 2 hr after meals and at bedtime to decrease the likelihood of vomiting or aspirating.

    - Administer a bronchodilator medication or nebulizer treatment 30 min to 1 hr prior to postural drainage if prescribed.

    - Offer the client an emesis basin and facial tissues.

- Intraprocedure

  o Nursing Actions

    - Perform hand hygiene, provide privacy, and explain the procedure to the client.

    - Ensure proper positioning of the client to promote drainage of specific areas of the lungs.

      □ Apical sections of the upper lobes – Fowler's position

      □ Posterior sections of the upper lobes – Side-lying position

      □ Right lobe – On the left side with a pillow under the chest wall

      □ Left lobe – Trendelenburg position

    - Apply manual percussion to the chest wall using cupped hands or a special device.

    - Place hands on the affected area, tense hand and arm muscles, and move the heel of the hands to create vibrations as the client exhales. Have the client cough after each set of vibrations.

    - Have the client remain in each position for 10 to 15 min to allow time for percussion, vibration, and postural drainage.

    - Discontinue the procedure if the client reports faintness or dizziness.

- Postprocedure

  - Nursing Actions

    - Perform lung auscultation and assess the amount, color, and character of expectorated secretions.

    - Document interventions and repeat the procedure as prescribed (typically two to three times per day).

- Complications

  - Hypoxia

    - Decrease in SaO_2

    - Nursing Actions

      - Monitor respiratory status during the procedure.

      - Discontinue the procedure if the client experiences dyspnea.

Suctioning

- Suctioning can be accomplished orally, nasally, or endotracheally.

- Indications

  - Potential Diagnoses

    - Hypoxemia

  - Client Presentation

    - Early signs of hypoxemia, such as restlessness, tachypnea, tachycardia, decreased SaO_2 levels, adventitious breath sounds, visualization of secretions, cyanosis, absence of spontaneous cough

  - Client Outcomes

    - The client maintains a patent airway.

    - The client maintains an SaO_2 of 95% to 100%.

- Preprocedure

  - Nursing Actions

    - Perform hand hygiene, provide privacy, and explain the procedure to the client.

    - Don the required personal protective equipment.

    - Assist the client to high-Fowler's or Fowler's position for suctioning if possible.

    - Encourage the client to breathe deeply and cough in an attempt to clear the secretions without artificial suction.

    - Obtain baseline breath sounds and vital signs, including SaO_2 by pulse oximeter. May monitor SaO_2 continually during the procedure.

- Oropharyngeal suctioning
  - Obtain baseline assessment data.
  - Use a Yankauer or tonsil-tipped rigid suction catheter.
- Nasopharyngeal and nasotracheal suctioning
  - Suctioning is performed with a flexible catheter.
  - Catheter size is based on the diameter of the client's nares and the thickness of the secretions.
  - Hyperoxygenate the client with an FiO_2 of 100% during equipment preparation.
  - Lubricate the distal 6 to 8 cm (2 to 3 in) of the suction catheter with a water-soluble lubricant.
  - Remove the oxygen delivery device with the nondominant hand, if applicable.
- Endotracheal suctioning (ETS)
  - Perform ETS through a tracheostomy or an endotracheal tube.
  - Ask for assistance if necessary.
  - Obtain a suction catheter with an outer diameter of no more than 1 cm (0.5 in) of the internal diameter of the endotracheal tube.
  - Hyperoxygenate the client using a bag-valve-mask (BVM) or specialized ventilator function with an FiO_2 of 100%.
- Client Education
  - Explain the procedure to all clients, conscious or unconscious.
- Intraprocedure
  - Nursing Actions
    - Use surgical asepsis when opening the suction catheter kit.
    - Use medical asepsis for suctioning the mouth.
    - Use surgical asepsis for all other types of suctioning.
    - Open the sterile suction package.
    - Place the sterile drape or towel on the client's chest.
    - Set up the container, touching only the outside.
    - Pour approximately 100 mL of sterile water or 0.9 % sodium chloride solution into the container.
    - Don sterile gloves.
    - The clean/nondominant hand holds the connecting tube; this glove protects the nurse.

- The sterile/dominant hand holds the sterile catheter; this glove protects the client.

- Connect the suction catheter to the wall unit's tubing.

- Set the suction pressure no higher than 120 mm Hg.

- Test the suction setup by aspirating sterile water/normal saline solution from the cup. If the unit is operating properly, continue with the procedure.

- Limit each suction attempt to no longer than 10 to 15 seconds to avoid hypoxemia and the vagal response. Limit suctioning to two to three attempts.

- Once suctioning is complete, clear the suction tubing by aspirating sterile water/ normal saline solution.

- Document pre- and post-assessment data (vital signs, SaO_2, breath sounds); how the client tolerated the procedure; and the color, consistency, and amount of secretions.

- Oropharyngeal suctioning

  □ Insert the catheter into the client's mouth.

  □ Apply suction and move the catheter around the mouth, gum line, and pharynx.

  □ Clear the catheter and tubing.

  □ Repeat as needed.

  □ Monitor the client's SaO_2 level.

- Nasopharyngeal and nasotracheal suctioning

  □ Insert the catheter into the naris during inhalation.

  □ Do not apply suction while inserting the catheter.

  □ Follow the natural course of the naris and slightly slant the catheter downward as it is advanced.

  □ Advance the catheter the approximate distance from the tip of the nose to the base of the earlobe.

  □ Apply suction intermittently by covering and releasing the suction port with the thumb for 10 to 15 seconds.

  □ Apply suction only while withdrawing the catheter and rotating it with the thumb and forefinger.

  □ Allow the client 20 to 30 seconds for recovery between sessions.

  □ Repeat as necessary, hyperoxygenating the client before each suctioning pass.

- Endotracheal suctioning (ETS)

  □ Remove the bag or ventilator from the tracheostomy or endotracheal tube and insert the catheter into the lumen of the airway. Advance the catheter until resistance is met. The catheter should reach the level of the carina (location of bifurcation into the mainstem bronchi).

  □ Pull the catheter back 1 cm (0.5 in) prior to applying suction to prevent mucosal damage.

  □ Apply suction intermittently by covering and releasing the suction port with the thumb for 10 to 15 seconds.

  □ Apply suction only while withdrawing the catheter and rotating it with the thumb and forefinger.

  □ Reattach the BVM or ventilator and supply the client with 100% inspired oxygen.

  □ Clear the catheter and tubing.

  □ Allow time for the client to recover between sessions.

  □ Repeat as necessary.

- ○ Client Education

  - Explain the procedure to all clients, conscious or unconscious.

- Postprocedure

  - ○ Nursing Actions

    - Oropharyngeal suctioning

      □ Replace the oxygen mask, if applicable.

      □ Store the catheter in a clean, dry place for reuse.

      □ Allow the client to perform his own suctioning if possible.

      □ Document the client's response.

    - Nasopharyngeal and nasotracheal suctioning

      □ Document the client's response.

      □ Do not reuse the suction catheter.

    - Endotracheal suctioning (ETS)

      □ Document the client's response.

- Complications

  - ○ Hypoxemia

    - Decrease in SaO_2 or cyanosis

- Nursing Actions
  - □ Stop the procedure. Limit each suction attempt to no longer than 10 to 15 seconds.
  - □ Limit suctioning to two to three attempts.
  - □ Allow the client 30 to 60 seconds for recovery between suction passes.

  - □ Hyperoxygenate the client before and after each suctioning pass. Decrease suctioning times for older adult clients.
- ○ Anxiety
  - Nursing Actions
    - □ Explain the procedure to all clients prior to suctioning.
    - □ Provide reassurance before, during, and after the procedure.
    - □ Maintain a calm manner.

ARTIFICIAL AIRWAYS AND TRACHEOSTOMY CARE

Overview

- A tracheotomy is a sterile surgical incision into the trachea through the skin and muscles for the purpose of establishing an airway.

- A tracheotomy can be performed as an emergency procedure or as a scheduled surgical procedure; it can be temporary or permanent.

- A tracheostomy is the stoma/opening that results from a tracheotomy to provide and secure a patent airway.

- Artificial airways can be placed orotracheally, nasotracheally, or through a tracheostomy to assist with respiration.

- Tracheostomy tubes vary in their composition (plastic, steel, silicone), number of parts, size (long vs. short), and shape (50° to 90° angles).

- There is no standard tracheostomy sizing system; however, the diameter of the tracheostomy tube must be smaller than the trachea.

- The outside cannula has a flange or neck plate that sits against the skin of the neck and has holes on each side for attaching ties around the client's neck to stabilize the tracheostomy tube.

- Airflow in and out of a tracheostomy without air leakage (a cuffed tracheostomy tube) bypasses the vocal cords, resulting in an inability to produce sound or speech.

- Uncuffed tubes and fenestrated tubes, in place or capped, allow the client to speak. Clients who have a cuffed tube can be off mechanical ventilation, can breathe around the tube, and can use a special valve to allow for speech. The cuff is deflated and the valve occludes the opening.

TUBES	CHARACTERISTICS	NURSING CONCERNS
Single lumen (cannula)	• Long, single-cannula tube • Used for clients who have long or thick necks	• Do not use with clients who have excessive secretions.
Double lumen (cannula)	• It has three major parts: ○ An outer cannula fits into the stoma and keeps the airway open. ○ An inner cannula fits snugly into the outer cannula and locks into place. ○ An obturator is a thin, solid tube placed inside the tracheostomy and is used as a guide for inserting the outer cannula. It is removed immediately after outer cannula insertion.	• This device allows for the inner cannula to be removed, cleaned, reused, or discarded, and replaced with a disposable inner cannula. • It is useful for clients who have excessive secretions.
Cuffed tube	• It has a balloon that is inflated around the outside of the distal segment of the tube to protect the lower airway by producing a seal between the upper and lower airway.	• A cuffed tube permits mechanical ventilation. • Cuffs do not hold the tube in place. • Cuff pressures must be monitored to prevent tracheal tissue necrosis. • The client is unable to speak.
Cuffless tube	• It has no balloon and is used for clients with long-term airway-management needs.	• The client must be at low risk for aspiration. • Cuffless tubes are not used for clients on mechanical ventilation. • This device allows the client to speak.
Fenestrated tube – With cuff	• One large or multiple openings (fenestrations) in the posterior wall of the outer cannula with a balloon around the outside of the distal segment of the tube • Also has an inner cannula	• This device allows for mechanical ventilation. • Removing the inner cannula allows the fenestrations to permit air to flow through the openings. • This device allows the client to speak.

TUBES	CHARACTERISTICS	NURSING CONCERNS
Fenestrated tube – Without cuff	• One larger or multiple openings (fenestrations) in the posterior wall of the outer cannula with no balloon • Also has an inner cannula	• The holes in the tube help wean the client from the tracheostomy. • Removing the inner cannula allows the fenestrations to permit air to flow through the openings. • This device allows the client to speak.

- Indications

    o Potential Diagnoses

        ▪ Indications for a tracheostomy

            □ Acute or chronic upper airway obstruction

            □ Edema (anaphylaxis, burns, trauma, head/neck surgery)

            □ Copious secretions

            □ The need for long-term mechanical ventilation

            □ The need for reconstruction after laryngeal trauma or laryngeal cancer surgery

            □ Obstructive sleep apnea refractory to conventional therapy

    o Client Outcomes

        ▪ The client maintains a patent airway.

        ▪ The client maintains an SaO_2 95% to 100%.

- Nursing Actions

    o Preparation of the Client

        ▪ Explain the procedure.

        ▪ Place in semi-Fowler's or Fowler's position.

        ▪ Keep the following at the client's bedside – Two extra tracheostomy tubes (one the client's size and one size smaller, in case of accidental decannulation), the obturator for the existing tube, an oxygen source, suction catheters and a suction source, and a manual resuscitation bag.

        ▪ Provide the client with methods to communicate with staff (paper and pen, dry-erase board).

        ▪ Provide the client with an emergency call system and a call light.

- o Ongoing Care
  - Assess/monitor:
    - Oxygenation and ventilation (respiratory rate, effort, SaO_2) and vital signs hourly
    - Thickness, quantity, odor, and color of mucus
    - Stoma and surrounding skin for signs of inflammation or infection (redness, swelling, drainage)
  - Provide adequate humidification and hydration to thin secretions and reduce the risk of mucous plugs.
  - Do not suction routinely, as this causes mucosal damage, bleeding, and bronchospasm.
  - Assess/monitor the need for suctioning. Suction on a PRN basis when assessment findings indicate it (audible/noisy secretions, crackles, restlessness, tachypnea, tachycardia, mucus in the airway).
  - Maintain surgical asepsis when suctioning to prevent infection.
  - Offer emotional support to the client and family.
  - Give frequent oral care, usually every 2 hr.
  - Provide tracheostomy care every 8 hr to reduce the risk of infection and skin breakdown.
    - Suction the tracheostomy tube, if necessary, using sterile suctioning supplies.
    - Remove soiled dressings and excess secretions.
    - Apply the oxygen source loosely if the client's SaO_2 decreases during the procedure.
    - Use cotton-tipped applicators and gauze pads to clean exposed outer cannula surfaces. Begin with hydrogen peroxide followed by 0.9% sodium chloride. Clean in a circular motion from the stoma site outward.
    - Use surgical asepsis to remove and clean the inner cannula (with half-strength or full-strength hydrogen peroxide and rinse it with sterile saline solution). Use a new inner cannula if it is disposable.
    - Clean the stoma site and then the tracheostomy plate with half-strength hydrogen peroxide followed by sterile saline.
    - Place a split 4 x 4 dressing around the tracheostomy.
    - Change tracheostomy ties if they are soiled. Secure the new ties before removing the soiled ones to prevent accidental decannulation.
    - If a knot is needed, tie a square knot that is visible on the side of the neck. Check that one or two fingers fit between the tie and the neck.
    - Document the type and amount of secretions, the general condition of the stoma and surrounding skin, the client's response to the procedure, and any teaching or learning.

- Change nondisposable tracheostomy tubes every 6 to 8 weeks or per protocol.

- Reposition the client every 2 hr to prevent atelectasis and pneumonia.

- Minimize dust in the client's room; do not shake bedding.

- If the client is permitted to eat, position him upright and tip his chin to his chest to enable swallowing. Assess for aspiration.

- Administer prescribed medications.

  □ Anti-inflammatory medications to reduce edema

  □ Antibiotics for prophylaxis or infection treatment

  □ Aerosolized bronchodilators to relieve bronchospasm

  □ Mucus-liquefying agents

- Interventions

  - Provide discharge teaching.

    □ Tracheostomy care

    □ Signs and symptoms to report immediately to the provider (signs of infection, copious secretions)

    □ Discuss ways to achieve good nutrition.

    □ Consider referring the client to a home health care agency and community support groups.

Complications

- Accidental Decannulation

  - Accidental decannulation in the first 72 hr after surgery is an emergency because the tracheostomy tract has not matured, and replacement may be difficult.

    - Ventilate the client with a manual resuscitation bag. Call for assistance.

  - Nursing Actions

    - Always keep the tracheostomy obturator and two spare tracheostomy tubes at the client's bedside.

    - If accidental decannulation occurs after the first 72 hr:

      □ Immediately hyperextend the neck and with the obturator inserted into the tracheostomy tube, quickly and gently replace the tube and remove the obturator.

      □ Secure the tube.

      □ Assess tube placement by auscultating for bilateral breath sounds.

    - If unable to replace the tracheostomy tube, administer oxygen through the stoma. If unable to administer oxygen through the stoma, occlude the stoma and administer oxygen through the client's nose and mouth.

- Damage to the Trachea

  o Tracheal wall necrosis is tissue damage that results when the pressure of the inflated cuff impairs blood flow to the tracheal wall.

  o Tracheal stenosis is the narrowing of the tracheal lumen due to scar formation resulting from irritation of the tracheal mucosa from the tracheal tube cuff.

    ▪ Keep the cuff pressure between 14 and 20 mm Hg.

    ▪ Check the cuff pressure at least once every 8 hr.

    ▪ Keep the tube in the midline position and prevent pulling or traction on the tracheostomy tube.

CHAPTER 53: RESPIRATORY MANAGEMENT

 Application Exercises

1. Match each of the following oxygen delivery systems with the appropriate description.

    _____ Nasal cannula   A. Delivers an FiO_2 of 24% to 55% at flow rates of 2 to 10 L/min via different size adaptors

    _____ Simple face mask   B. Delivers an FiO_2 of 24% to 100% at flow rates of at least 10 L/min and requires high humidification of oxygen

    _____ Nonrebreather mask   C. Delivers an FiO_2 of 24% to 44% at a flow rate of 1 to 6 L/min via tubing with two small prongs for insertion into the nares

    _____ Venturi mask   D. Delivers an FiO_2 of 40% to 60% at flow rates of 5 to 8 L/min for short-term oxygen therapy

    _____ Face tent   E. Delivers an FiO_2 of 80% to 95% at flow rates of 10 to 15 L/min to keep the reservoir bag two-thirds full during inspiration and expiration

2. Which of the following can cause a low pulse oximetry reading? (Select all that apply.)

    _____ Nail polish

    _____ Inadequate peripheral circulation

    _____ Hyperthermia

    _____ Increased hemoglobin level

    _____ Edema

3. Differentiate between early (E) and late (L) signs of hypoxemia.

    _____ Confusion and stupor

    _____ Pale skin and mucous membranes

    _____ Bradycardia

    _____ Hypotension

    _____ Elevated blood pressure

    _____ Restlessness

    _____ Cyanotic skin and mucous membranes

4. A nurse is caring for a client who is having difficulty breathing. The nurse should place the client in which of the following positions?

    A. Supine

    B. Dorsal recumbent

    C. Fowler's

    D. Lateral

5. Which of the following oxygen delivery systems should be used when a precise amount of oxygen needs to be delivered?

    A. Nonrebreather mask

    B. Venturi mask

    C. Nasal cannula

    D. Simple face mask

6. Place the following steps for obtaining a sputum specimen in the correct order.

    _____   Place the client in Fowler's position.

    _____   Have the client expectorate the sputum into a sterile cup without contamination.

    _____   Check for a provider's order.

    _____   Deliver the specimen to the laboratory within 30 min.

    _____   Have the client rinse his mouth.

    _____   Maintaining sterility, place the lid on the specimen cup, label it, and place it in the biohazard bag.

    _____   Assess the client's ability to cough and expectorate secretions.

    _____   Obtain the necessary equipment.

    _____   Instruct the client to breathe deeply two to four times and then cough deeply to raise the sputum from the lung.

    _____   Perform hand hygiene, provide privacy, and explain the procedure to the client.

7. A nurse is preparing to perform endotracheal suctioning for a client. Which of the following are appropriate guidelines to be followed? (Select all that apply.)

    _____   Apply suction while withdrawing the catheter.

    _____   Perform suctioning on a routine basis, every 2 to 3 hr.

    _____   Maintain medical asepsis.

    _____   Use a new tube each time suctioning is performed.

    _____   Limit suctioning to two to three attempts.

8. Which of the following interventions is appropriate when caring for a client who has a tracheostomy tube?

    A. Use medical asepsis when performing tracheostomy care.

    B. Change the tracheostomy ties each time tracheostomy care is given.

    C. Keep the cuff pressure between 14 and 20 mm Hg.

    D. Clean the stoma site with the prescribed antibiotic solution.

CHAPTER 53: RESPIRATORY MANAGEMENT

Ⓐ Application Exercises Answer Key

1. Match each of the following oxygen delivery systems with the appropriate description.

<u>C</u>   Nasal cannula

A. Delivers an FiO_2 of 24% to 55% at flow rates of 2 to 10 L/min via different size adaptors

<u>D</u>   Simple face mask

B. Delivers an FiO_2 of 24% to 100% at flow rates of at least 10 L/min and requires high humidification of oxygen

<u>E</u>   Nonrebreather mask

C. Delivers an FiO_2 of 24% to 44% at a flow rate of 1 to 6 L/min via tubing with two small prongs for insertion into the nares

<u>A</u>   Venturi mask

D. Delivers an FiO_2 of 40% to 60% at flow rates of 5 to 8 L/min for short-term oxygen therapy

<u>B</u>   Face tent

E. Delivers an FiO_2 of 80% to 95% at flow rates of 10 to 15 L/min to keep the reservoir bag two-thirds full during inspiration and expiration

Ⓝ NCLEX® Connection: Physiological Adaptation, Alterations in Body Systems

2. Which of the following can cause a low pulse oximetry reading? (Select all that apply.)

<u>X</u>   **Nail polish**
<u>X</u>   **Inadequate peripheral circulation**
_____   Hyperthermia
_____   Increased hemoglobin level
<u>X</u>   **Edema**

Nail polish, inadequate peripheral circulation, and edema can all generate a low reading. Hypothermia rather than hyperthermia and decreased hemoglobin level rather than increased hemoglobin level can result in a low reading.

Ⓝ NCLEX® Connection: Reduction of Risk Potential, Diagnostic Tests

3. Differentiate between early (E) and late (L) signs of hypoxemia.

<u>L</u>   Confusion and stupor
<u>E</u>   Pale skin and mucous membranes
<u>L</u>   Bradycardia
<u>L</u>   Hypotension
<u>E</u>   Elevated blood pressure
<u>E</u>   Restlessness
<u>L</u>   Cyanotic skin and mucous membranes

Ⓝ NCLEX® Connection: Reduction of Risk Potential, System Specific Assessment

4. A nurse is caring for a client who is having difficulty breathing. The nurse should place the client in which of the following positions?

    A. Supine

    B. Dorsal recumbent

    C. Fowler's

    D. Lateral

Fowler's position facilitates maximal lung expansion and thus optimizes breathing. Supine, dorsal recumbent, and lateral positions will not facilitate breathing.

 NCLEX® Connection: Physiological Adaptation, Alterations in Body Systems

5. Which of the following oxygen delivery systems should be used when a precise amount of oxygen needs to be delivered?

    A. Nonrebreather mask

    B. Venturi mask

    C. Nasal cannula

    D. Simple face mask

A Venturi mask incorporates an adaptor that allows a precise amount of oxygen to be delivered. The other oxygen delivery systems deliver an approximated amount of oxygen.

NCLEX® Connection: Physiological Adaptation, Alterations in Body Systems

6. Place the following steps for obtaining a sputum specimen in the correct order.

    __4__   Place the client in Fowler's position.

    __8__   Have the client expectorate the sputum into a sterile cup without contamination.

    __1__   Check for a provider's order.

    __10__   Deliver the specimen to the laboratory within 30 min.

    __5__   Have the client rinse his mouth.

    __9__   Maintaining sterility, place the lid on the specimen cup, label it, and place it in the biohazard bag.

    __6__   Assess the client's ability to cough and expectorate secretions.

    __2__   Obtain the necessary equipment.

    __7__   Instruct the client to breathe deeply two to four times and then cough deeply to raise the sputum from the lung.

    __3__   Perform hand hygiene, provide privacy, and explain the procedure to the client.

 NCLEX® Connection: Physiological Adaptation, Alterations in Body Systems

7. A nurse is preparing to perform endotracheal suctioning for a client. Which of the following are appropriate guidelines to be followed? (Select all that apply.)

__X__	**Apply suction while withdrawing the catheter.**
_____	Perform suctioning on a routine basis, every 2 to 3 hr.
_____	Maintain medical asepsis.
__X__	**Use a new tube each time suctioning is performed.**
__X__	**Limit suctioning to two to three attempts.**

Suction should be applied only while the catheter is withdrawn. Endotracheal suctioning requires surgical asepsis, so the catheter should not be reused (unless an inline suctioning system is in place). To prevent hypoxemia, each suctioning session is limited to two to three attempts. Suctioning should be performed only when indicated, not on a routine basis.

 NCLEX® Connection: Physiological Adaptation, Alterations in Body Systems

8. Which of the following interventions is appropriate when caring for a client who has a tracheostomy tube?

A. Use medical asepsis when performing tracheostomy care.

B. Change the tracheostomy ties each time tracheostomy care is given.

C. Keep the cuff pressure between 14 and 20 mm Hg.

D. Clean the stoma site with the prescribed antibiotic solution.

Suction pressure should be kept between 14 and 20 mm Hg to prevent tracheal wall necrosis. Surgical asepsis is mandatory when performing tracheostomy care. Ties are changed only when they are soiled. It is not appropriate to clean the stoma site with an antibiotic solution. Half-strength hydrogen peroxide and normal saline solution are routinely used.

 NCLEX® Connection: Physiological Adaptation, Alterations in Body Systems

UNIT 4	PHYSIOLOGICAL INTEGRITY
Section	Reduction of Risk Potential
Chapter 54	Nasogastric Intubation and Enteral Feedings

Overview

- Nasogastric intubation is the insertion of a nasogastric (NG) tube to manage gastrointestinal dysfunction and provide enteral nutrition.

- In addition to NG tubes, enteral tube feedings can be delivered via jejunal or gastric tubes.

- The insertion and maintenance of nasogastric/enteral feeding tubes is the nurse's responsibility.

Nasogastric Intubation

- A nasogastric (NG) tube is a hollow, flexible, cylindrical device inserted through the nasopharynx into the stomach.

- Indications

  o Decompression

    ▪ Removal of gases or stomach contents to relieve distention, nausea, or vomiting

    ▪ Tube types – Salem sump, Miller-Abbott, Levin

  o Feeding

    ▪ Route of administering nutritional supplements when oral/esophageal passageways cannot be used

    ▪ Tube types – Duo, Levin, Dobbhoff

  o Lavage

    ▪ Washing out the stomach to treat overdose or ingestion of poison

    ▪ Tube types – Ewald, Levin, Salem sump

  o Compression

    ▪ Applied pressure using an internal balloon to prevent hemorrhage

    ▪ Tube type – Sengstaken-Blakemore

(M) View Media Supplement:

- Enteral Feeding Tube (Image)
- Sengstaken-Blakemore Tube (Image)

- Preprocedure
    - Nursing Actions
        - Review the prescription and purpose, plan for drainage or suction, and understand the need for placement for diagnostic purposes.
        - Identify the client and explain the procedure.
        - Evaluate the client's ability to assist and/or cooperate.
        - Perform hand hygiene.
        - Set up the equipment.
            - Nasogastric tube – selected according to the indication
            - Tape to secure the dressing
            - Gloves
            - Water-soluble lubricant
            - Topical anesthetic if prescribed
            - Cup of water and straw
            - Catheter-tipped syringe, usually 30- to 60-mL
            - Basin – to prepare for gag-induced nausea
            - pH test strip or meter – to measure gastric secretions for acidity
            - Stethoscope – to check placement
            - Disposable towel – to maintain a clean environment
            - Clamp or plug – to close the tubing after insertion
            - Suction apparatus – if continuous or intermittent suction is needed
            - Gauze square – to cleanse the outside of the tubing after insertion
            - Safety pin and elastic band – to secure the tubing and prevent erroneous removal
        - Position a disposable towel and basin.
        - Provide privacy.
- Intraprocedure
    - Nursing Actions
        - The nurse may require assistance with clients who are confused or disoriented.
        - Assist the client to high-Fowler's position (if possible).
        - Assess the nares for the best position/route.
            - Assess whether or not the client has had any nasopharyngeal surgery or septal deviation to determine which naris to use.
        - Administer topical anesthetic.

- Measure the tubing – from the tip of the nose, to the tip of the ear lobe, to the tip of the xiphoid, and mark it with adhesive tape.

- Put on gloves.

- Lubricate the tip of the tubing.

- If the client is able, have her hold the cup of water with a straw in place, and tell her that she will be told when to drink.

- Have the client hyperextend her head back.

- Gradually insert the tube.

- When resistance is met, apply gentle pressure downward, and proceed beyond the curve of the nasopharynx.

- Have the client lean her head forward and begin sipping as insertion continues. Swallowing helps feed the tubing downward toward the stomach.

- When the tubing reaches the mark, anchor the tube using tape or a nasogastric clamp.

- Placement check

  □ Ask the client to talk.

  □ Inspect the posterior pharynx for coiled tubing.

  □ Aspirate gently to collect gastric contents and observe the color.

  □ Test pH (4 or less is expected.).

  □ Confirm placement with an x-ray as prescribed.

  □ Injecting air into the tube and then listening over the abdomen is not an acceptable practice.

- If the tube is not in the stomach, advance it 5 cm and repeat the placement check.

- When placement is confirmed, secure the tube to the nose using tape.

- Secure the lower end of the tube by wrapping a rubber band around the tube and pinning it to the client's gown.

- Clamp the nasogastric tube or connect it to the appropriate suction device.

- If the client vomits, clear the airway and provide comfort prior to continuing.

- Salem sump tubing has a blue pigtail for negative air release. Do not insert any substance into the blue pigtail, as it will break the seal and the tubing will leak.

- Postprocedure

  o Nursing Actions

    - The insertion and maintenance of a nasogastric tube is a nursing responsibility; but measuring output, providing comfort, and giving oral care can be delegated.

- Discontinuation/removal

  □ Inform the client of the order and process, emphasizing that removal is less stressful than placement.

  □ Perform hand hygiene and don gloves.

  □ Remove the safety pin from the gown, and remove the tape anchoring the tube to the nose.

  □ Disconnect the tubing from suction and clamp it.

  □ Provide facial tissues for the client.

  □ Instruct the client to take and hold a deep breath.

  □ Remove the tubing with a steady continuous pull while the client is holding her breath.

  □ Measure and record any drainage.

  □ Clean the nares and provide oral care.

  □ Ensure the client's comfort.

  □ Dispose of the equipment.

  □ Document all relevant information, including:

    ▸ Tubing removal and condition of the tube

    ▸ Volume and description of the drainage

    ▸ Abdominal assessment, including inspection, auscultation, palpation, and percussion

    ▸ Last and next bowel movement and urine output

- Complications

  ○ Excoriation of nares and stomach

    - Apply lubricant to the nares as needed.

    - Assess the color of the nasogastric tube drainage. Report dark "coffee-ground" or blood-streaked drainage to the provider immediately.

  ○ Discomfort

    - Rinse the client's mouth with water for dryness.

    - Throat lozenges may be helpful.

    - Provide oral hygiene frequently.

  ○ Occlusion of the NG tube leading to distention

    - Irrigate the tube per facility protocol to unclog blockages. Tap water may be used with enteral feedings. Have the client change position in case the tube is against the stomach wall.

Enteral Feedings

- Enteral feeding is a method of providing nutrients to clients who cannot consume foods orally.

  o Enteral formulas

    ▪ Polymeric – (1.0 to 2.0 kcal/mL) milk-based, blenderized foods

      □ Whole-nutrient formulas prepared by hospital dietary staff or are commercially prepared

      □ Only used if the client's gastrointestinal (GI) tract can absorb whole nutrients

    ▪ Modular formulas – (3.8 to 4.0 kcal/mL) single macronutrient preparation

      □ Not nutritionally complete

      □ Added to other foods for supplemental nutrition

    ▪ Elemental formulas – (1.0 to 3.0 kcal/mL) predigested nutrients

      □ Not nutritionally complete

      □ Easier for a partially dysfunctional GI tract to absorb

    ▪ Specialty formulas – (1.0 to 2.0 kcal/mL) created to meet specific nutritional needs

      □ Not nutritionally complete

      □ Primarily for clients who have hepatic failure, respiratory disease, or HIV infection

- Enteral access tubes

  ▪ Nasogastric or nasointestinal

    □ Therapy duration shorter than 4 weeks

    □ Inserted via the nose

  ▪ Gastrostomy or jejunostomy

    □ Therapy duration longer than 4 weeks

    □ Inserted surgically

  ▪ Percutaneous endoscopic gastrostomy (PEG) or jejunostomy (PEJ)

    □ Therapy duration longer than 4 weeks

    □ Inserted endoscopically

  ▪ Gastroparesis, esophageal reflux, or a history of aspiration pneumonia generally requires intestinal placement.

- Indications

  o Critical illness/trauma

  o Neurological and muscular disorders – brain neoplasm, cerebrovascular accident, dementia, myopathy, Parkinson's disease

  o Gastrointestinal disorders – enterocutaneous fistula, inflammatory bowel disease, mild pancreatitis

  o Respiratory failure with prolonged intubation

  o Inadequate oral intake

- Nursing Actions

  o Preparation of the Client

    ■ Review the client's prescription.

      □ The type of tube feeding formula is usually determined by the primary care provider in consultation with dietary staff.

    ■ Set up the equipment.

      □ Feeding bag

      □ Tubing

      □ 30- to 60-mL syringe (compatible with the tubing)

      □ Stethoscope

      □ pH indicator strip

      □ Infusion pump (if not a gravity drip)

      □ Appropriate enteral formula

      □ Irrigant solution: sterile or tap water, according to facility policy

      □ Gloves

      □ Supplies for blood glucose (if protocol or orders indicate)

  o Ongoing Care

    ■ Prepare the formula, tubing, and infusion device.

      □ Check expiration dates and note the content of the formula.

      □ Assure that the formula is at room temperature.

      □ Set up the feeding system via gravity or pump.

      □ Mix or shake the formula, fill the container, prime the tubing, and clamp it.

    ■ Assist the client to Fowler's position or elevate the head of the bed to a minimum of 30°.

- Monitor tube placement.
  - □ Check gastric contents for pH. A good indication of appropriate placement is obtaining gastric contents with a pH between 0 and 4.
  - □ Aspirate for residual volume; intestinal residual should be less than 10 mL, and gastric residual less than 100 mL.
  - □ Note the appearance of the aspirate.
  - □ Return aspirated contents or follow facility protocol.
- Flush the tubing with 30 to 60 mL of tap water.
- Administer the formula.
  - □ Intermittent feeding
    - ▸ Have the formula and a 60-mL syringe prepared.
    - ▸ Remove the plunger from the syringe.
    - ▸ Hold the tubing above the instillation site.
    - ▸ Open the stopcock on the tubing, and insert the barrel of the syringe with the end up.
    - ▸ Fill the syringe with 40 to 50 mL of formula.
    - ▸ If using a feeding bag, fill the bag with the total amount of formula prescribed for one feeding, and hang it to drain via gravity until empty (about 30 min).
    - ▸ If using a syringe, hold it high enough for the formula to empty gradually via gravity.
    - ▸ Continue to refill the syringe until the amount prescribed for the feeding is instilled.
    - ▸ Follow with 60 to 100 mL of tap water (or the amount prescribed) to flush the tube and prevent clogging.
  - □ Continuous-drip feeding
    - ▸ Connect the feeding bag system to the feeding tube.
    - ▸ If using a pump, program the instillation rate as prescribed, and set the total volume to instill.
    - ▸ Start the pump.
    - ▸ Flush the enteral tubing with 30 to 60 mL of irrigant, usually tap water, every 4 to 6 hr, and check tube placement again.
- Monitor intake and output and include 24-hr totals.
- Monitor capillary blood glucose every 6 hr until the maximum administration rate is reached and maintained for 24 hr.
- An infusion pump is required for intestinal tube feedings.

- Follow the manufacturer's recommendations for formula hang time. Unused formula should be refrigerated and discarded after 24 hr.

- Gastric residual should be checked every 4 to 8 hr. Facility protocol specifies the actions to take based on the amount of residual obtained.

- Delegation of this skill to assistive personnel is inappropriate.

- Complications

  - When gastric residual exceeds 100 mL (10 mL for intestinal placement)
    - Withhold the feeding.
    - Notify the provider.
    - Maintain semi-Fowler's position.
    - Recheck residual in 1 hr or as prescribed.

  - Diarrhea three times or more in a 24-hr period
    - Notify the provider.
    - Confer with the dietitian.
    - Provide skin care and protection.

  - Nausea or vomiting
    - Withhold the feeding.
    - Turn the client to the side.
    - Notify the provider.
    - Check the tube's patency.
    - Aspirate for residual.
    - Auscultate for bowel sounds.

  - Aspiration of formula
    - Withhold the feeding.
    - Turn the client to the side.
    - Suction the airway.
    - Provide oxygen if indicated.
    - Monitor the client's vital signs for elevated temperature.
    - Auscultate breath sounds for increased congestion.
    - Notify the provider.
    - Obtain a chest x-ray.

  - Skin irritation around the tubing site
    - Provide a skin barrier from any drainage at the site.
    - Monitor the tube's placement.

CHAPTER 54: NASOGASTRIC INTUBATION AND ENTERAL FEEDINGS

(A) Application Exercises

1. Which of the following formulas is nutritionally complete?

    A. Polymeric

    B. Modular

    C. Elemental

    D. Specialty

2. The enteral access tube best suited for short-term use (less than 4 weeks) is a

    A. nasogastric tube.

    B. gastrostomy tube.

    C. jejunostomy tube.

    D. PEG tube.

3. The purpose of flushing a tube after an enteral feeding is given is to

    A. provide adequate fluid intake.

    B. dilute the concentration of the formula.

    C. clear the tubing to prevent clogging.

    D. ensure that the placement of the tube is maintained.

4. The highest priority nursing assessment before initiating an enteral feeding is determining

    A. if the client is alert and oriented.

    B. that the tube is correctly placed.

    C. how long the feeding container has been open.

    D. if the client has diarrhea.

5. A nurse is caring for a client receiving continuous enteral feedings. Which of the following nursing interventions is the highest priority if aspiration of tube feeding is suspected?

    A. Auscultate breath sounds.

    B. Stop the feeding.

    C. Obtain a chest x-ray.

    D. Provide oxygen.

6. The proper way to secure a nasogastric tube is to apply

    A. tape from the client's nose to the nasogastric tube.

    B. a safety pin through the nasogastric tube to the client's gown.

    C. tape to the client's cheek with a short length of tubing looped on the nose.

    D. tape around the connection of the nasogastric tube and the suction tubing.

CHAPTER 54: NASOGASTRIC INTUBATION AND ENTERAL FEEDINGS

 Application Exercises Answer Key

1. Which of the following formulas is nutritionally complete?

   A. Polymeric

   B. Modular

   C. Elemental

   D. Specialty

   Polymeric formulas are nutritionally complete. Modular formulas provide a single macronutrient. Elemental formulas are composed of predigested nutrients, and specialty formulas are designed to meet specific nutritional needs and are not nutritionally complete.

   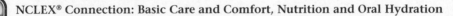 **NCLEX® Connection: Basic Care and Comfort, Nutrition and Oral Hydration**

2. The enteral access tube best suited for short-term use (less than 4 weeks) is a

   A. nasogastric tube.

   B. gastrostomy tube.

   C. jejunostomy tube.

   D. PEG tube.

   Nasogastric tubes are used short-term and can be inserted through the nose. Insertion of a gastrostomy or jejunostomy tube is done by a surgical procedure, and a percutaneous endoscopic gastrostomy (PEG) tube is inserted endoscopically. Surgical and endoscopic insertion presents an increased risk for injury and infection; therefore, they are only indicated for long-term use.

   NCLEX® Connection: Basic Care and Comfort, Nutrition and Oral Hydration

3. The purpose of flushing a tube after an enteral feeding is given is to

   A. provide adequate fluid intake.

   B. dilute the concentration of the formula.

   C. clear the tubing to prevent clogging.

   D. ensure that the placement of the tube is maintained.

   Flushing the tube after the feeding has been given helps maintain patency by clearing any excess formula from the tube. If the client requires additional fluids, the small amount used for flushing will not be adequate. If formula is to be diluted, it should be done before instilling the feeding. Flushing the tube does not maintain placement of the tube.

   NCLEX® Connection: Basic Care and Comfort, Nutrition and Oral Hydration

4. The highest priority nursing assessment before initiating an enteral feeding is determining

 A. if the client is alert and oriented.

 B. that the tube is correctly placed.

 C. how long the feeding container has been open.

 D. if the client has diarrhea.

The greatest risk to the client receiving enteral feedings is injury from aspiration. Therefore, the priority nursing assessment before initiating an enteral feeding is to determine proper place of the tube. Assessing the client's level of consciousness, the presence of any complications of tube feeding (diarrhea), and the freshness of the formula are important but are not the highest priority for this client.

 NCLEX® Connection: Basic Care and Comfort, Nutrition and Oral Hydration

5. A nurse is caring for a client receiving continuous enteral feedings. Which of the following nursing interventions is the highest priority if aspiration of tube feeding is suspected?

 A. Auscultate breath sounds.

 B. Stop the feeding.

 C. Obtain a chest x-ray.

 D. Provide oxygen.

The greatest risk to the client is aspiration pneumonia. Therefore, the first action the nurse should take is to stop the feeding so that no more formula can travel to the lungs. Auscultating for breath sounds, obtaining a chest x-ray, and providing oxygen are all important actions, but none of them is the highest priority.

 NCLEX® Connection: Basic Care and Comfort, Nutrition and Oral Hydration

6. The proper way to secure a nasogastric tube is to apply

 A. tape from the client's nose to the nasogastric tube.

 B. a safety pin through the nasogastric tube to the client's gown.

 C. tape to the client's cheek with a short length of tubing looped on the nose.

 D. tape around the connection of the nasogastric tube and the suction tubing.

Tape from the client's nose to the nasogastric tube secures the placement. Safety pins pose a risk for piercing the tubing. The tubing is too bulky to create a loop. Applying tape to the connection of the nasogastric tube and suction tubing does not secure the tube.

 NCLEX® Connection: Reduction of Risk Potential, Potential for Complications of Diagnostic Tests/Treatments/Procedures

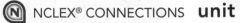

UNIT 4: PHYSIOLOGICAL INTEGRITY

Section: Physiological Adaptation

- Pressure Ulcers, Wounds, and Wound Management
- Fluid and Electrolyte Imbalances
- Cardiac Arrest, CPR, and Defibrillation

NCLEX® CONNECTIONS

When reviewing the chapters in this section, keep in mind the relevant sections of the NCLEX® outline, in particular:

CLIENT NEEDS: REDUCTION OF RISK POTENTIAL

Relevant topics/tasks include:
- Changes/Abnormalities in Vital Signs
  - Assess and respond to changes in the client's vital signs.
- Potential for Complications of Diagnostic Tests/Treatments/Procedures
  - Perform a focused assessment and reassessment.

CLIENT NEEDS: PHYSIOLOGICAL ADAPTATION

Relevant topics/tasks include:
- Alterations in Body Systems
  - Monitor wounds for signs and symptoms of infection.
- Fluid and Electrolyte Imbalances
  - Identify signs and symptoms of the client's fluid and/or electrolyte imbalance.
- Medical Emergencies
  - Perform emergency care procedures.
- Pathophysiology
  - Understand general principles of pathophysiology.

UNIT 4	PHYSIOLOGICAL INTEGRITY
Section	Physiological Adaptation
Chapter 55	Pressure Ulcers, Wounds, and Wound Management

Overview

- Wounds are a result of injury to the skin. Although there are many different methods and degrees of injury, the basic phases of healing are essentially the same for most wounds.

- A pressure ulcer (formerly called a decubitus ulcer) is a specific type of tissue injury caused by unrelieved pressure that results in ischemia and damage to the underlying tissue.

- Pressure ulcers are classified according to a staging system developed by the National Pressure Ulcer Advisory Panel. The stages are:

  o Suspected deep tissue injury – Discolored but intact skin caused by damage to underlying tissue.

  o Stage I – Intact skin with an area of persistent, non-blanchable redness, typically over a bony prominence, that may feel warm or cool to touch. The tissue is swollen and congested, with possible discomfort at the site. With darker skin tones, the ulcer may appear blue or purple.

  o Stage II – Partial-thickness skin loss involving the epidermis and the dermis. The ulcer is visible and superficial and may appear as an abrasion, blister, or shallow crater. Edema persists, and the ulcer may become infected, possibly with pain and scant drainage.

  o Stage III – Full-thickness tissue loss with damage to or necrosis of subcutaneous tissue. The ulcer may extend down to, but not through, underlying fascia. The ulcer appears as a deep crater with or without undermining of adjacent tissue and without exposed muscle or bone. Drainage and infection are common.

  o Stage IV – Full-thickness tissue loss with destruction, tissue necrosis, or damage to muscle, bone, or supporting structures. There may be sinus tracts, deep pockets of infection, tunneling, undermining, eschar (black scab-like material), or slough (tan, yellow, or green scab-like material).

  o Unstageable – Ulcers whose stage cannot be determined because eschar or slough obscures the wound.

 View Media Supplement: Stages of Pressure Ulcers (Image)

Wound Healing and Management

- Stages of Wound Healing

  - The inflammatory stage is the first 3 days after the initial trauma. Attempts are made at the site to:

    - Control bleeding with clot formation.

    - Deliver oxygen, white blood cells, and nutrients to the area via the blood supply.

  - The proliferative stage lasts the next 3 to 24 days. Effects to the wound include:

    - Replacing lost tissue with connective or granulated tissue.

    - Contracting the wound's edges.

    - Resurfacing of new epithelial cells.

  - The maturation or remodeling stage involves the strengthening of the collagen scar and the restoration of a more normal appearance. It can take more than 1 year to complete, depending on the extent of the original wound.

- Healing Processes

TYPE OF HEALING	CHARACTERISTICS	WOUND TYPE
Primary intention	• Little or no tissue loss • Edges are approximated, as with a surgical incision	• Heals rapidly • Low risk of infection • No or minimal scarring
Secondary intention	• Loss of tissue • Wound edges widely separated (pressure ulcers, stab wounds)	• Longer healing time • Increased risk of infection • Scarring
Tertiary intention	• Widely separated • Deep • Spontaneous opening of a previously closed wound • Risk of infection	• Extensive drainage and tissue debris • Closed later • Long healing time

- Factors Affecting Wound Healing

  - Increased age delays healing because of:

    - Loss of skin turgor

    - Skin fragility

    - Decreased peripheral circulation and oxygenation

    - Slower tissue regeneration

    - Decreased absorption of nutrients

    - Decreased collagen

    - Impaired function of the immune system

- o Overall wellness – A compound fracture of the femur in a client with a head injury will present greater healing problems.

- o Immune function is the body's ability to fight infection by destroying invading pathogens.

- o Medications may interfere with the body's ability to respond to and/or prevent infection.

- o Nutrition provides energy and elements required for wound healing.

- o Tissue perfusion provides circulation that delivers the required elements for tissue repair and infection control.

- o Obesity – Fatty tissue lacks blood supply.

- o Chronic diseases, such as diabetes mellitus, place additional stress on the body's healing mechanisms.

- o Chronic stress further impedes healing.

- o Smoking impairs oxygenation and clotting.

- o Wound stress, such as from vomiting or coughing, puts pressure on the suture line and disrupts the wound healing process.

- • General Principles of Wound Management

- o Wounds impair skin integrity.

- o Inflammation is a localized protective response triggered by injury or destruction of tissue.

- o Wounds heal by various processes and in stages.

- o Wounds may become infected by the invasion of pathogenic micro-organisms.

- o Principles of wound care include assessment, cleansing, and protection.

- o Wound care is a nursing responsibility that has a significant impact on wound healing.

Assessment/Data Collection

- • Appearance

- o Note the color of open wounds. The following colors reflect the wound's condition:

- ▪ Red – Healthy regeneration of tissue.

- ▪ Yellow – Presence of purulent drainage and slough.

- ▪ Black – Presence of eschar that hinders healing and must be removed.

- o Closed wounds – Skin edges should be well-approximated.

- • Drainage is a normal result of the healing process and occurs during the inflammatory and proliferative phases of healing.

- o Note the amount of drainage from a drain or on a dressing.

- o With each cleansing, observe the skin around a drain for irritation and breakdown.

- o The character of drainage is distinguished by consistency, color, and odor.

  - ▪ Serous drainage is the portion of the blood (serum) that is watery and clear or slightly yellow in appearance.

  - ▪ Sanguineous drainage contains serum and red blood cells. It is thick and appears reddish.

  - ▪ Serosanguineous drainage contains both serum and blood. It is watery and appears blood-streaked or blood-tinged.

  - ▪ Purulent drainage is the result of infection. It is thick and contains white blood cells, tissue debris, and bacteria. It may have a foul odor, and its color reflects the type of organism present (green for a *Pseudomonas aeruginosa* infection).

- Wound closure (staples, sutures, wound-closure strips [Steri-strips])

- Pain

  - o Note – Location, quality, intensity, timing, setting, associated symptoms, and aggravating/relieving factors

Nursing Interventions

- Provide adequate hydration and meet protein and calorie needs.

  - o Encourage an intake of 2,000 to 3,000 mL of fluid/day, from food and beverage sources if not contraindicated (heart failure, renal failure).

  - o Provide education about good sources of protein (meat, fish, poultry, eggs, dairy products, beans, nuts, whole grains).

  - o Note if serum albumin levels are low (below 3.5 g/dL), because a lack of protein puts the client at greater risk for delayed wound healing and infection.

  - o Provide nutritional support as indicated (vitamin and mineral supplements, nutritional supplements, enteral nutrition, parenteral nutrition).

- Perform wound cleansing.

  - o Cleanse in a direction from the least contaminated toward the most contaminated.

  - o Use gentle friction when cleansing or applying solutions to the skin to avoid bleeding or further injury to the wound.

  - o While other mild cleansing agents may be prescribed, isotonic solutions remain the preferred cleansing agents.

  - o Never use the same gauze to cleanse across an incision or wound more than once.

  - o Irrigation with a solution-filled syringe held 2.5 cm (1 in)1 inch above the wound may be used.

- For wound dressings, use:

  - o Woven gauze (sponges) – Absorbs exudate from the wound.

  - o Nonadherent material – Does not adhere to the wound bed.

       Self-adhesive, transparent film – A temporary "second skin" ideal for small, superficial wounds.

- ○ Hydrocolloid – An occlusive dressing that swells in the presence of exudate.
    - Used to maintain a granulating wound bed
    - May be left in place up to 5 days
- ○ Hydrogel (Aquasorb)
    - May be used on infected, deep wounds
    - Provides a moist wound bed

- Use the negative pressure of a wound vacuum-assisted closure if prescribed.

- Remove sutures/staples as prescribed.

- Administer analgesics as prescribed.

- Administer antimicrobials (topical and/or systemic) as prescribed.

- Document the location and type of wound/incision, the status of the wound and type of drainage, the type of dressing and materials used, client teaching provided, and how the client tolerated the procedure.

Complications and Nursing Implications

- Dehiscence is a partial or total rupture (separation) of a sutured wound, usually with separation of underlying skin layers. Evisceration is a dehiscence that involves the protrusion of visceral organs through a wound opening. It is usually caused by the increased flow of serosanguineous fluid about 3 to 11 days postoperatively.

    - ○ Signs/symptoms of dehiscence include:
        - A significant increase in the flow of serosanguineous fluid on the wound dressings.
        - Immediate history of sudden straining (coughing, sneezing, vomiting).
        - The client reporting a change or "popping" or "giving way" in the wound area.
        - Visualization of viscera.
    - ○ Risk factors include:
        - Chronic disease
        - Advanced age
        - Obesity
        - Invasive abdominal cancer
        - Vomiting

- Dehydration/malnutrition
- Ineffective suturing
- Abdominal surgery

○ Evisceration/dehiscence requires emergency treatment.

- Call for help.
- Stay with the client.
- Cover the wound and any protruding organs with sterile towels or dressings that have been soaked in sterile normal saline solution. Do not attempt to reinsert the organs.
- Position the client supine with the hips and knees bent.
- Observe the client for signs of shock.
- Maintain a calm environment.

- Infection

  ○ Risk factors

  - Extremes in age (immature immune system, decreased immune function)
  - Impaired circulation and oxygenation (COPD, peripheral vascular disease)
  - Wound condition/nature (gunshot wound vs. surgical incision)
  - Impaired/suppressed immune system
  - Malnutrition, such as with alcoholism
  - Chronic disease
  - Poor wound care, such as breaches in aseptic technique

  ○ Signs and symptoms are usually apparent within 2 to 7 days of injury/surgery.

  - Purulent drainage
  - Pain
  - Redness and edema (in and around the wound)
  - Fever
  - Chills
  - Increased pulse and respiratory rate
  - Increase in WBC count

  ○ Interventions

  - Prevent infection by using appropriate asepsis when performing dressing changes.
  - Provide optimal nutrition to promote the immune response.
  - Provide for adequate rest to promote healing.
  - Administer antibiotic therapy as prescribed.

PRESSURE ULCERS

- Pressure ulcers range from non-blanchable tissue redness to full-thickness skin loss with damage to underlying muscle and bone.

- Excellent nursing care is the primary factor in the prevention of pressure ulcers.

- The primary focus of prevention and treatment is to relieve the pressure and provide optimal nutrition and hydration.

- All clients must be assessed regularly for skin-integrity status and evaluated regularly for risk factors that contribute to impaired skin integrity.

- Ⓖ   Pressure ulcers are a significant source of morbidity and mortality among older adults and those who have limited mobility.

- Risk factors for developing pressure ulcers include:

    o   Skin changes related to aging

    o   Immobility

    o   Incontinence or excessive moisture

    o   Skin friction and shearing

    o   Vascular disorders

    o   Obesity

    o   Inadequate nutrition and/or hydration

    o   Anemia

    o   Fever

    o   Impaired circulation

    o   Edema

    o   Sensory deficits

    o   Impaired cognitive functioning, neurological disorders

    o   Chronic diseases (diabetes mellitus, chronic renal failure, congestive heart disease, chronic lung disease)

    o   Sedation that impairs spontaneous repositioning

Nursing Interventions

- Prevention

  ○ Maintain clean, dry skin and wrinkle-free linens.

    ■ Appropriately use pressure-reducing surfaces and pressure-relieving devices.

    ■ Inspect the skin frequently and document the client's risk using a tool such as the Braden scale.

    ■ Clean and dry the skin immediately following urine or stool incontinence.

    ■ Apply moisture barrier creams to the skin of clients who are incontinent.

    ■ Use tepid water (not hot), minimal scrubbing, and pat the skin dry.

  ○ Reposition the client in bed at least every 2 hr and every 1 hr in a chair. Document position changes.

    ■ Place pillows strategically between bony surfaces.

    ■ Maintain the head of the bed at or below a 30° angle (or flat), unless contraindicated, to relieve pressure on the sacrum, buttocks, and heels.

    ■ Keep the client from sliding down in bed, as this increases shearing forces that pull tissue layers apart and cause damage.

    ■ Lift, rather than pull, the client up in bed or in a chair, because pulling creates friction that can damage the outer layer of skin (epidermis).

    ■ Raise the client's heels off of the bed to prevent pressure on the heels.

    ■ Ambulate the client as soon as possible and as often as possible.

    ■ Implement active/passive exercises for immobile clients.

    ■ Do not massage bony prominences.

  ○ Provide adequate hydration (2,000 to 3,000 mL/day) and meet protein and calorie needs.

    ■ Note if serum albumin levels are low (below 3.5 g/dL), because a lack of protein puts the client at greater risk for skin breakdown, slowed healing, and infection.

    ■ Provide nutritional support as indicated, such as vitamin and mineral supplements, nutritional supplements, enteral nutrition, and parenteral nutrition.

- Treatment

STAGE	INTERVENTIONS
Suspected deep tissue injury and Stage I	<ul><li>Relieve pressure.</li><li>Encourage frequent turning/repositioning.</li><li>Use pressure-relieving devices, such as an air-fluidized bed.</li><li>Implement pressure-reduction surfaces (air mattress, foam mattress).</li><li>Keep the client dry, clean, well-nourished, and hydrated.</li></ul>
Stage II	<ul><li>Maintain a moist healing environment (saline or occlusive dressing).</li><li>Promote natural healing while preventing the formation of scar tissue.</li><li>Provide nutritional supplements as prescribed.</li><li>Administer analgesics as prescribed.</li></ul>
Stage III	<ul><li>Clean and/or debride:<ul><li>Prescribed dressing</li><li>Surgical intervention</li><li>Proteolytic enzymes</li></ul></li><li>Provide nutritional supplements as prescribed.</li><li>Administer analgesics as prescribed.</li><li>Administer antimicrobials (topical and/or systemic) as prescribed.</li></ul>
Stage IV	<ul><li>Clean and/or debride:<ul><li>Prescribed dressing</li><li>Surgical intervention</li><li>Proteolytic enzymes</li></ul></li><li>Perform nonadherent dressing changes every 12 hr.</li><li>Treatment may include skin grafts.</li><li>Provide nutritional supplements as prescribed.</li><li>Administer analgesics as prescribed.</li><li>Administer antimicrobials (topical and/or systemic) as prescribed.</li></ul>
Unstageable	<ul><li>Debride as prescribed until the ulcer can be staged.</li></ul>

(M) **View Media Supplement:** Pressure-Relieving Device (Image)

Complications and Nursing Implications

- Deterioration to a Higher Stage Ulceration and/or Infection

  o Assess/monitor the ulcer frequently and report increases in the size or depth of the lesion, changes in granulation tissue (color, texture), and changes in exudates (color, quantity, odor).

  o Follow the facility's protocol for ulcer treatment.

- Systemic Infection

  o Assess/monitor the client for signs of sepsis (changes in level of consciousness, persistent recurrent fever, tachycardia, tachypnea, hypotension, oliguria, increased WBC count).

  o Prevent infection by using appropriate asepsis when performing ulcer treatment and dressing changes.

  o Provide optimal nutrition to promote the immune response.

  o Provide for adequate rest to promote healing.

  o Administer antibiotic therapy as prescribed.

CHAPTER 55: PRESSURE ULCERS, WOUNDS, AND WOUND MANAGEMENT

 Application Exercises

1. An adolescent client who has diabetes mellitus is 2 days postoperative following an appendectomy. The client is tolerating a regular diet well. He has ambulated successfully around the unit with assistance and requests pain medication every 6 to 8 hr while reporting pain at a 2 on a scale of 0 to 10 after the medication is given. His incision is approximated and free of redness with scant serous drainage noted on the dressing. Which of the following risk factors for poor wound healing does this client have? (Select all that apply.)

_____ Extremes in age

_____ Impaired circulation

_____ Impaired/suppressed immune system

_____ Malnutrition

_____ Poor wound care such as breaches in aseptic technique

2. An entry in a client's chart states the wound drainage is "sanguineous." That means it is

A. watery in appearance.

B. green-tinged or yellow.

C. bright red.

D. foul-smelling.

3. Which of the following is an example of a wound or injury healing by secondary intention?

A. An open burn area

B. A bone fracture that is casted

C. A sprained ankle

D. A sutured surgical incision

Scenario: An older adult woman is 6 days postoperative following surgery for a bowel obstruction. During the last 24 hr, she has reported nausea, and she vomited small amounts of clear liquid three times in the last 8 hr. Her vital signs are stable. Currently, her incision is well approximated and free of redness, tenderness, and swelling.

4. Which of the following findings would indicate development of a wound infection?

A. Decreased pulse rate

B. Increased pain

C. Decreased WBC count

D. Increased thirst

5. Later that day, the client becomes confused and pulls off her surgical dressing. The nurse enters the room and finds the client's wound separated with viscera protruding. Which of the following nursing interventions are appropriate? (Select all that apply.)

_____ Repack the wound.

_____ Call for help.

_____ Assist the client to a chair.

_____ Cover the wound with a sterile dressing moistened with 0.9% sodium chloride.

_____ Stay with the client.

Scenario: An older adult client who has diabetes mellitus must now use a wheelchair after a cerebrovascular accident (CVA) 2 years ago that affected her right side. She does not respond to pain on the right side of her body. Her fluid and food intake is good, but she needs help with eating.

6. Which of the following risk factors for developing pressure ulcers does this client have?

A. Dehydration

B. Limited mobility

C. Nutritional impairment

D. Incontinence

7. Which of the following can the nurse do to prevent skin breakdown?

A. Massage the client's bony prominences frequently.

B. Keep the client in high-Fowler's position while in bed.

C. Have the client sit on a donut-shaped cushion.

D. Encourage repositioning every 15 min while the client is in the wheelchair.

8. Which of the following statements describes a stage III pressure ulcer?

A. The skin is reddened and does not blanch with pressure.

B. The ulcer is an abrasion or a blister.

C. The bone is exposed at the center of the ulcer.

D. The ulcer extends past the subcutaneous tissue to the muscle.

CHAPTER 55: PRESSURE ULCERS, WOUNDS, AND WOUND MANAGEMENT

 Application Exercises Answer Key

1. An adolescent client who has diabetes mellitus is 2 days postoperative following an appendectomy. The client is tolerating a regular diet well. He has ambulated successfully around the unit with assistance and requests pain medication every 6 to 8 hr while reporting pain at a 2 on a scale of 0 to 10 after the medication is given. His incision is approximated and free of redness with scant serous drainage noted on the dressing. Which of the following risk factors for poor wound healing does this client have? (Select all that apply.)

    _____ Extremes in age
    __X__ **Impaired circulation**
    __X__ **Impaired/suppressed immune system**
    _____ Malnutrition
    _____ Poor wound care such as breaches in aseptic technique

    Diabetes mellitus places this client at risk for impaired circulation and immune system function. The client is not at either extreme of the age spectrum, and there is no indication that he is malnourished or that there have been any breaches in aseptic technique during wound care.

 NCLEX® Connection: Reduction of Risk Potential, System Specific Assessment

2. An entry in a client's chart states the wound drainage is "sanguineous." That means it is

    A. watery in appearance.
    B. green-tinged or yellow.
    C. bright red.
    D. foul-smelling.

    Sanguineous drainage is bright red and the result of active bleeding. A watery appearance is characteristic of serous or serosanguineous drainage. Green-tinged or yellow and foul-smelling are characteristics of purulent drainage.

 NCLEX® Connection: Reduction of Risk Potential, System Specific Assessment

3. Which of the following is an example of a wound or injury healing by secondary intention?

    A. An open burn area
    B. A bone fracture that is casted
    C. A sprained ankle
    D. A sutured surgical incision

    A burn has loss of tissue, and the skin edges are not together. A fractured bone and sprained ankle are injuries to underlying structures and do not require healing of the skin. A sutured surgical incision heals by primary intention.

 NCLEX® Connection: Reduction of Risk Potential, System Specific Assessment

Scenario: An older adult woman is 6 days postoperative following surgery for a bowel obstruction. During the last 24 hr, she has reported nausea, and she vomited small amounts of clear liquid three times in the last 8 hr. Her vital signs are stable. Currently, her incision is well approximated and free of redness, tenderness, and swelling.

4. Which of the following findings would indicate development of a wound infection?

    A. Decreased pulse rate

    B. Increased pain

    C. Decreased WBC count

    D. Increased thirst

An increase in incisional pain is a sign of a possible wound infection. With infection, the pulse rate and WBC count increase. Increased thirst has many possible causes and does not necessarily indicate an infectious process.

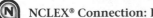 NCLEX® Connection: Physiological Adaptation, Alterations in Body Systems

5. Later that day, the client becomes confused and pulls off her surgical dressing. The nurse enters the room and finds the client's wound separated with viscera protruding. Which of the following nursing interventions are appropriate? (Select all that apply.)

    _____ Repack the wound.

    __X__ **Call for help.**

    _____ Assist the client to a chair.

    __X__ **Cover the wound with a sterile dressing moistened with 0.9% sodium chloride.**

    __X__ **Stay with the client.**

It is appropriate for the nurse to call for help, cover the wound with a sterile dressing moistened with 0.9% sodium chloride, and stay with the client. The nurse should not attempt to reinsert the organs or repack the wound. The nurse should have the client lie supine with her hips and knees bent.

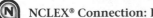 NCLEX® Connection: Physiological Adaptation, Alterations in Body Systems

Scenario: An older adult client who has diabetes mellitus must now use a wheelchair after a cerebrovascular accident (CVA) 2 years ago that affected her right side. She does not respond to pain on the right side of her body. Her fluid and food intake is good, but she needs help with eating.

6. Which of the following risk factors for developing pressure ulcers does this client have?

   A. Dehydration

   B. Limited mobility

   C. Nutritional impairment

   D. Incontinence

   The client's limited mobility as a result of the CVA puts her at risk for skin breakdown. She is well-hydrated and nourished, and there are no data to indicate that she has urinary or fecal incontinence.

 NCLEX® Connection: Reduction of Risk Potential, System Specific Assessment

7. Which of the following can the nurse do to prevent skin breakdown?

   A. Massage the client's bony prominences frequently.

   B. Keep the client in high-Fowler's position while in bed.

   C. Have the client sit on a donut-shaped cushion.

   D. Encourage repositioning every 15 min while the client is in the wheelchair.

   It is essential to encourage and help the client alter her position every 15 min while seated to prevent sustained pressure on any skin areas. While in bed, the head of the client's bed should be elevated no more than 30° to prevent skin breakdown from shearing forces in the sacral area. Donut-shaped cushions increase pressure on the sacral area. A gel foam or air cushion would be a better choice.

NCLEX® Connection: Reduction of Risk Potential, Potential for Alterations in Body Systems

8. Which of the following statements describes a stage III pressure ulcer?

   A. The skin is reddened and does not blanch with pressure.

   B. The ulcer is an abrasion or a blister.

   C. The bone is exposed at the center of the ulcer.

   D. The ulcer extends past the subcutaneous tissue to the muscle.

   A stage III ulcer may extend past all the layers of skin and subcutaneous tissue to the muscle. Reddened skin that does not blanch is characteristic of stage I. An abrasion or a blister is seen with stage II. Exposed bone is characteristic of stage IV.

NCLEX® Connection: Reduction of Risk Potential, System Specific Assessment

UNIT 4	PHYSIOLOGICAL INTEGRITY
Section	Physiological Adaptation
Chapter 56	Fluid and Electrolyte Imbalances

Overview

- Fluids

  - Body fluids are distributed between intracellular (ICF) and extracellular (ECF) compartments.

  - Fluid can move between compartments (through selectively permeable membranes) by a variety of methods (diffusion, active transport, filtration, osmosis) in order to maintain homeostasis.

- Electrolytes

  - Electrolytes are minerals (sometimes called salts) that are present in all body fluids. They regulate fluid balance and hormone production, strengthen skeletal structures, and act as catalysts in nerve response, muscle contraction, and the metabolism of nutrients.

  - When dissolved in water or another solvent, electrolytes separate into ions and then conduct either a positive (cations – magnesium, potassium, sodium, calcium) or negative (anions – phosphate, sulfate, chloride, bicarbonate) electrical current.

  - Electrolytes are distributed between ICF and ECF compartments. While laboratory tests can accurately reflect the electrolyte concentrations in plasma, it is not possible to directly measure electrolyte concentrations within cells.

  - Fluid imbalances that the nurse should be familiar with are:

    - Fluid volume deficits
    - Fluid volume excess

Fluid Volume Deficits

- Fluid volume deficits (FVDs) include hypovolemia-isotonic (loss of water and electrolytes from the ECF) and dehydration-osmolar (loss of water with no loss of electrolytes).

- Hemoconcentration occurs with dehydration, resulting in increases in Hct, serum electrolytes, and urine specific gravity.

- Note – Compensatory mechanisms include sympathetic nervous system responses of increased thirst, antidiuretic hormone (ADH) release, and aldosterone release.

- Hypovolemia can lead to hypovolemic shock.

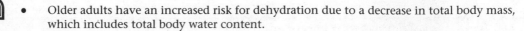

- Older adults have an increased risk for dehydration due to a decrease in total body mass, which includes total body water content.

Assessment

- Risk Factors

  - Causes of Hypovolemia

    - Abnormal gastrointestinal (GI) losses – Vomiting, nasogastric suctioning, diarrhea

    - Abnormal skin losses – Diaphoresis

    - Abnormal renal losses – Diuretic therapy, diabetes insipidus, renal disease, adrenal insufficiency, osmotic diuresis

    - Third spacing – Peritonitis, intestinal obstruction, ascites, burns

    - Hemorrhage

    - Altered intake, such as nothing by mouth (NPO)

  - Causes of Dehydration

    - Hyperventilation

    - Diabetic ketoacidosis

    - Enteral feeding without sufficient water intake

- Subjective and Objective Data

  - Vital signs – Hyperthermia, tachycardia, thready pulse, hypotension, orthostatic hypotension, decreased central venous pressure, tachypnea (increased respirations), hypoxia

  - Neuromusculoskeletal – Dizziness, syncope, confusion, weakness, fatigue

  - GI – Thirst, dry furrowed tongue, nausea/vomiting, anorexia, acute weight loss

  - Renal – Oliguria (decreased production of urine)

  - Other signs – Diminished capillary refill, cool clammy skin, diaphoresis, sunken eyeballs, flattened neck veins

- Laboratory Findings

  - Hct

    - Hypovolemia – Increased Hct

    - Dehydration – Increased hemoconcentration but not present when dehydration is caused by hemorrhage

- Serum osmolarity

  - Dehydration – Increased hemoconcentration osmolarity (greater than 300 mOsm/L) – Increased protein, BUN, electrolytes, glucose

- Urine specific gravity and osmolarity

  - Dehydration – Increased concentration

- Serum sodium

  - Dehydration – Increased hemoconcentration

Collaborative Care

- Nursing Care

  - Assess respiratory rate, symmetry, and effort.

  - Monitor for shortness of breath and dyspnea.

  - Check urinalysis, oxygen saturation (SaO_2), CBC, and electrolytes.

  - Administer supplemental oxygen as prescribed.

  - Measure the client's weight daily at same time of day using the same scale.

  - Observe for nausea and vomiting.

  - Assess and monitor the client's vital signs. (check for hypotension and orthostatic hypotension).

  - Check neurological status to determine level of consciousness.

  - Assess heart rhythm (may be irregular or tachycardic).

  - Initiate and maintain IV access.

  - Place the client in shock position (on the back with the legs elevated).

  - Fluid replacement: Administer IV fluids as prescribed (isotonic solutions such as lactated Ringer's, 0.9% sodium chloride; blood transfusions).

  - Monitor I&O. Alert the provider to a urine output less than 30 mL/hr.

  - Monitor level of consciousness and ensure client safety.

  - Assess level of gait stability.

  - Encourage the client to use the call-light and ask for assistance.

  - Encourage the client to change positions slowly (rolling from side to side or standing up).

  - Check capillary refill (expected reference range less than 2 seconds).

Fluid Volume Excesses

- Fluid volume excesses (FVEs) include hypervolemia-isotonic (water and sodium retained in abnormally high proportions) and overhydration-osmolar (more water gained than electrolytes).

- Severe hypervolemia can lead to pulmonary edema and heart failure.

- Hemodilution occurs with overhydration, resulting in decreases in Hct, serum electrolytes, and protein.

- Note – Compensatory mechanisms include an increased release of natriuretic peptides, resulting in increased loss of sodium and water by the kidneys, and a decreased release of aldosterone.

Assessment

- Risk Factors

  o Causes of Hypervolemia

    ■ Chronic stimulus to the kidney to conserve sodium and water (heart failure, cirrhosis, increased glucocorticosteroids)

    ■ Abnormal renal function with reduced excretion of sodium and water (renal failure)

    ■ Interstitial to plasma fluid shifts (hypertonic fluids, burns)

    ■ Age-related changes in cardiovascular and renal function

    ■ Excessive sodium intake

  o Causes of Overhydration

    ■ Water replacement without electrolyte replacement (strenuous exercise with profuse diaphoresis)

- Subjective and Objective Data

  o Vital signs – Tachycardia, bounding pulse, hypertension, tachypnea, increased central venous pressure

  o Neuromusculoskeletal – Confusion, muscle weakness

  o GI – Weight gain, ascites

  o Respiratory – Dyspnea, orthopnea, crackles

  o Other signs – Edema, distended neck veins

- Laboratory Findings

  - Hct

    - Hypervolemia – Decreased Hct

    - Overhydration – Decreased Hct = hemodilution

  - Serum osmolarity

    - Overhydration – Decreased hemodilution (osmolarity less than 270 mOsm/L)

  - Serum sodium

    - Hypervolemia – Sodium within expected reference range

  - Electrolytes, BUN, and creatinine

    - Overhydration/hypervolemia – Decreased electrolytes, BUN, and creatinine

  - Arterial blood gases

    - Respiratory alkalosis – Decreased $PaCO_2$ (less than 35 mm Hg), increased pH (greater than 7.45)

- Diagnostic Procedures

  - Chest x-rays may indicate pulmonary congestion.

Collaborative Care

- Nursing Care

  - Assess respiratory rate, symmetry, and effort.

  - Assess breath sounds in all lung fields. Lung sounds may be diminished with crackles.

  - Monitor for shortness of breath and dyspnea.

  - Check ABGs, SaO_2, CBC, and chest x-ray results.

  - Position the client in semi-Fowler's position.

  - Measure the client's weight daily.

  - Monitor I&O.

  - Administer supplemental oxygen as needed.

  - Reduce IV flow rates.

  - Administer diuretics (osmotic, loop) as prescribed.

    - Limit fluid and sodium intake as prescribed.

    - Monitor and document edema (pretibial, sacral, periorbital).

- Monitor and document circulation to the extremities.

- Reposition the client at least every 2 hr.

- Support arms and legs to decrease dependent edema as appropriate.

Electrolytes

- Major electrolytes in the body include sodium, potassium, chloride, magnesium, phosphorus, and calcium. Nurses monitor the client's laboratory values to identify any electrolyte imbalances.

Ⓖ • It is important to recognize the signs and symptoms of electrolyte imbalance. Clients at greatest risk for electrolyte imbalance are infants and children, older adults, clients with cognitive disorders, and clients who are chronically ill.

Sodium Imbalances

- Sodium (Na+) is the major electrolyte found in ECF.

- Sodium is essential for maintenance of acid-base balance, active and passive transport mechanisms, and irritability and conduction of nerve and muscle tissue.

- Expected serum sodium levels are between 136 and 145 mEq/L.

Hyponatremia

- Hyponatremia is a serum sodium level less than 136 mEq/L.

- Hyponatremia is a net gain of water or loss of sodium-rich fluids.

- Hyponatremia delays and slows the depolarization of membranes.

- Water moves from the ECF into the ICF, which causes cells to swell (cerebral edema).

- Serious complications can result from untreated acute hyponatremia (coma, seizures, respiratory arrest).

Assessment

- Risk Factors

  o Causes of Hyponatremia (loss of sodium)

    - Deficient ECF volume

    - Abnormal GI losses – Vomiting, nasogastric suctioning, diarrhea, tap water enemas

    - Renal losses – Diuretics, kidney disease, adrenal insufficiency, excessive sweating

    - Skin losses – Burns, wound drainage, gastrointestinal obstruction, peripheral edema, ascites.

- Increased or normal ECF volume – Excessive oral water intake, syndrome of inappropriate antidiuretic hormone (SIADH), which is the excess secretion of antidiuretic hormone (ADH)

- Edematous states – Heart failure, cirrhosis, nephrotic syndrome

- Excessive hypotonic IV fluids

- Inadequate sodium intake (NPO status)

- Age-related risk factors – Older adult clients are at greater risk due to an increased incidence of chronic illnesses, use of diuretic medications, and risk for insufficient sodium intake.

- Subjective and Objective Data

  - Physical assessment findings – Vary with a normal, decreased, or increased ECF volume

  - Vital signs – Hypothermia, tachycardia, rapid thready pulse, hypotension, orthostatic hypotension

  - Neuromusculoskeletal – Headache, confusion, lethargy, muscle weakness with possible respiratory compromise, fatigue, decreased deep tendon reflexes (DTR)

  - GI – Increased motility, hyperactive bowel sounds, abdominal cramping, nausea

- Laboratory Findings

  - Serum sodium

    - Decreased – Less than 136 mEq/L

  - Serum osmolarity

    - Decreased – Less than 280 mOsm/L

Collaborative Care

- Nursing Care

  - Report abnormal laboratory findings to the provider.

  - Fluid overload – Restrict water intake as prescribed.

  - Acute hyponatremia:

    - Administer hypertonic oral and IV fluids as prescribed.

    - Encourage foods and fluids high in sodium (cheese, milk, condiments).

  - Restoration of normal ECF volume – Administer isotonic IV therapy (0.9% sodium chloride, lactated Ringer's).

  - Monitor I&O and weigh the client daily.

  - Monitor vital signs and level of consciousness, reporting abnormal findings.

  - Encourage the client to change positions slowly.

  - Follow any prescribed fluid restrictions.

Hypernatremia

- Hypernatremia is a serum sodium level that is greater than 145 mEq/L.

- Hypernatremia is a serious electrolyte imbalance. It can cause significant neurological, endocrine, and cardiac disturbances.

- Increased sodium causes hypertonicity of the serum. This causes a shift of water out of the cells, making the cells dehydrated.

Assessment

- Risk Factors

  o Water deprivation (NPO)

  o Excessive sodium intake – Dietary sodium intake, hypertonic IV fluids, bicarbonate intake

  o Excessive sodium retention – Renal failure, Cushing's syndrome, aldosteronism, some medications (glucocorticosteroids)

  o Fluid losses – Fever, diaphoresis, burns, respiratory infection, diabetes insipidus, hyperglycemia, watery diarrhea

  o Age-related changes, specifically decreased total body water content and inadequate fluid intake related to an altered thirst mechanism

  o Compensatory mechanisms – Increased thirst and increased production of ADH.

- Subjective and Objective Data

  o Vital signs – Hyperthermia, tachycardia, orthostatic hypotension

  o Neuromusculoskeletal – Restlessness, irritability, muscle twitching, muscle weakness, seizures, coma, reduced to absent DTRs

  o GI – Thirst, dry mucous membranes, increased motility, hyperactive bowel sounds, abdominal cramping, nausea

  o Other signs – Edema, warm flushed skin, oliguria

- Laboratory Findings

  o Serum sodium

    ▪ Increased – Greater than 145 mEq/L

  o Serum osmolarity

    ▪ Increased – Greater than 300 mOsm/L

Collaborative Care

- Nursing Care
    - Report abnormal laboratory findings to the provider.
    - Fluid loss – Based on serum osmolarity
        - Administer hypotonic IV fluids (0.45% sodium chloride).
        - Administer isotonic IV fluids (0.9% sodium chloride).
    - Excess sodium
        - Encourage water intake and discourage sodium intake.
        - Administer diuretics (loop diuretics).
    - Monitor level of consciousness and ensure safety.
    - Provide oral hygiene and other comfort measures to decrease thirst.
    - Monitor I&O, and alert the provider if renal output is inadequate.

Potassium Imbalances

- Potassium (K+) is the major cation in ICF.
- Potassium plays a vital role in cell metabolism; transmission of nerve impulses; functioning of cardiac, lung, and muscle tissues; and acid-base balance.
- Potassium has reciprocal action with sodium.
- Expected serum potassium levels are 3.5 to 5 mEq/L.

Hypokalemia

- Hypokalemia is a serum potassium level below 3.5 mEq/L.
- Hypokalemia is the result of an increased loss of potassium from the body or movement of potassium into the cells.

Assessment

- Risk Factors
    - Causes of hypokalemia (loss of potassium)
    - Abnormal GI losses – Vomiting, nasogastric suctioning, diarrhea, inappropriate laxative use
    - Renal losses – Excessive use of diuretics such as furosemide (Lasix), corticosteroids
    - Skin losses – Diaphoresis, wound losses
    - Insufficient potassium
    - Inadequate dietary intake (rare)

- o Prolonged administration of non-electrolyte-containing IV solutions such as 5% dextrose in water

- o ICF – Metabolic alkalosis, after correction of acidosis, during periods of tissue repair (burns, trauma, starvation), total parenteral nutrition

- o Age-related risk factors – Older adult clients are at greater risk due to increased use of diuretics and laxatives.

- Subjective and Objective Data

  - o Vital signs – Hyperthermia, weak irregular pulse, hypotension, respiratory distress

  - o Neuromusculoskeletal – Weakness with respiratory collapse and paralysis, muscle cramping, decreased muscle tone and hypoactive reflexes, paresthesias, mental confusion

  - o ECG – Premature ventricular contractions (PVCs), bradycardia, blocks, ventricular tachycardia, inverted T waves, and ST depression

  - o GI – Decreased motility, abdominal distention, constipation, ileus, nausea, vomiting, anorexia

  - o Other signs – Polyuria (excretion of dilute urine)

- Laboratory Findings

  - o Serum potassium

    - ▪ Decreased – Less than 3.5 mEq/L

  - o Arterial blood gases

    - ▪ Metabolic alkalosis – pH greater than 7.45

- Diagnostic Procedures

  - o Electrocardiogram (ECG)

    - ▪ Will show findings of dysrhythmias, such as PVCs, ventricular tachycardia, inverted T waves, and ST depression

Collaborative Care

- Nursing Care

  - o Report abnormal findings to the provider.

  - o Treat the underlying cause.

  - o Replace potassium.

    - ▪ Encourage foods high in potassium (avocados, broccoli, dairy products, dried fruit, cantaloupe, bananas).

    - ▪ Provide oral potassium supplementation.

- o   IV potassium supplementation

  - ▪   Never IV bolus (high risk of cardiac arrest)

  - ▪   The maximum recommended rate is 5 to 10 mEq/hr.

- o   Monitor for phlebitis (tissue irritant).

- o   Monitor for and maintain an adequate urine output.

- o   Monitor for shallow, ineffective respirations and diminished breath sounds.

- o   Monitor the client's cardiac rhythm and intervene promptly as needed.

- o   Monitor clients receiving digoxin. Hypokalemia increases the risk for digoxin toxicity.

- o   Monitor level of consciousness and ensure safety.

- o   Monitor bowel sounds and abdominal distention and intervene as needed.

Hyperkalemia

- •   Hyperkalemia is a serum potassium level greater than 5.0 mEq/L.

- •   Hyperkalemia is the result of an increased intake of potassium, movement of potassium out of the cells, or inadequate renal excretion.

Assessment

- •   Risk Factors

  - o   Increased total body potassium – IV potassium administration, salt substitutes

  - o   ECF shift – Decreased insulin, acidosis (diabetic ketoacidosis), tissue catabolism (sepsis, trauma, surgery, fever, myocardial infarction)

  - o   Hypertonic states – Uncontrolled diabetes mellitus

  - o   Decreased excretion of potassium – Renal failure, severe dehydration, potassium-sparing diuretics, ACE inhibitors, NSAIDs, adrenal insufficiency

  - o   Older adult clients – At greater risk due to increased use of salt substitutes, angiotensin-converting enzyme inhibitors, and potassium-sparing diuretics

- •   Subjective and Objective Data

  - o   Vital signs – Slow, irregular pulse; hypotension

  - o   Neuromusculoskeletal – Restlessness, irritability, weakness with ascending flaccid paralysis, paresthesias

  - o   ECG – Ventricular fibrillation, peaked T waves, widened QRS

  - o   GI – Nausea, vomiting, increased motility, diarrhea, hyperactive bowel sounds

  - o   Other signs – Oliguria

- Laboratory Findings

  o Serum potassium

    ▪ Increased – Greater than 5 mEq/L

  o Arterial blood gases

    ▪ Metabolic alkalosis – pH less than 7.45

- Diagnostic Procedures

  o ECG

    ▪ Will show dysrhythmias (ventricular fibrillation, peaked T waves, widened QRS)

Collaborative Care

- Nursing Care

  o Report abnormal findings to the provider.

  o Decrease potassium intake:

    ▪ Stop infusion of IV potassium.

    ▪ Withhold oral potassium.

    ▪ Provide a potassium-restricted diet (avoiding avocados, broccoli, dairy products, dried fruit, cantaloupe, bananas).

    ▪ If potassium levels are extremely high, dialysis may be required.

  o Promote the movement of potassium from ECF to ICF:

    ▪ Administer IV fluids with dextrose and regular insulin.

    ▪ Administer sodium bicarbonate to reverse acidosis.

  o Monitor the client's cardiac rhythm and intervene promptly as needed.

  o Medications to increase potassium excretion:

    ▪ Administer loop diuretics, such as furosemide (Lasix), if renal function is adequate. Loop diuretics increase the depletion of potassium from the renal system.

  o Maintain IV access.

  o Prepare the client for dialysis if prescribed.

Calcium Imbalances

- Calcium is found in the bones and the teeth. It is plentiful in the body. The expected calcium level is 9 to 10.5 mg/dL or 4.5 mg/dL for ionized calcium.

- Calcium balance is essential for proper functioning of the cardiovascular, neuromuscular, and endocrine systems, as well as blood clotting and bone and teeth formation.

Hypocalcemia

- Hypocalcemia is a serum calcium level less than 9 mg/dL.

- Risk Factors

  - Malabsorption syndromes, such as Crohn's disease

  - End-stage renal disease

  - Post thyroidectomy

  - Hypoparathyroidism

  - Repeated transfusion

- Subjective and Objective Data

  - Muscle twitches/tetany

    - Frequent, painful muscle spasms at rest

    - Hyperactive DTRs

    - Positive Chvostek's sign (tapping on the facial nerve triggering facial twitching)

    - Positive Trousseau's sign (hand/finger spasms with sustained blood pressure cuff inflation)

  - Cardiovascular

    - Decreased myocardial contractility (decreased heart rate and hypotension)

  - GI – Hyperactive bowel sounds, diarrhea, abdominal cramping

  - Central nervous system – Seizures due to overstimulation of the CNS

- Laboratory Findings

  - Calcium level less than 9 mg/dL

- Diagnostic Procedures

  - ECG

    - Prolonged QT interval

Collaborative Care

- Nursing Care

  - Administer oral or IV calcium supplements.

  - Initiate seizure precautions.

  - Keep emergency equipment on standby.

  - Encourage foods high in calcium, including dairy products and dark green vegetables.

Magnesium Imbalances

- Most of the body's magnesium is found in the bones. Magnesium in smaller amounts is found within the body cells. A very small amount is found in ECF. The expected magnesium level is 1.3 to 2.1 mEq/L

Hypomagnesemia

- Hypomagnesemia is a serum magnesium level less than 1.3 mg/dL.

Assessment

- Risk Factors

    o Causes of hypomagnesemia

    o Malnutrition (insufficient magnesium intake)

    o Alcohol ingestion (magnesium excretion)

- Subjective and Objective Data

    o Neuromuscular – Increased nerve impulse transmission (hyperactive DTRs, paresthesias, muscle tetany), positive Chvostek's and Trousseau's signs

    o GI – Hypoactive bowel sounds, constipation, abdominal distention, paralytic ileus.

- Nursing Care

    o Discontinue magnesium-losing medications (loop diuretics).

    o Administer oral or IV magnesium sulfate following safety protocols. IV route is used because IM can cause pain and tissue damage. Oral magnesium can cause diarrhea and increase magnesium depletion. Monitor closely.

    o Encourage foods high in magnesium, including dairy products and dark green vegetables.

CHAPTER 56: FLUID AND ELECTROLYTE IMBALANCES

 Application Exercises

1. A nurse is collecting data from an older adult client who states he has had vomiting and diarrhea for the last 48 hr. Which of the following findings should indicate to the nurse that the client is hypovolemic? (Select all that apply.)

_____ Bradycardia

_____ Hypertension

_____ Tachypnea

_____ Furrowed tongue

_____ Sunken eyeballs

2. A nurse is providing teaching about a healthy lifestyle for a group of young adults who are training for a marathon. Which of the following should the nurse include in the teaching session?

A. Decrease fluid intake after training.

B. Decrease fluid intake in high altitudes.

C. Increase fluid intake in dry climates.

D. Increase intake of fluids containing caffeine.

3. A nurse is caring for a client who was admitted to the hospital for peritonitis and has signs of dehydration. Which of the following laboratory findings would be expected for this client? (Select all that apply.)

_____ Increased Hct

_____ Decreased serum osmolarity

_____ Increased serum sodium

_____ Decreased urine specific gravity

_____ Increased urine osmolarity

4. A nurse on a medical-surgical unit has been assigned to care for four clients. Which of the following clients is at risk for fluid volume excess (hypervolemia)?

A. A client who is receiving a high-ceiling loop diuretic.

B. A client who has heart failure.

C. A client who lost 500 mL of blood during surgery.

D. A client who is 4 hr postoperative and is receiving nasogastric suction.

5. A nurse is reviewing the laboratory findings for a group of clients. Which of the following findings should be reported to the provider?

A. Serum sodium 143 mEq/L

B. Serum potassium 4 mEq/L

C. Serum calcium 8.5 mg/dL

D. Serum chloride 99 mEq/L

6. A nurse on a medical-surgical unit is caring for a client who is hypernatremic. Which of the following should be included in the plan of care?

    A. Infuse hypotonic IV fluids.

    B. Restrict oral intake of water.

    C. Increase sodium intake.

    D. Administer a loop diuretic.

CHAPTER 56: FLUID AND ELECTROLYTE IMBALANCES

 Application Exercises Answer Key

1. A nurse is collecting data from an older adult client who states he has had vomiting and diarrhea for the last 48 hr. Which of the following findings should indicate to the nurse that the client is hypovolemic? (Select all that apply.)

	Bradycardia
	Hypertension
X	**Tachypnea**
X	**Furrowed tongue**
X	**Sunken eyeballs**

A client who has altered intake is at risk for hypovolemia. Older adults are at greater risk than younger adults. In the presence of hypovolemia, tachycardia, hypotension, tachypnea, a furrowed dry tongue, and sunken eyeballs may be seen.

 NCLEX® Connection: Physiological Adaptation, Fluid and Electrolyte Imbalances

2. A nurse is providing teaching about a healthy lifestyle for a group of young adults who are training for a marathon. Which of the following should the nurse include in the teaching session?

A. Decrease fluid intake after training.

B. Decrease fluid intake in high altitudes.

C. Increase fluid intake in dry climates.

D. Increase intake of fluids containing caffeine.

Fluid intake should be increased with excessive, vigorous exercise in high altitudes. Fluid intake should also be increased in dry climates. Caffeine should be avoided because excessive intake may lead to dehydration.

 NCLEX® Connection: Physiological Adaptation, Fluid and Electrolyte Imbalances

3. A nurse is caring for a client who was admitted to the hospital for peritonitis and has signs of dehydration. Which of the following laboratory findings would be expected for this client? (Select all that apply.)

X	**Increased Hct**
	Decreased serum osmolarity
X	**Increased serum sodium**
	Decreased urine specific gravity
X	**Increased urine osmolarity**

In the presence of dehydration (not related to hemorrhage), urine osmolarity and urine specific gravity are increased. Due to hemoconcentration, serum osmolarity and serum sodium are increased.

 NCLEX® Connection: Physiological Adaptation, Fluid and Electrolyte Imbalances

4. A nurse on a medical-surgical unit has been assigned to care for four clients. Which of the following clients is at risk for fluid volume excess (hypervolemia)?

    A. A client who is receiving a high-ceiling loop diuretic.

    B. A client who has heart failure.

    C. A client who lost 500 mL of blood during surgery.

    D. A client who is 4 hr postoperative and is receiving nasogastric suction.

A client who has heart failure is at risk for fluid retention and fluid volume excess. The other clients are at risk for hypovolemia.

 NCLEX® Connection: Physiological Adaptation, Fluid and Electrolyte Imbalances

5. A nurse is reviewing the laboratory findings for a group of clients. Which of the following findings should be reported to the provider?

    A. Serum sodium 143 mEq/L

    B. Serum potassium 4 mEq/L

    C. Serum calcium 8.5 mg/dL

    D. Serum chloride 99 mEq/L

A serum calcium level of 8.5 mg/dL is below the expected reference range and should be reported to the provider. The other findings are within the expected reference range.

 NCLEX® Connection: Physiological Adaptation, Fluid and Electrolyte Imbalances

6. A nurse on a medical-surgical unit is caring for a client who is hypernatremic. Which of the following should be included in the plan of care?

    A. Infuse hypotonic IV fluids.

    B. Restrict oral intake of water.

    C. Increase sodium intake.

    D. Administer a loop diuretic.

The plan of care for a client who is hypernatremic should include hypotonic or isotonic fluids. Water intake is encouraged. Sodium intake is restricted. A loop diuretic will increase the excretion of sodium.

NCLEX® Connection: Physiological Adaptation, Fluid and Electrolyte Imbalances

UNIT 4	PHYSIOLOGICAL INTEGRITY
Section	Physiological Adaptation
Chapter 57	Cardiac Arrest, CPR, and Defibrillation

 Overview

- Cardiac Arrest

  o Cardiac arrest, the sudden cessation of cardiac function, is characterized by the absence of a carotid pulse in adults and children 1 year of age to adolescence, and the absence of a brachial pulse in infants up to 1 year. If no brachial pulse is detected, check the carotid. (Brachial is checked first because the carotid may be difficult to palpate due to the fatty tissue of the neck.)

  o Ashen appearance of the skin.

  o Absence of respirations.

  o Dilated pupils.

  o Ventricular tachycardia, ventricular fibrillation, or asystole are the most common causes of cardiac arrest. Cardiac arrest may also occur following respiratory arrest. Sometimes electrical activity is present but is not sufficient to stimulate effective cardiac contractions. This condition is called pulseless electrical activity (PEA).

  View Media Supplement: Ventricular Tachycardia (Animation)

  o In children and infants, cardiac arrest is most often secondary to hypoxemia or shock.

  o Without sufficient cardiac output, brain cell anoxia (cell death) develops within 4 to 6 min, with death following shortly thereafter.

  o Management of cardiac arrest depends on prompt recognition of signs and symptoms and the introduction of therapeutic interventions directed at artificially sustaining circulation and ventilation.

  o After identification, the goals for management of a cardiac arrest include:

    ▪ Quick initiation of both circulatory and respiratory support.

    ▪ Activation of the emergency medical system (EMS).

    ▪ Use of emergency equipment and cardiac monitoring.

    ▪ Stabilization of the client following the arrest.

    ▪ Diagnosis and treatment of the cause of the cardiac arrest.

o CPR is the process of externally supporting the circulation and respiration of an individual who has just had a cardiac arrest. Defibrillation is used in the presence of ventricular fibrillation and ventricular tachycardia. Neither of these rhythms provides sufficient cardiac output to support life. CPR and defibrillation significantly increase the chances of survival when initiated immediately.

o Prehospital care greatly improves the chance of survival for cardiac arrest victims.

- CPR

   o CPR is a combination of basic interventions designed to sustain oxygen and circulation to vital organs until more advanced interventions can be initiated to correct the root cause of the cardiac arrest.

   o Basic interventions can be delivered by trained individuals, but advanced interventions require more sophisticated training and certification and the use of emergency equipment.

   o CPR is a series of emergency procedures directed at artificially providing a client with circulation (chest compressions) and oxygenation (ventilations) in the absence of cardiac output.

   o CPR is a component of basic life support (BLS) and advanced cardiac life support (ACLS).

   o The goal of BLS is to provide oxygen to the vital organs until appropriate advanced resuscitation measures can be initiated or until resuscitative efforts are ordered to be stopped. BLS involves the ABCs of CPR:

      - Airway

         □ Confirm the absence or presence of spontaneous respirations.

         □ Establish a patent airway.

         □ Use the Heimlich maneuver if the airway is obstructed with a foreign object.

         □ Use abdominal thrusts for unconscious clients.

      - Breathing

         □ Provide artificial respiration (ventilation) to deliver oxygen into the blood in an attempt to prevent cell anoxia.

      - Circulation

         □ Confirm the absence or presence of a pulse.

         □ Provide external support of circulation (chest compressions) to transport oxygenated blood to the brain.

- o The goal of ACLS is the return of spontaneous breathing and circulation. In addition to the ABCs of BLS, ACLS involves:

  - Diagnosis of underlying cardiac dysrhythmias. Pharmacological interventions vary with the rhythm identified. Defibrillation may be required. This involves delivering a pre-measured shock to the heart in order to interrupt the aberrant rhythm and allow the natural pacemaker of the heart to initiate beats.

  - Insertion of an oropharyngeal or endotracheal airway with bag ventilation and supplemental oxygen.

  - Administration of IV fluids.

  - Administration of IV antidysrhythmic drugs.

  - o The chain of survival is a series of interventions directed at the resuscitation of the cardiac arrest victim. It involves:

    - Early activation of emergency medical services

    - Early CPR/defibrillation

    - Early ACLS care

- Nursing Responsibilities during a Cardiac Arrest

  - o Nurses assisting during a cardiac arrest must:

    - Be knowledgeable about the facility's procedure for alerting members of the code team to the emergency.

    - Use the current BLS and ACLS guidelines from the American Heart Association (AHA).

    - Be knowledgeable about institutional policies/procedures and the location and operation of emergency equipment (crash cart).

    - Have current certification for BLS and/or ACLS skills.

    - Know the client's status regarding resuscitation (whether or not the client has a current do-not-resuscitate order.).

    - Maintain airway patency.

    - Assess the depth and rate of respirations.

    - Provide chest compressions at the appropriate rate and depth for age.

    - Assess vital signs for effectiveness of chest compressions and ventilations.

    - Defibrillate the client when indicated.

    - Initiate and maintain IV access.

    - Provide medications as prescribed.

    - Monitor laboratory values (ABGs, CBC, electrolytes).

    - Document all interventions and medications.

- American Heart Association guidelines for basic life support and advanced life support are updated on a regular basis. These updates are based on research and aggregate client outcomes.

- Because most cases of adult cardiac arrest are caused by ventricular fibrillation or ventricular tachycardia, early defibrillation is essential. When a defibrillator is immediately available and ventricular fibrillation or ventricular tachycardia is confirmed, the client is defibrillated prior to the initiation of CPR. A standard defibrillator or an automated external defibrillator (AED) may be used. Although cardiac arrest is rare in children, nurses must also be prepared to used a defibrillator when indicated in a pediatric situation.

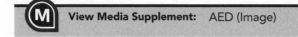

View Media Supplement: AED (Image)

CHAPTER 57: CARDIAC ARREST, CPR, AND DEFIBRILLATION

 Application Exercises

1. When caring for an infant during cardiac arrest, which of the following pulses should the nurse palpate to determine cardiac function?

    A. Radial

    B. Pedal

    C. Carotid

    D. Brachial

2. Identify the goal of BLS.

3. A nurse in the emergency department is caring for a client who has chest pain and is diaphoretic. The client becomes unresponsive and the ECG monitor reveals ventricular fibrillation. Which of the following resuscitation steps should the nurse take first?

    A. Open the airway.

    B. Initiate rescue breathing.

    C. Deliver chest compressions.

    D. Provide defibrillation.

CHAPTER 57: CARDIAC ARREST, CPR, AND DEFIBRILLATION

 Application Exercises Answer Key

1. When caring for an infant during cardiac arrest, which of the following pulses should the nurse palpate to determine cardiac function?

    A. Radial

    B. Pedal

    C. Carotid

    D. Brachial

    The nurse should palpate the brachial pulse to determine cardiac function in an infant because it is the most accessible pulse. The radial and pedal pulses may not be reliable indicators of cardiac function, and the carotid pulse may be difficult to palpate in an infant due to the fatty tissue surrounding the neck.

 NCLEX® Connection: Physiological Adaptation, Alterations in Body Systems

2. Identify the goal of BLS.

    The goal of BLS is to provide oxygen to the vital organs until appropriate advanced resuscitation measures can be initiated or until resuscitative efforts are ordered to be stopped.

 NCLEX® Connection: Physiological Adaptation, Alterations in Body Systems

3. A nurse in the emergency department is caring for a client who has chest pain and is diaphoretic. The client becomes unresponsive and the ECG monitor reveals ventricular fibrillation. Which of the following resuscitation steps should the nurse take first?

    A. Open the airway.

    B. Initiate rescue breathing.

    C. Deliver chest compressions.

    D. Provide defibrillation.

    The treatment for ventricular fibrillation is defibrillation. It should be provided prior to the initiation of CPR (airway, rescue breathing, and chest compressions).

 NCLEX® Connection: NCLEX® Connection: Physiological Adaptation, Alterations in Body Systems

Berman, A., Snyder, S. J., Kozier, B., & Erb, G. (2008). *Fundamentals of nursing: Concepts, process, and practice* (8th ed.). Upper Saddle River, NJ: Pearson Prentice Hall.

Dudek, S. G. (2010). *Nutrition essentials for nursing practice* (6th ed.). Philadelphia, PA: Lippincott Williams & Wilkins.

Ebersole, P., Hess, P., Touhy, T. A., Jett, K., & Schmidt Luggen, A. (2008). *Toward healthy aging: Human needs & nursing response* (7th ed.). St. Louis, MO: Mosby Elsevier.

Eliopoulos, C. (2010). *Gerontological nursing* (7th ed.). Philadelphia, PA: Lippincott Williams & Wilkins.

Grodner, M., Long, S., & Walkingshaw, B. C. (2007). *Foundations and clinical applications of nutrition: A nursing approach* (4th ed.). St. Louis, MO: Mosby Elsevier.

Ignatavicius, D. D., & Workman, M. L. (2010). *Medical-surgical nursing: Patient-centered collaborative care* (6th ed.). St. Louis, MO: Saunders Elsevier.

Lehne, R. A. (2010). *Pharmacology for nursing care* (7th ed.). St. Louis, MO: Saunders.

Potter, P. A., & Perry, A. G. (2009). *Fundamentals of nursing* (7th ed.). St. Louis, MO: Mosby Elsevier.

Townsend, M. C. (2008). *Essentials of psychiatric mental health nursing: Concepts of care in evidence-based practice* (4th ed.). Philadelphia, PA: F. A. Davis.

Varcarolis, E. M., Carson, V. B., & Shoemaker, N. C. (2006). *Foundations of psychiatric mental health nursing: A clinical approach* (5th ed.). St. Louis, MO: Saunders Elsevier.

Wilson, B. A., Shannon, M. T., & Shields, K. M. (2010). *Pearson nurse's drug guide 2010.* Upper Saddle River, NJ: Pearson Education, Inc.